# SLEEP MEDICINE ESSENTIALS

Edited by

**Teofilo L. Lee-Chiong**

Division of Sleep Medicine, Department of Medicine, National Jewish Health, University
of Colorado Denver School of Medicine, Denver, Colorado

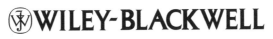

**WILEY-BLACKWELL**

A John Wiley & Sons, Inc., Publication

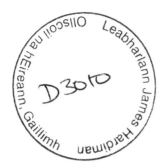

Published by John Wiley & Sons, Inc., Hoboken, New Jersey
Published simultaneously in Canada

For general information on our other products and services or for technical support, please contact our Customer Care Department within the United States at (800) 762-2974, outside the United States at (317) 572-3993 or fax (317) 572-4002.

Wiley also publishes its books in a variety of electronic formats. Some content that appears in print may not be available in electronic formats. For more information about Wiley products, visit our web site at www.wiley.com.

*Library of Congress Cataloging-in-Publication Data is available.*

ISBN   978-0-470-19566-6

Printed in the United States of America
10 9 8 7 6 5 4 3 2 1

# CONTENTS

# PREFACE

*Sleep Medicine Essentials* is designed with the busy clinician in mind. It can serve both as an independent, practical, and portable book on sleep medicine as well as a complementary compendium to its larger companion textbook, the *Wiley Comprehensive Handbook of Sleep Medicine*, which has the most extensive coverage of sleep medicine among all the current textbooks in the field. Carefully chosen from the chapters of the *Comprehensive Handbook*, the topics in this guide provide the essential information that the clinician would need in the day-to-day management of patients with sleep-related disorders. Thus, whereas the *Comprehensive Handbook* may be read unhurriedly in the solitude of the medical library or office, this guide can be brought into the clinic, sleep laboratory, or wherever else patients are being cared for.

Advances in the understanding of the complex biology and physiology of sleep and of the various sleep disorders will continue to transform the multidisciplinary science of sleep medicine. As the disciplines of sleep and dreaming evolve, new discoveries will be incorporated in future editions of this book.

I wish to thank the many authors for their excellent chapters and counsel. As with the *Comprehensive Handbook*, *Sleep Medicine Essentials* is dedicated to my wife, Dolores Grace Zamudio, and my daughter, Zoë Lee-Chiong.

TEOFILO L. LEE-CHIONG JR.

# CONTRIBUTORS

**Sonia Ancoli-Israel**, Department of Psychiatry, University of California, San Diego and Veterans Affairs San Diego Healthcare System, San Diego, California

**Roseanne Armitage**, University of Michigan, Ann Arbor, Michigan

**J. Todd Arnedt**, University of Michigan, Ann Arbor, Michigan

**Liat Ayalon**, Department of Psychiatry, University of California San Diego and Veterans Affairs San Diego Healthcare System, San Diego, California

**Dennis R. Bailey**, Englewood, Colorado

**Preetam Bandla**, The Children's Hospital of Philadelphia, University of Pennsylvania, Philadelphia, Pennsylvania

**Joshua Baron**, Department of Pediatric Neurology, Tufts-New England Medical Center, Boston, Massachusetts

**Philip M. Becker**, Sleep Medicine Fellowship Program, Department of Psychiatry, University of Texas Southwestern Medical Center at Dallas, Dallas, Texas and Sleep Medicine Associates of Texas, Dallas, Texas

**David A. Beuther**, National Jewish Health and University of Colorado Health Sciences Center, Denver, Colorado

**Bradley F. Boeve**, Mayo Sleep Disorders Center and Department of Neurology, Mayo Clinic College of Medicine, Rochester, Minnesota

**Katy Borodkin**, Department of Psychology, Bar Ilan University, Ramat Gan, Israel

**Stephen N. Brooks**, Austin, Texas

**W. David Brown**, Sleep Diagnostics of Texas, The Woodlands, Texas

**Daniel J. Buysse**, Sleep and Chronobiology Center, Department of Psychiatry, University of Pittsburgh, Pittsburgh, Pennsylvania

**Melynda D. Casement**, University of Michigan, Ann Arbor, Michigan

**Keith Cavanaugh**, Rocky Mountain Pediatric Sleep Disorders, The Children's Hospital, Aurora, Colorado

**Amanda Charlesworth**, Center for Translational Neuroscience, Department of Neurobiology and Developmental Sciences, College of Medicine, University of Arkansas for Medical Sciences, Little Rock, Arkansas

**S. Charles Cho**, Stanford Sleep Disorders Clinic, Stanford University, Stanford, California

**George P. Chrousos**, Pediatric and Reproductive Endocrinology Branch, National Institutes of Health, Bethesda, Maryland

**Nancy A. Collop**, Johns Hopkins University, Baltimore, Maryland

**Cynthia Crowder**, Sleep Medicine Fellowship Program, Department of Psychiatry, University of Texas Southwestern Medical Center at Dallas, Dallas, Texas

**Yaron Dagan**, Institute for Sleep Medicine, Assuta Medical Center, Tel Aviv, Israel and Department of Medical Education, Sackler Faculty of Medicine, Tel Aviv University, Tel Aviv, Israel

**Carolyn D'Ambrosio**, Division of Pulmonary, Critical Care, and Sleep Medicine, Tufts-New England Medical Center, Tufts University School of Medicine, Boston, Massachusetts

**Helen S. Driver**, Sleep Disorders Laboratory, Kingston General Hospital, Departments of Medicine and Psychology, Queen's University, Kingston, Ontario, Canada

**Jack D. Edinger**, Department of Veterans Affairs Medical Center, Durham, North Carolina and Duke University Medical Center, Durham, North Carolina

**Norman R. Friedman**, Rocky Mountain Pediatric Sleep Disorders, The Children's Hospital, Aurora, Colorado

**Edgar Garcia-Rill**, Center for Translational Neuroscience, Department of Neurobiology and Developmental Sciences, College of Medicine, University of Arkansas for Medical Sciences, Little Rock, Arkansas

**Erik Garpestad**, Division of Pulmonary, Critical Care, and Sleep Medicine, Tufts-New England Medical Center, Tufts University School of Medicine, Boston, Massachusetts

**Indira Gurubhagavatula**, Division of Sleep Medicine and the Center for Sleep and Respiratory Neurobiology and Division of Pulmonary and Critical Care Medicine, Department of Medicine, Hospital of the University of Pennsylvania, Philadelphia, Pennsylvania and Pulmonary, Critical Care, and Sleep Section, Philadelphia VA Medical Center, Philadelphia, Pennsylvania

**Peter Y. Hahn**, Mayo Clinic College of Medicine, Rochester, Minnesota

**David G. Harper**, McLean Hospital and Harvard Medical School, Belmont, Massachusetts

**David Heister**, Center for Translational Neuroscience, Department of Neurobiology and Developmental Sciences, College of Medicine, University of Arkansas for Medical Sciences, Little Rock, Arkansas

**Nicholas S. Hill**, Division of Pulmonary, Critical Care, and Sleep Medicine, Tufts-New England Medical Center, Tufts University School of Medicine, Boston, Massachusetts

**Max Hirshkowitz**, Baylor College of Medicine, Houston, Texas and Department of Medicine and Department of Psychiatry, Michael E. DeBakey VAMC Sleep Center, Houston, Texas

**Maren Hyde**, Henry Ford Health System, Sleep Disorders and Research Center, Detroit, Michigan

**Conrad Iber**, University of Minnesota, Minneapolis, Minnesota

**Shahrokh Javaheri**, College of Medicine, University of Cincinnati, Cincinnati, Ohio and Sleepcare Diagnostics, Mason, Ohio

**Kyle Johnson**, Department of Psychiatry, Oregon Health Science University, Portland, Oregon

**Wajahat Khalil**, University of Minnesota, Minneapolis, Minnesota

**James M. Krueger**, Washington State University, Pullman, Washington

**Clete A. Kushida**, Stanford Sleep Disorders Clinic, Stanford University, Stanford, California

**Teofilo Lee-Chiong**, National Jewish Medical and Research Center, Denver, Colorado

**Maria Cecilia Lopes**, Stanford Sleep Disorders Clinic, Stanford University, Stanford, California

**Jeannine A. Majde**, Washington State University, Pullman, Washington

**Carole L. Marcus**, The Children's Hospital of Philadelphia, University of Pennsylvania, Philadelphia, Pennsylvania

**Gerald A. Marks**, University of Texas Southwestern Medical Center, Dallas, Texas and Dallas Veterans Affairs Medical Center, Dallas, Texas

**Richard J. Martin**, National Jewish Health and University of Colorado Health Sciences Center, Denver, Colorado

**Emilio Mazza**, Allergy and Pulmonary Associates, Trenton, New Jersey

**Melanie K. Means**, Department of Veterans Affairs Medical Center, Durham, North Carolina and Duke University Medical Center, Durham, North Carolina

**Reena Mehra**, Case School of Medicine, Cleveland, Ohio and University Hospitals Case Medical Center, Cleveland, Ohio

**Mark Mennemeier**, Center for Translational Neuroscience, Department of Neurobiology and Developmental Sciences, College of Medicine, University of Arkansas for Medical Sciences, Little Rock, Arkansas

**Timothy H. Monk**, Human Chronobiology Research Program, Western Psychiatric Institute and Clinic, University of Pittsburgh Medical Center, Pittsburgh, Pennsylvania

**William H. Moorcroft**, Northern Colorado Sleep Consultants, Fort Collins, Colorado

**Timothy I. Morgenthaler**, Mayo Sleep Disorders Center and Department of Internal Medicine, Division of Pulmonary and Critical Care Medicine, Mayo Clinic College of Medicine, Rochester, Minnesota

**Douglas E. Moul**, Sleep and Chronobiology Center, Department of Psychiatry, University of Pittsburgh, Pittsburgh, Pennsylvania

**Rachel J. Norwood**, National Jewish Health, Denver, Colorado

**Lyle J. Olson**, Mayo Clinic College of Medicine, Rochester, Minnesota

**William C. Orr**, Lynn Institute for Healthcare Research, Oklahoma City, Oklahoma

**John G. Park**, Center for Sleep Medicine, Division of Pulmonary and Critical Care Medicine, Mayo Clinic College of Medicine, Rochester, Minnesota

**Kathy P. Parker**, Nell Hodgson Woodruff School of Nursing and Department of Neurology, Emory University, Atlanta, Georgia

**Slobodanka Pejovic**, Department of Psychiatry, Penn State College of Medicine, Hershey, Pennsylvania

**Rafael Pelayo**, Stanford Sleep Disorders Clinic, Stanford University, Stanford, California

**Christophe Perrin**, Division of Pulmonary, Critical Care, and Sleep Medicine, Tufts-New England Medical Center, Tufts University School of Medicine, Boston, Massachusetts

**Anil Natesan Rama**, Stanford Sleep Disorders Clinic, Stanford University, Stanford, California

**Gary S. Richardson**, Henry Ford Hospital, Detroit, Michigan

**Timothy A. Roehrs**, Henry Ford Health System, Sleep Disorders and Research Center, Detroit, Michigan and Department of Psychiatry and Behavioral Neurosciences, School of Medicine, Wayne State University, Detroit, Michigan

**Gerald Rosen**, Sleep Disorders Center, Hannepin County Medical Center, Minneapolis, Minnesota

**Leon Rosenthal**, Sleep Medicine Associates of Texas, Dallas, Texas

**Thomas Roth**, Henry Ford Health System, Sleep Disorders and Research Center, Detroit, Michigan and Department of Psychiatry and Behavioral Neurosciences, School of Medicine, Wayne State University, Detroit, Michigan

**Robert L. Sack**, Department of Psychiatry, Oregon Health Science University, Portland, Oregon

**Michael Sateia**, Sleep Disorders Center, Dartmouth-Hitchcock Medical Center, Lebanon, New Hampshire

**Stephen H. Sheldon**, Feinberg School of Medicine, Northwestern University and Sleep Medicine Center, Children's Memorial Hospital, Chicago, Illinois

**Margaret N. Shouse**, Department of Neurobiology, UCLA School of Medicine, Los Angeles, California

**Michael H. Silber**, Mayo Sleep Disorders Center and Center for Sleep Medicine and Department of Neurology, Mayo Clinic College of Medicine, Rochester, Minnesota

**Daniel Smith**, National Jewish Medical and Research Center, Denver, Colorado

**Virend K. Somers**, Mayo Clinic College of Medicine, Rochester, Minnesota

**Edward J. Stepanski**, Accelerated Community Oncology Research Network, Memphis, Tennessee

**Kingman P. Strohl**, Case School of Medicine, Cleveland, Ohio, University Hospitals Case Medical Center, Cleveland, Ohio, and Department of Veterans Affair Medical Center, Cleveland, Ohio

**Maja Tippmann-Peikert**, Mayo Sleep Disorders Center and Department of Neurology, Mayo Clinic College of Medicine, Rochester, Minnesota

**Alexandros N. Vgontzas**, Department of Psychiatry, Penn State College of Medicine, Hershey, Pennsylvania

**Michael V. Vitiello**, Department of Psychiatry and Behavioral Sciences, University of Washington, Seattle, Washington

**Tiffany Wallace-Huitt**, Center for Translational Neuroscience, Department of Neurobiology and Developmental Sciences, College of Medicine, University of Arkansas for Medical Sciences, Little Rock, Arkansas

**Michael Weissberg**, Department of Psychiatry, University of Colorado School of Medicine, Denver, Colorado

**Alexander White**, Division of Pulmonary, Critical Care, and Sleep Medicine, Tufts-New England Medical Center, Tufts University School of Medicine, Boston, Massachusetts

**Merrill S. Wise**, Methodist Healthcare Sleep Disorders Center, Memphis, Tennessee

**Charlotte Yates**, Center for Translational Neuroscience, Department of Neurobiology and Developmental Sciences, College of Medicine, University of Arkansas for Medical Sciences, Little Rock, Arkansas

**Meijun Ye**, Center for Translational Neuroscience, Department of Neurobiology and Developmental Sciences, College of Medicine, University of Arkansas for Medical Sciences, Little Rock, Arkansas

# 1

## NORMAL HUMAN SLEEP

Anil Natesan Rama, S. Charles Cho, and Clete A. Kushida
Stanford Sleep Disorders Clinic, Stanford University, Stanford, California

## INTRODUCTION

Normal human sleep is comprised of two distinct states, known as nonrapid eye movement (NREM) and rapid eye movement (REM) sleep. NREM sleep is subdivided into four stages, namely stages 1, 2, 3, and 4, which have been recently reclassified to stages N1, N2, and N3. REM sleep may also be further subdivided into two stages, phasic and tonic.

## ADULT SLEEP ARCHITECTURE

### NREM Sleep

Nonrapid eye movement sleep accounts for 75–80% of total sleep time:

- Stage 1 (N1) sleep comprises 3–8% of total sleep time. N1 sleep occurs most frequently in the transition from wakefulness to the other sleep stages or following arousals from sleep. In N1 sleep, alpha activity (8–13 Hz), which is characteristic of wakefulness, diminishes and a low-voltage, mixed-frequency pattern emerges. The highest amplitude electroencephalography (EEG) activity is generally in the theta range (4–8 Hz). Electromyography (EMG) activity decreases and electro-oculography (EOG) demonstrates slow rolling eye movements. Vertex sharp waves (50–200 ms) are noted toward the end of N1 sleep
- Stage 2 (N2) sleep begins after approximately 10–12 min of N1 sleep and comprises 45–55% of total sleep time. The characteristic EEG findings of N2 sleep include sleep spindles and K complexes. A sleep spindle is described as a 12 to 14-Hz waveform lasting at least 0.5 s and having a "spindle"-shaped appearance. A K complex is a waveform with two components, a negative wave followed by a positive wave, both lasting more than 0.5 s. Delta

waves (0.5–4 Hz) in the EEG may first appear in N2 sleep but are present in small amounts. The EMG activity is diminished compared to wakefulness.
- Stage 3 and 4 (N3) sleep occupy 15–20% of total sleep time and constitute slow-wave sleep. N3 sleep is characterized by greater than 20% of high-amplitude, slow-wave activity. EOG does not register eye movements in N2 or N3 sleep. Muscle tone is decreased compared to wakefulness or N1 sleep.

### REM Sleep

Rapid eye movement sleep accounts for 20–25% of total sleep time. The first REM sleep episode occurs 60–90 min after the onset of NREM sleep. EEG tracings during REM sleep are characterized by a low-voltage, mixed-frequency activity with slow alpha (defined as 1–2 Hz slower than wake alpha) and theta waves:

- Based on EEG, EMG, and EOG characteristics, REM sleep can be divided into two stages, tonic and phasic. Characteristics of the tonic stage include a desynchronized EEG, atonia of skeletal muscle groups, and suppression of monosynaptic and polysynaptic reflexes. Phasic REM sleep is characterized by rapid eye movements in all directions as well as by transient swings in blood pressure, heart rate changes, irregular respiration, tongue movements, and myoclonic twitching of chin and limb muscles. Sawtooth waves, which have a frequency in the theta range and have the appearance of the teeth on the cutting edge of a saw blade, often occur in conjunction with rapid eye movements.

### NREM–REM Cycle

The NREM–REM sleep cycle occurs about every 90 min, and approximately four to six cycles occur per major

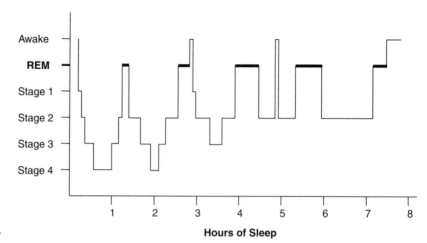

**Figure 1.1**  Young adult hypnogram.

sleep episode. The ratio of NREM sleep to REM sleep in each cycle varies during the course of the night:

- The early cycles are dominated by slow-wave sleep and REM sleep dominates the later cycles. The first episode of REM sleep may last only a few minutes and subsequent REM episodes progressively lengthen in duration during the course of the major sleep period.
- N3 sleep is prominent in the first third of the night and REM sleep is prominent in the last third of the night. The temporal arrangement of sleep type is described graphically by a hypnogram (Fig. 1.1).

## SLEEP IN NEWBORNS AND INFANTS

Adult sleep stages and features are not evident until 6 months of age. Newborn sleep states are characterized as quiet, active, or indeterminate:

- Quiet sleep is analogous to NREM sleep. EEG demonstrates a discontinuous pattern with intermittent bursts of electrical activity alternating with quiescent periods. Heart rate and respirations are regular, body movements are few, and EMG activity is sustained.
- Active sleep is analogous to REM sleep. EEG demonstrates a low-voltage, irregular pattern. Rapid eye movements, body movements, grimaces, and twitches are frequent. Muscle tone, heart rate, and respirations are variable.
- Indeterminate sleep is disorganized and cannot be classified as either active or quiet sleep.
- Vertex sharp waves develop between 0 and 6 months of age. Sleep spindles develop between 4 and 8 weeks of age. K complexes develop between 4 and 6 months of age.
- The newborn sleep cycle is about 60 min. The cycle starts with active sleep. At term, over 50% of a newborn's sleep is active. Sleep-onset REM periods are normal until 10–12 weeks of age. During the first 6 months of life, there is a decrease in the amount of active sleep and a simultaneous rise in the amount

of quiet sleep. The sleep cycle gradually increases to the adult average of 90 min by adolescence.

## CHANGES IN SLEEP WITH AGING

Sleep patterns change during life. Newborns may spend more than 16 h of the day asleep but intermittently sleep and awaken throughout the 24-h period. At the age of 3 months, infants may sleep throughout the course of the night and may take two or more daytime naps. As the child first enters school, sleep is consolidated into a major nocturnal period with a single daytime nap. As the child ages into adulthood, the major nocturnal sleep is not accompanied by a daytime nap. Age-associated deterioration of the sleep pattern results in fragmented sleep in the elderly in whom more time is spent in bed but less time asleep.

Slow-wave sleep and REM sleep patterns also change during life. Slow-wave sleep declines after adolescence and continues to decline as a function of aging. REM sleep decreases from more than 50% at birth to 20–25% during adolescence and middle age.

## SLEEP NEUROPHYSIOLOGY

### NREM Sleep

The transition from wakefulness to NREM sleep is associated with altered neurotransmission at the level of the thalamus whereby incoming messages are inhibited and the cerebral cortex is deprived of signals from the outside world. NREM sleep is characterized by three major oscillations (Fig. 1.2).

- Spindles (7–14 Hz) are generated within thalamic reticular neurons that impose rhythmic inhibitory sequences onto thalamocortical neurons. However, the widespread synchronization of this rhythm is governed by corticothalamic projections.
- There are two types of delta activity. The first type are clocklike waves (1–4 Hz) generated in thalamocortical neurons and the second type are cortical waves (1–4 Hz) that persist despite extensive thalamectomy.

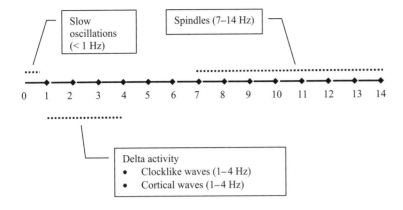

**Figure 1.2** NREM sleep oscillations.

However, the hallmark of NREM sleep is the slow oscillation (<1 Hz), which is generated intracortically and has the ability to group the thalamically generated spindles as well as thalamically and cortically generated delta oscillations, leading to a coalescence of the different rhythms.

## REM Sleep

Transection studies demonstrate that the pontomesencephalic region is critical for REM sleep generation. When the mesopontine region is connected to rostral structures, REM sleep phenomena such as a desynchronized EEG and ponto–geniculo–occipital (PGO) spikes are seen in the forebrain. When the mesopontine region is continuous with the medulla and spinal cord, REM sleep phenomena such as skeletal muscle atonia can be seen.

- The pontomesencephalic area contains the so-called cholinergic "REM-on" nuclei, specifically the laterodorsal tegmental (LDT) and pedunculopontine tegmental (PPT) nuclei. The LDT and PPT nuclei project through the thalamus to the cortex, which produces desynchronization of REM sleep. The LDT and PPT nuclei project caudally via the ventral medulla to alpha motor neurons in the spinal cord where skeletal muscle tone is inhibited during REM sleep by the release of glycine.

- PGO spikes are precursors to the rapid eye movements seen in REM sleep, are formed in the cholinergic mesopontine nuclei, and propagate rostrally through the lateral geniculate and other thalamic nuclei to the occipital cortex.

- In addition, as NREM sleep transitions to REM sleep, tonic inhibition of REM-generating cholinergic pontomesencephalic nuclei by brainstem serotoninergic and adrenergic nuclei decreases, thereby allowing the development of PGO spikes and muscle atonia. Thus, the cholinergic REM-on nuclei of the PPT and LDT slowly activate the monoaminergic "REM-off" nuclei of the dorsal raphe and locus ceruleus that in turn inhibit REM-on nuclei (Fig. 1.3).

- Hypocretin has an important role in the modulation of wakefulness and REM sleep. Hypocretin neurons are located in the perifornical region of the lateral hypothalamus and widely project to brainstem and forebrain areas, densely innervating monoaminergic and cholinergic cells. Hypocretin neurons promote wakefulness and inhibit REM sleep. Elevated levels of hypocretin during active waking and in REM sleep compared to quiet waking and slow-wave sleep suggest a role for hypocretin in the central programming of motor activity. Hypocretin projections to the nucleus pontis oralis may play a role in the generation of active (REM) sleep and muscle atonia.

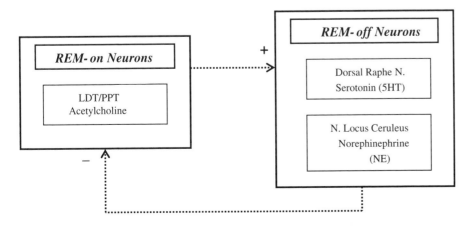

**Figure 1.3** NREM–REM reciprocal interaction model.

**Table 1.1  Autonomic Nervous System Fluctuations During Normal Human Sleep**

|  | Parasympathetic Nervous System | Sympathetic Nervous System |
|---|---|---|
| **NREM sleep** | Increase | Decrease |
| **REM sleep** |  |  |
| Tonic | Increases further | Decreases further |
| Phasic |  | Intermittent increases |

## AUTONOMIC NERVOUS SYSTEM

The autonomic nervous system (ANS) regulates the vital functions of internal homeostasis. The ANS is comprised of the sympathetic nervous system and parasympathetic nervous system.

- The essential autonomic feature of NREM sleep is increased parasympathetic activity and decreased sympathetic activity.
- The essential autonomic feature of REM sleep is an additional increase in parasympathetic activity and an additional decrease in sympathetic activity, with intermittent increases in sympathetic activity occurring during phasic REM (Table 1.1) For example, pupilloconstriction is seen during NREM sleep and is maintained during REM sleep with phasic dilatations noted during phasic REM sleep.

## MODEL OF SLEEP REGULATION

Several models have been proposed to explain the regulation of sleep and wakefulness. One such model proposes that two processes govern the regulation of the sleep–wake cycle: a sleep-dependent homeostatic process (process S) and a sleep-independent circadian process (process C).

*Process S* is a homeostatic process that is dependent upon the duration of prior sleep and waking. This process shows an exponential rise during waking and a decline during sleep. In other words, the longer a person stays awake, the sleepier he or she becomes; conversely, the longer a person sleeps, the lower the pressure to remain asleep.

*Process C* is a circadian process that is independent of duration of prior sleep and waking. This process is

under the control of the suprachiasmatic nucleus, which determines the rhythmic propensity to sleep and awaken. Each person has an endogenous drive to fall asleep and awaken at a certain time regardless of the duration of prior sleep or wake.

- The two-process model posits that the timing of sleep and waking is determined by the interaction between process S and process C. Sleep onset is thought to occur when both the homeostatic and circadian drive to sleep intersect.
- Other models have also been proposed, such as the opponent-process model and the three-process model of alertness regulation; however, further work is necessary to determine the biological substrates of the elements of these models and the pathways by which they interact.

## KEY POINTS

1. The adult NREM–REM sleep cycle occurs every 90 min with early cycles dominated by slow-wave sleep and the later cycles dominated by REM sleep.
2. Until the age of 6 months, newborn sleep states are characterized as quiet, active, or indeterminate. Quiet sleep is analogous to NREM sleep; whereas, active sleep is analogous to REM sleep.
3. The essential autonomic feature of NREM sleep is increased parasympathetic activity and decreased sympathetic activity. The essential autonomic feature of REM sleep is an additional increase in parasympathetic activity and an additional decrease in sympathetic activity, with intermittent increases in sympathetic activity occurring during phasic REM sleep.

## BIBLIOGRAPHY

Borbely AA. A two process model of sleep regulation. *Hum Neurobiol* 1982; 1:195–204.

Holmes CJ, et al. Importance of cholinergic, GABAergic, serotonergic and other neurons in the medial medullary reticular formation for sleep-wake states studied by cytotoxic lesions in the cat. *Neuroscience* 1994; 62:1179–1200.

Rechtschaffen A, Kales A (Eds). *A Manual of Standardized Terminology, Techniques and Scoring System for Sleep Stages of Human Subjects.* BIS/BRI, UCLA, Los Angeles, 1968.

# 2

# NEUROBIOLOGY OF SLEEP

GERALD A. MARKS

University of Texas Southwestern Medical Center, Dallas, Texas, and Dallas Veterans Affairs Medical Center, Dallas, Texas

## INTRODUCTION

Rational questions on the nature of sleep behavior have a long published history and, with little doubt, extend to prehistory. It is not surprising that much attention would be paid to a prominent human endeavor such as sleep. Yet, the current condition of our knowledge of how, and for what purpose, we sleep is far from complete. The paucity of technology through most of the past to observe the operation of the central nervous system has resulted in a relatively short history of efforts to identify neural mechanisms underlying the generation and maintenance of sleep and wakefulness. A limitation of time as it impacts the capriciousness of the process of discovery is one factor. Another critical factor, which has become apparent with the accumulation of knowledge, is the complexity of the problem.

- A large body of knowledge has accumulated on sleep–wake behavior including natural observation, pathological alterations, and experimental manipulation. The conclusion that constitutes the basic tenet of the neurobiology of sleep is that sleep is a product of the central nervous system. To understand how the brain produces sleep is to identify those neural mechanisms necessary and sufficient to produce it.

- Early investigations employing the emerging technology of modern neuroscience conceived of a brain made up of centers of localized function. Thus, destruction of the "sleep center" would result in the elimination of sleep and serve to identify the structure and its function. Inasmuch as the use of this approach has yet to yield a consensus as to what structure constitutes the sleep center, a concept of interacting, distributed systems has emerged as a more plausible mechanism of this process.

- While mechanisms within the brain produce sleep and wakefulness, brain mechanisms also are the targets of their influence, and these various mechanisms need not be mutually exclusive. Alterations in brain activity accompanying changes in state of arousal are so widespread and global in nature that they can be viewed as constituting a reorganization in the whole brain. In every region of the brain, neurons alter their rate or pattern of firing with changes in state.

## PROBLEM OF DEFINITION

Defining sleep–wake behavior is not a trivial matter nor is a single definition appropriate for all cases. Definitions based on overt, gross behavior suffer from an inability to distinguish several conditions generally not recognized as sleep. The problem of definition is most acute when applied across species. Circadian patterns of rest and activity are observed across phyla, including single-celled organisms and plants. Conservation through evolution may provide a clue to the adaptive value of temporally regulating activity and also indicates that the mechanisms subserving this behavior probably vary with the complexity of the organism expressing them. From the viewpoint of neurobiology, definitions of sleep are couched in subservience to a nervous system. This requires that the subject not only posses a nervous system but also that the behavior be dependent upon its operation.

- Neurobiological investigations of sleep–wake mechanisms have been conducted almost exclusively with mammalian species. This has generated a definition of sleep based on a confluence of several electrophysiologic correlates of brain activity. It should be pointed out that these indicators of state are defining properties and are not chosen because of any relationship to fundamental saliency or functional significance. Or is the definition invariant. For example, a specific pattern in the cortical electroencephalogram (EEG) is used to define sleep, yet other measures of neural activity clearly indicate the presence of sleep in a cat with its neocortex removed. This flexibility in defining sleep can result in a high

*Sleep Medicine Essentials*, edited by Teofilo L. Lee-Chiong
Copyright © 2009 John Wiley & Sons, Inc.

degree of ambiguity interpreting effects of experimental manipulations and pathological conditions. There is no absolute agreement on how many indicators are required to identify sleep. Problems also arise when neurobiological definitions of sleep are applied to other than mammalian and avian species. Current investigations are revealing many similarities between the inactive states of the fruit fly and mammalian sleep. Electrophysiologic correlates of neural activity may be uncovered, but brain mechanisms implicated in the control of sleep- wake behavior in the mammalian brain do not exist in the fly. If the fly sleeps, then it will have to be defined differently than mammalian sleep. Inasmuch as the functions of sleep are currently unknown, it remains to be determined whether the sleep states of mammals and flies are even analogous, and if so, on what basis.

- Among mammalian species, there appears to be a high degree of similarity in both expression and mechanism. Differences exist in daily amounts and temporal distribution of sleep. Certain species' specializations exist, such as the unihemispheric sleep of some cetaceans and the single, consolidated, sleep period of some primates, including humans. Consensus among workers in the field is that the basic neural mechanisms identified in work on cats and rats likely apply to humans and other mammals.

## DEFINING CHARACTERISTICS OF SLEEP AND WAKEFULNESS

In the third decade of the twentieth century, the application of the newly discovered EEG began to yield insights into the altered brain activity associated with the sleep–wake cycle. Initial findings recognized clear distinctions in the EEG during wake and sleep. The low–amplitude, high–frequency activity characteristic of wakefulness increases in amplitude and decreases in frequency during sleep. At first, degrees of slowing and increased amplitude within sleep were viewed along a single dimension, depth, with the lightest sleep being most similar to wake. With hindsight, many subsequent observations on sleeping subjects report data indicating multidimensional aspects to sleep. It was not, however, until the midtwentieth century that Aserinski and Kleitman reported the cyclic appearance of a distinct stage of sleep associated with dreaming and characterized by a wakelike EEG in the presence of rapid eye movements.

- The pioneering work of Dement, Jouvet, and their colleagues utilizing cats identified the presence of rapid eye movement (REM) sleep, also called paradoxical sleep for the wakelike brain activity present. Several defining characteristics differentiated this state from that of the rest of sleep or what is now referred to as nonrapid eye movement (NREM) sleep. In addition to the low-voltage, fast EEG and rapid eye movements absent from NREM sleep, there appears an inhibition of muscle activity

between paroxysmal muscle movements, wakelike activity in the hippocampus, and a unique spindling activity in the pons, now recognized as ponto-geniculo–occipital (PGO) waves. Based on threshold to arousal by the presentation of sensory stimuli, REM sleep is a deep sleep; thus the association of EEG amplitude and frequency with sleep depth had to be revised. Work on animals permitted neurophysiological investigations that initially took the form of gross brain lesions. Results of these studies confirmed the individual identities of the two stages of sleep by indicating reliance upon different neural mechanisms for their generation.

- In all adult therian mammals studied, the general organization of sleep and wakefulness assume a similar form. In addition to a cyclic alternation of sleep and wake states, there is a more rapid alternation within sleep between NREM and REM. The occurrence of REM sleep is always preceded by NREM. The distribution of sleep–wake episodes repeats daily, thus expressing a circadian rhythm shared by many physiological functions under a common temporal influence. The faster ultradian rhythm of the sleep cycle also may be served by mechanisms independent of sleep. Many observations support a basic, rest–activity cycle, with relatively fixed period, underlying several physiological functions. Sleep stage amounts, temporal daily distributions, and the period of the ultradian sleep cycle are species-specific traits. The period of the sleep cycle is highly correlated to the size of the species and, inversely, to its basal metabolic rate.

- In addition to temporal factors controlling sleep–wake behavior, total sleep time and time in the individual stages also express homeostatic types of regulation. That is, when sleep, or a specific stage, is not permitted to be expressed, the amount lost tends to be recovered, as if a quota was being maintained. Time lost, however, is usually greater than time recovered, giving rise to the concept that sleep intensity increases, permitting recovered sleep to be more efficient. The amplitude of slow-wave activity in the EEG is an indicator of intensity of NREM sleep, whereas density of phasic activity such as eye movements or PGO waves has been used to reflect REM sleep intensity. The rates of incurring a sleep debt and of recovery appear not only to be species specific but also characteristic of strains within a species, indicating a high degree of heritability. The inverse dependence of sleep, or stage amounts, on prior expression creates another factor contributing to the oscillation among states of arousal, making up the cyclic nature of sleep–wake behavior.

## NATURE OF SLEEP–WAKE MECHANISMS

Two of the major characteristics of sleep are its reversibility and sensitivity to modulation by a variety of influences. In addition to inducing arousal from sleep by stimuli in any sensory modality of sufficient magnitude, amounts of sleep are affected by many factors such as ambient temperature, lighting conditions, level of oxygen in the air, as well as a host of wake experiences, including stress and learning. These would indicate that neural mechanisms whose primary function is not the generation of sleep and wake can control sleep and wake behavior. This raises a question as to how a sleep mechanism can be identified. Does the observation that loud sounds inhibit sleep make the auditory system a sleep mechanism? On some levels the answer is yes. Yet we know that the auditory system is not necessary for the production of sleep and wakefulness. Is necessity then the criteria for judging primacy? In a system of distributed, interactive mechanisms, it may be that no one mechanism is necessary.

- Historically, it was thought that the withdrawal of sensory input produced sleep by removing excitation to the neural systems of the brain that give rise to wakefulness. Studies utilizing brain transections and lesions were not successful at proving this hypothesis. They did, however, provide the antecedents to the discovery of Marouzzi and Magoun that the reticular core of the brain, when stimulated electrically, was sufficient to induce arousal. This led to the concept of the ascending reticular activating system as a primary mechanism of conscious wakefulness. Additional work utilizing lesion techniques, found that destruction of certain regions resulted in decreased sleep. The conclusion was that there existed mechanisms within the brain opposed to the arousal induced by the activating system. The sleep process, then and now, is no longer viewed as a passive result of disfacilitation but rather as an active process subserved by active mechanisms. The discovery of the neurally active REM sleep stage firmly entrenched this view as doctrine in sleep research.

- Differences in neural activity, as well as in behavior, among wake, NREM, and REM sleep are so great that they appear to constitute discrete states of arousal. If each state is actively produced, then there may exist mechanisms exclusively subserving each state. Evidence supports such a division, and most of the putatively identified brain mechanisms are categorized as such. The individual states, however, are not completely independent of each other. As mentioned previously, there is a dependence of REM sleep on prior NREM sleep. With only three states, an increase or decrease in one will, by necessity, tend to have a reciprocal effect on time spent in the other states. A decrease in the efficacy of a wake-inducing mechanism, for example, may reduce wakefulness, but also will result in more sleep. There are circumstances under experimental and pathological conditions in which other than the three normal states can occur, such as coma or dissociated states, which do not conform to the definitions of any one state. However, the common, and most often repeated, finding with experimental destruction or pharmacological intervention of brain function is the tenacity with which only the three

states appear, though possibly at altered levels, as well as the trend toward complete recovery of preintervention amounts.

- Although the action potential of a single neuron can be considered an all-or-none event, neural interactions within networks are graded phenomena. The fact that neural networks produce the discrete states of arousal with rare instances of dissociation is an important clue to their organization. This has been likened to a switch that is only stable within one of the configurations of the confluence of processes attendant to one of the three states of arousal. Historically, this function was performed by "executive mechanisms" centralizing decision making by integrating input from multiple sources. A more egalitarian alternative consists of relatively equipotent mechanisms interacting through reciprocal connectivity. The process suggested for the "switch" is mutual inhibition. This type of interaction favors stable configurations in which only one mutually inhibitory influence dominates at one time. Inasmuch as the executive mechanisms of sleep and wakefulness have not been found and evidence is accumulating for the reciprocal connectivity of sleep and arousal centers, a view of interacting, distributed mechanisms is currently in favor. Such a system is also consistent with the difficulty with which selective destruction of individual components of the system fail to chronically eliminate any state of arousal. Putative sleep–wake mechanisms are segmentally distributed through the brain. Determination of the specific roles played by each mechanism will be needed to understand the whole.

## MECHANISMS OF WAKEFULNESS

Since the original proposal of the ascending reticular activating system to account for wakefulness, several systems have been implicated in contributing to this function. With the introduction of sophisticated immunological and histochemical techniques, certain aminergic systems in the brainstem were differentiated from the diffuse reticular core of the brain. These systems share several properties that include widespread projections and utilization of neurotransmitters associated with neuromodulation, making these systems appealing candidates for control over the global alterations accompanying state changes. The noradrenergic system of the locus coeruleus and the serotonergic midline, raphe system have been speculated to play various roles, but the current consensus is that these wake-active neurons are involved in setting a general preparedness for wake activity associated with alertness and sensory–motor function. These monoaminergic systems are virtually silent in REM sleep. The brainstem also contains a population of cholinergic neurons in the lateral dorsal tegmental nucleus and the pedunculopontine tegmental nucleus, in which the majority are most active during wake and REM sleep. This system is thought to contribute to the activation associated with both these states. While sharing many targets with the adrenergic and serotonergic systems, cholinergic brainstem neurons differ in that they do not project directly to the neocortex. Their influence on cortical activation is relayed through the thalamus and extrathalamic pathways of the hypothalamus and basal forebrain. The brainstem cholinergic and monoaminergic systems also innervate the reticular formation.

- Although much has been discovered, it is ironic that the least progress has been made in specifically identifying mechanisms of the reticular formation itself. Extending from the medulla oblongata to the midbrain, the complex structure has been resistant to revealing its secrets. Early stimulation and lesion experiments implicated the more rostral aspects of the reticular formation, and it was shown later that neurons residing in this region of the midbrain projecting to the midline thalamus discharge at their highest rates during the states of cortical activation, wake, and REM sleep. In that the majority of reticular neurons utilize the excitatory transmitter, glutamate, as do the thalamic neurons that relay to the neocortex, this mechanism provides another path for cortical activation. Reticular influences also can be relayed through the extrathalamic pathways. Most sensory and motor systems collaterally innervate the reticular formation. Excitation of the reticular formation by sensory, or electrical, stimulation probably is responsible for the rapid arousal from sleep following their presentation.

- The reticular formation is not a homogeneous mass with respect to its innervation, projections, or local circuitry; however, one property characteristic of its structure is the high degree of intraconnectivity. As one moves more caudal, fewer and fewer long, ascending projections of reticular neurons reach the thalamus, but rather end in more rostral regions of the reticular formation. There also is a high degree of local interconnectivity. The structure of the reticular formation is well suited for the propagation of ascending as well as descending influences. This is consistent with the findings of focal electrical stimulation and local microinjection of drugs into the reticular formation inducing global changes in arousal. The specific role played by the reticular formation in behavior during wakefulness is not clear at this time. Its intraconnectivity may aid in the integration of multiple systems.

- Characteristic of the distributed nature of structures controlling states of arousal, wake mechanisms are located rostral to the brainstem, in the diencephalon, thalamus, and hypothalamus, and the telencephalon, basal forebrain, and neocortex. A population of neurons in the posterior lateral hypothalamus, tuberomammallary nucleus, utilizes histamine as a neurotransmitter. Shared with the aminergic cell groups of the brainstem, these neurons have widespread projections and activity patterns selective to wakefulness. Antagonism of this arousal system produces the hypnotic effects of antihistamines.

- Also found in the posterior hypothalamus are neurons that synthesize a newly discovered peptide transmitter, orexin, also know as hypocretin. Deficiency in this system is associated with narcolepsy. Current evidence links this system to maintenance of wakefulness; the finding of excitatory inputs to other known arousal mechanisms also supports this.

- The medial nuclei of the thalamus link, though not exclusively, brainstem activation to widespread areas of the neocortex. This region has been considered a rostral extension of the reticular formation. It is, at least, a major target of it. The entire thalamus, as well as the neocortex, undergoes profound alterations in activity with changes in state. The specific alterations are dependent upon mutual interactions between these structures and provide many of the defining characteristics of each state. Excitation of the thalamus is critical to the accurate relay of sensory information to the cortex during wakefulness.

- Cortically projecting cholinergic neurons are distributed within several nuclei of the basal forebrain and include the nucleus of the diagonal band of Broca, substantia inominata, and the magnocellular preoptic nucleus. This appears to be a major activation system of the neocortex achieved through the release of acetylcholine and other neurotransmitters. More caudal arousal systems project to this region, the cholinergic neurons discharge at their highest rates during states of cortical activation, and antagonism of cholinergic transmission in the cortex is sufficient to block spontaneous activation. The role of the basal forebrain is not solely to relay excitation to the cortex. Stimulation, lesion, and drug manipulation can have great effects on the time spent in individual states. This is probably accomplished through the reciprocal connections the basal forebrain neurons make with many other arousal-related systems.

## MECHANISMS OF NREM SLEEP

Despite the original premise that inhibition of reticular activation is the basis for the presence of active sleep mechanisms, identification of specific neural circuitry in the inhibition of the reticular formation has not been forthcoming. By some estimates, 20–25% of reticular neurons utilize the inhibitory transmitter, gamma aminobutyric acid (GABA). One possibility is that excitatory inputs to inhibitory neurons are at work; however, injection of GABA receptor agonists into the pontine reticular formation induces wakefulness. Evidence in support of other active NREM sleep mechanisms is compelling.

- Several sources of evidence implicate the presence of a sleep-generating mechanism in the anterior hypothalamus-basal forebrain region. The finding of neurons that are selectively active during sleep has identified several mechanisms. One of these mechanisms is comprised of a collection of neurons in the ventrolateral preoptic (VLPO) nucleus in which the vast majority contain GABA and the inhibitory peptide transmitter, galanin. Small excitotoxic lesions of these neurons cause a reduction in sleep correlated to the amount of cell loss. Reciprocal connections have been observed between the VLPO and several wake-related structures, including the histaminergic and orexinergic neurons, locus coeruleus, dorsal raphe, and cholinergic regions of the brainstem and basal forebrain. It has been hypothesized that reciprocal inhibitory connections between wake-active centers and the sleep-active VLPO constitutes the sleep-switch preventing the expression of mixed or disassociated states of arousal. Additional sleep-active neurons are found throughout the hypothalamic preoptic area with a more dense aggregation in the median preoptic nucleus. These neurons share many of the properties of VLPO in connectivity and utilization of GABA. An additional property is that they are warm sensitive and are posited to mediate the relationships between sleep and temperature.

- Just anterior to the preoptic area lies the basal forebrain, which in addition to being a wake mechanism, also serves NREM sleep. Distributed among the cholinergic neurons of these nuclei is a large population of GABA-containing cells. NREM sleep-active neurons are found in this region and evidence indicates that at least some are GABAergic. Some of these GABAergic neurons are projection neurons with one target being the neocortex. Thus, sleep-active GABAergic neurons of the basal forebrain may serve to inhibit the wake-active cholinergic neurons and directly inhibit cortical activity in the production of NREM sleep. The GABAergic nature of sleep promoting neurons is probably responsible for the hypnotic effects of systemically administered agents that potentiate GABA transmission such as the benzodiazepines.

- A role for the basal forebrain in sleep production has been supported further by the action of adenosine in this region to increase sleep. Adenosine is a product of cellular energy utilization. Levels of adenosine increase with the sustained increase in activity accompanying prolonged wakefulness. The basal forebrain may be one site of this action. Sleep-active neurons of the preoptic area also are excited by adenosine. Both these regions may mediate the wake-promoting effects of caffeine, an adenosine receptor antagonist.

## MECHANISMS OF REM SLEEP

The results of brain transections that isolate the medulla oblongata and pons from the rest of the brain clearly indicate that structures sufficient to produce REM sleep lie within these regions of the brainstem. Communication between these two regions is necessary for the appearance of REM sleep.

- The many physiological phenomena occurring during REM sleep can be separated into two categories, namely *phasic* events occurring discontinuously and sporadically, and *tonic* events occurring rather continuously throughout a REM sleep episode.

- Phasic events include autonomic irregularities, muscle twitches, rapid eye movements, and field potentials recorded at various places along the neuraxis called PGO waves. Phasic events tend to occur at the same time within REM periods, which has raised speculation of a phasic event system with a single or few central generators. An area in the caudal pontine reticular formation, in the subceruleus (below the locus ceruleus), has been putatively identified as a generator of PGO wave activity.

- The major tonic events of REM sleep are muscle atonia and widespread neural activation, which includes a wakelike EEG. During NREM sleep, there is a diminution of muscle activity; however, during REM sleep, there is an increase in activity in the motor centers of the brain while an active inhibition is exerted upon motor neurons. The result is paralysis and atonia in the majority of the skeletal musculature. This phenomenon appears to be dependent on the activation of a population of neurons in the caudal pontine reticular formation projecting to, and facilitating activity in, the medial medullary reticular formation that provides the inhibition to the motor neurons. Bilateral lesions in the subceruleus area of the pons, can result in REM sleep without muscle atonia, whereby animals express a variety of integrated behaviors during this sleep state.

- The wakelike activation of REM sleep recruits many of the mechanisms involved in wakefulness. Neurons of the reticular formation, brainstem, and forebrain cholinergic neurons, thalamus, and neocortex all exhibit firing rates and levels of excitability equal to, or greater in, REM sleep as compared to wakefulness. One notable exception is the aminergic system, which is almost completely silent. Some investigators have speculated that the absence of the widespread neuromodulatory influences of norepinephrine, serotonin, and histamine are the basis for the differences between REM sleep and wakefulness.

- It has been suggested that the brainstem cholinergic system is the substrate of the ascending reticular activating system. In the cat, microinjection of agents that potentiate cholinergic transmission into the pontine reticular formation induces a dramatic and rapid onset of long-lasting REM sleep episodes. While some of the cholinergic neurons fire selectively in REM sleep, most discharge at their highest rates in REM sleep and wake. It has been suggested that a reciprocal inhibition between cholinergic REM-on cells and aminergic REM-off cells provides the mechanism for reciprocal activities and state oscillations. This has not been totally supported experimentally.

- Acetylcholine levels are highest in the reticular formation during REM sleep. This may be due to reticular formation projections from cholinergic REM-on cells or inhibition of cholinergic release during wake. Evidence supports a role for the REM-off (or wake-on) noradrenergic neurons in producing this inhibition through projections to presynaptic, cholinergic terminals in the reticular formation. Wake-on/REM-on cholinergic neurons provide ascending activation in REM sleep as in wakefulness, and levels of acetylcholine are high in the thalamus during both states.

- It would appear that the release of acetylcholine in the pontine reticular formation is a condition sufficient to induce REM sleep. Directly or indirectly, brainstem cholinergic neurons may excite the reticular formation initiating ascending activation, excite the pontine neurons responsible for muscle inhibition, inhibit serotonin release responsible for the appearance of PGO waves, and provide additional ascending activation via thalamic and extrathalamic relays to the cortex. However, acetylcholine in the pontine reticular formation is *not* sufficient to induce REM sleep when the pons is separated from the medulla, and there is still some undisclosed mechanism in the medulla required for REM sleep.

- It is not clear that the integrity of brainstem cholinergic neurons is necessary for REM sleep. Excitotoxic lesions of the region produce a long-lasting decrease in REM sleep amounts that correlates with the number of cholinergic cells lost, and the size of the lesion, the effectiveness of large size being consistent with a distributed system of multiple mechanisms in the region, including the rostral pontine reticular formation.

- While evidence supports the brainstem as sufficient in the generation of REM sleep, additional structures are implicated in its control. In the preoptic area of the hypothalamus, known as the extended VLPO, there is a population of GABAergic neurons projecting to brainstem aminergic nuclei that appear to selectively fire in REM sleep, possibly contributing to the inhibition of aminergic neurons. Pharmacological manipulations of the basal forebrain can effect all states; microinjection of cholinergic agonists in the basal forebrain blocks the REM sleep induction by injections in the pontine reticular formation. Thus, mechanisms of REM sleep also appear to be distributed and interactive.

## KEY POINTS

1. The neurobiology of sleep and wakefulness involves mechanisms distributed along the neuraxis from the medulla oblongata to the neocortex. The high degree of interaction among components of the system gives rise to the unique and interdependent expression of the states of arousal.

2. Sleep–wake mechanisms appear so highly integrated in the brain that a complete understanding of them will require an advanced knowledge of basic brain function.

## BIBLIOGRAPHY

Aston-Jones G, et al. Role of locus coeruleus in attention and behavioral flexibility. *Biol Psychiatry* 1999; 46:1309–1320.

Datta S. Cellular basis of pontine ponto-geniculo-occipital wave generation and modulation. *Cell Mol Neurobiol* 1997; 17:341–365.

Datta S, et al. Single cell activity patterns of pedunculopontine tegmentum neurons across the sleep-wake cycle in the freely moving rats. *J Neurosci Res* 2002; 70:611–621.

Franken P, et al. The homeostatic regulation of sleep need is under genetic control. *J Neurosci* 2001; 21:2610–2621.

Jacobs BL, et al. Serotonin and motor activity. *Curr Opin Neurobiol* 1997; 7:820–825.

Jones BE. Arousal systems. *Front Biosci* 2003; 8:s438–451.

Jones BE. Activity, modulation and the role of basal forebrain cholinergic neurons innervating the cerebral cortex. *Prog Brain Res* 2004; 145:157–169.

Lu J, et al. Selective activation of the extended ventrolateral preoptic nucleus during rapid eye movement sleep. *J Neurosci* 2002; 22:4568–4576.

McCormick DA, et al. Sleep and arousal: Thalamocortical mechanisms. *Annu Rev Neurosci* 1997; 20:185–215.

McGinty D, et al. Brain structures and mechanisms involved in the generation of NREM sleep: Focus on the preoptic hypothalamus. *Sleep Med Rev* 2001; 5:323–342.

Mignot E, et al. The role of cerebrospinal fluid hypocretin measurement in the diagnosis of narcolepsy and other hypersomnias. *Arch Neurol* 2002; 59:1553–1562.

Peyron C, et al. Neurons containing hypocretin (orexin) project to multiple neuronal systems. *J Neurosci* 1998; 18:9996–10015.

Saper CB, et al. The sleep switch: Hypothalamic control of sleep and wakefulness. *Trends Neurosci* 2001; 24:726–731.

Semba K, et al. Noradrenergic presynaptic inhibition of acetylcholine release in the rat pontine reticular formation: An *in vitro* electrophysiological and *in vivo* microdialysis study. *Soc Neurosci Abstr* 1997; 23:1065.

Shaw PJ, et al. Correlates of sleep and waking in *Drosophila melanogaster*. Science 2000; 287:1834–1837.

Strecker RE, et al. Adenosinergic modulation of basal forebrain and preoptic/anterior hypothalamic neuronal activity in the control of behavioral state. *Behav Brain Res* 2000; 115:183–204.

Turek FW. Circadian rhythms. *Horm Res* 1998; 49:109–113.

Xi MC, et al. Evidence that wakefulness and REM sleep are controlled by a GABAergic pontine mechanism. *J Neurophysiol* 1999; 82:2015–2019.

# 3

## PHYSIOLOGIC PROCESSES DURING SLEEP

Leon Rosenthal
Sleep Medicine Associates of Texas, Dallas, Texas

### INTRODUCTION

Sleep is a highly organized, complex behavior characterized by a relative disengagement from the outer world and variable but specific brain activity. Under normal conditions, sleep is associated with little muscular activity, a stereotypic posture, and reduced response to environmental stimuli. Sleep is indispensable for the survival of the species. As such, it is endogenously generated, homeostatically regulated, and reversible.

#### Physiologic Characteristics of Adult Human Sleep

Endogenously generated

Regulated by homeostatic and circadian factors

Modulated by environmental factors

Sleep rebound follows sleep loss

Functional impairment produced by sleep loss/deprivation

### CIRCADIAN AND HOMEOSTATIC DETERMINANTS OF SLEEP

Sleep, as other physiological variables, is regulated by the circadian timing system. The suprachiasmatic nucleus in the hypothalamus serves as the central neural pacemaker of the circadian timing system.

- The dominant synchronizing input to the human circadian pacemaker is environmental light. The retino-hypothalamic tract links the retina to the suprachiasmatic nucleus, conveying photic information that enables synchronization to the light–dark cycle. Humans are usually synchronized to the 24-h day with most adult humans sleeping at night. It is the temporal interplay of the circadian pacemaker and the sleep homeostatic drive that determine alertness, neurobehavioral performance, and sleep.

- The propensity to fall asleep follows a biphasic pattern during the 24-h day. Two peaks of sleepiness have been characterized, one during nocturnal hours (2–6 AM) and another during daytime hours (2–4 PM). The sleepiness rhythm parallels the circadian variation in body temperature, with shortened sleep latencies occurring in conjunction with temperature reduction. Likewise, more difficulty falling and staying asleep is associated with the rising phase of the temperature curve.

- Sleep per se is considered a basic physiologic need state. The homeostatic drive for sleep increases during wakefulness and decreases during sleep. Acute sleep deprivation is followed by an increase in the propensity to fall asleep and stay asleep. The homeostatic drive to sleep is impacted by the oscillations of the circadian rhythm (e.g., enhanced alertness in the early evening, even after a sleepless night).

### AUTONOMIC CHANGES IN SLEEP

Many of the physiologic changes occurring during sleep are associated to changes in the level of activity of the autonomic nervous system.

- Nonrapid eye movement (NREM) sleep is characterized by a period of relative autonomic stability with sympathetic activity remaining at about the same level as during relaxed wakefulness, and parasympathetic activity increasing through vagus nerve dominance and heightened baroreceptor gain.

- During tonic rapid eye movement (REM) sleep, a relative increase in parasympathetic activation is noted (mostly as a result of a decline in sympathetic input).

*Sleep Medicine Essentials*, edited by Teofilo L. Lee-Chiong
Copyright © 2009 John Wiley & Sons, Inc.

- Phasic REM sleep is characterized by an increase of both sympathetic and parasympathetic activity.
- The status of autonomic activity during sleep can be summarized as reflecting prevalent parasympathetic influence during NREM sleep (associated with quiescence of sympathetic activity), and great variability in sympathetic activity (associated with phasic changes in tonic parasympathetic discharge) during REM sleep.

## CARDIAC PHYSIOLOGY

Nonrapid eye movement sleep is usually characterized by brief heart rate acceleration during normal inspiration to accommodate venous return. During expiration, there is a progressive decrease in heart rate. This variability in cardiac rhythm is considered a marker of cardiac health. During REM sleep, heart rate becomes variable with episodes of tachycardia and bradycardia. Phasic REM sleep might be associated with significant increases in heart rate as a result of bursts of sympathetic activity, and this might lead to significant arrhythmias. Likewise, striking changes in coronary blood flow may occur during REM sleep and sleep-state transitions.

- Individuals with heart disease may experience life-threatening arrhythmias and myocardial ischemia (and/or infarction) during REM sleep as a result of sympathetic nerve activity, which is concentrated in short, irregular bursts. These bursts trigger momentary and intermittent increases in heart rate and arterial blood pressure to levels similar to wakefulness.

## RESPIRATORY PHYSIOLOGY

Sleep does not only modify the neural control of ventilation but also impacts its mechanical and chemical control.

- Nonrapid eye movement sleep is characterized by regularity of both respiratory frequency and amplitude. There is a decrease in alveolar ventilation with a concomitant decrease in arterial $PaO_2$ and increase in $PaCO_2$.
- During REM sleep, there is a further decline in tidal volume, and minute ventilation drops to its lowest level. Central apneas and periodic breathing are more frequent during REM sleep, and these are mostly associated with phasic REM sleep.
- Hypoxic ventilatory response is lower during NREM sleep when compared to wakefulness, although some studies have described gender differences in this response. Both men and women experience a similar decline in the hypoxic ventilatory response during REM sleep. Increases in end-tidal $PaCO_2$ during sleep results in an increase in ventilation. However, this response is variable. Likewise, hypocapnia has

an important inhibitory effect on respiration during sleep.
- Sleep results in a general decrease in muscle tone. This is particularly relevant to the muscles of the upper airway, which, in turn, have an impact on ventilation. The genioglossal muscle activity pulls the tongue down and forward, enabling the airway to remain open. NREM sleep results in decreased discharge activity with further reductions noted during REM sleep. The potential result of this physiological change is the obstruction of the upper airway, which might result in obstructive sleep apnea.

## CEREBRAL BLOOD FLOW

Cerebral blood flow (CBF) mostly decreases during NREM sleep when compared to wakefulness. During REM sleep there are significant regional changes in CBF. In general, a significant increase in CBF is associated with REM sleep. Certain areas of the brain have been described as experiencing significant increases in CBF. Among these, the pontine tegmentum, the dorsal mesencephalon, thalamic nuclei, the amygdala, the anterior cingulate cortex, and the enthorhinal cortex.

- A decrease of CBF in cortical and limbic structures during postsleep wakefulness has been described (when compared to presleep wakefulness). It has been speculated that such a change might be a reflection of a resetting process by which the circulatory and metabolic activity of the brain is set at a lower level of activity.

## TEMPERATURE REGULATION

Core body temperature ($T_{core}$) shows a circadian variation. The $T_{core}$ cycle is a sinusoidal-like function with a maximum in the early evening and a minimum in the early morning. The amplitude of temperature variation is of about $1°C$.

- The circadian $T_{core}$ variation is independent of muscular activity.
- Under normal conditions, the drop in $T_{core}$ during nocturnal sleep is accomplished by two separate mechanisms. One is the sleep-related reduction in the body's thermal set point (the result of increased heat dissipation and decreased heat generation) and the second is the intrinsic circadian temperature variation (which is independent of sleep).
- The preoptic-anterior hypothalamic area is critical to the regulation of $T_{core}$. During NREM sleep, $T_{core}$ is regulated at a lower set point when compared to the wake state. In contrast, $T_{core}$ is not regulated during REM sleep, which represents a poikilothermic state. As a result, the body temperature during REM sleep drifts toward environmental temperature.

## ENDOCRINE FUNCTION

Sleep in humans is associated with prominent changes in the function of virtually every endocrine system in the body. It is through the various hormones secreted in the body that tissue growth is promoted, sexual development and activity are regulated, the absorption of sodium is synchronized, and perhaps, most importantly, the response to stress is modulated to preserve homeostatic balance.

- The plasma concentrations of many hormones display sleep-related variations. Circadian regulation synchronizes these events in many instances. The endocrine hormones that undergo sleep-related changes include the adrenocorticotropic hormone, thyrotropin, growth hormone, gonadotropic hormones, prolactin, and melatonin.
- Sleep duration might have an effect on endocrine function. Specifically, short sleep duration is associated with decreased leptin levels (which suppresses food intake) and a concurrent increase in ghrelin levels (which stimulates appetite). These findings suggest a possible association between poor sleep (specifically insufficient sleep) and obesity.

## GENITAL FUNCTION

Penile erections are a naturally occurring phenomenon associated with REM sleep. This phenomenon has been demonstrated to be present in all healthy males from infancy to old age. Clitoral erections and vaginal engorgement have been documented in women during REM sleep. These physiologic events are the result of increased parasympathetic activity, which results in local vasodilation, decreased venous outflow, and increased bulbocavernosus muscular activity.

- Few changes in genital function are present during NREM sleep.

## FUNCTION OF SLEEP

The available research provides strong evidence that sleep is critical to the survival of the species. While no widespread agreement exists on why sleep is important, it is clear sleep deprivation (or chronic insufficient sleep) results in increased sleepiness and decreased functioning.

- Chronic sleep deprivation in rats has shown that these animals die after 2–3 weeks. REM-deprived rats survive for longer periods but end up dying as well. Unfortunately, a clear cause for the death of these animals has not been identified.
- Several hypotheses about the function of sleep have been advanced, including thermoregulation, conservation of metabolic energy, and cognition (neural maturation and memory consolidation).

## KEY POINTS

1. Sleep is an endogenously generated, homeostatically regulated and a reversible behavioral state characterized by a relative disengagement from the outer world and variable but specific brain activity.
2. Sleep is regulated by the circadian timing system, and the homeostatic drive for sleep.
3. Many of the physiologic changes occurring during sleep are associated with changes in the level of activity of the autonomic nervous system.
4. The available evidence has established that sleep serves an important function, as evidenced by the rebound of sleep following sleep loss and the developmental, functional, and metabolic impairments produced by sleep deprivation. While no unitary theory of sleep function has explained the wealth of data on available sleep phenomena, the evidence suggests that the function of sleep is likely multidimensional and differential depending on the organism's stage of development.

## BIBLIOGRAPHY

Shaffery JP, et al. Ponto-geniculo-occipital wave suppression amplifies lateral geniculate nucleus cell-size changes in monocularly deprived kittens. *Dev Brain Res* 1999; 114: 109–119.

Spiegel K, et al. Sleep curtailment in healthy young men is associated with decreased leptin levels, elevated ghrelin levels, and increased hunger and appetite. *Ann Intern Med* 2004; 141:846–850.

Taheri S, et al. Short sleep duration is associated with reduced leptin, elevated ghrelin, and increased body mass index. *Plos Med* 2004; 1:210–217.

Tung A, et al. Anesthesia and sleep. *Sleep Med* 2004; 8:213–226.

# 4

# NEUROPHARMACOLOGY OF SLEEP AND WAKEFULNESS

Edgar Garcia-Rill, Tiffany Wallace-Huitt, Mark Mennemeier, Amanda Charlesworth, David Heister, Meijun Ye, and Charlotte Yates
Center for Translational Neuroscience, Department of Neurobiology, and Developmental Sciences, College of Medicine, University of Arkansas for Medical Sciences, Little Rock, Arkansas

## INTRODUCTION

The major sleep–wake control centers consist of the reticular activating system, intralaminar thalamus, hypothalamus, and basal forebrain.

- There are two main regions that modulate our sleep–wake cycles, the mesopontine reticular activating system (RAS) and the hypothalamus. In addition, the intralaminar thalamus and the basal forebrain are modulated by the RAS and hypothalamus and participate in the process of arousal and alertness, as well as in the modulation of sleep states. Neuroactive agents that modulate these regions will also modulate the level of arousal. Disorders that manifest changes in sleep–wake states and/or affect arousal, alertness, and sleep can be expected, of necessity, to include dysregulation in the above-named regions.
- Many neurologic and psychiatric disorders involve, and may even be presaged by, disruption of sleep–wake control regions. For example, many patients with Parkinson's disease exhibit sleep dysregulation years before the clinical signs of the disease, and almost half of rapid eye movement (REM) sleep behavior disorder (RBD) patients will develop Parkinson's disease as many as 13 years after developing the symptoms of RBD. Sleep dysregulation mainly due to an increase in REM sleep drive is a hallmark of psychiatric disorders such as schizophrenia, anxiety disorders and depression. The hallucinations in schizophrenia have been equated with REM sleep intrusion into waking, that is, dreaming while awake.
- Because the process of arousal is essential to attention, and attention to learning and memory, disruption of arousal-related systems has profound effects on higher cognitive functions. Sleep–wake disorders, or the effects of psychoactive agents on these systems, may be at the root of decrements in cognitive performance.

## CONNECTIVITY

The RAS is composed of three main nuclei, the cholinergic pedunculopontine nucleus (PPN) (and its medial partner, the laterodorsal tegmental nucleus), the noradrenergic locus ceruleus (LC), and the serotonergic raphe nucleus (RN) (see Figure 4.1).

- The RN sends inhibitory projections to the PPN and LC, and the LC inhibits the PPN while the PPN activates the LC. The RAS sends the majority of its ascending cholinergic and monoaminergic projections to the thalamus and hypothalamus, while also synapsing on other regions.
- During waking, all three cell groups are active while, in slow-wave sleep, the cholinergic cells decrease firing while monoaminergic cells remain active. However, in REM sleep, the cholinergic cells are highly active while monoaminergic cells decrease their firing rates markedly. Cholinergic RAS neurons are active during waking and REM sleep, that is, during synchronization of fast cortical rhythms (states of increased vigilance and REM sleep drive), but slow their firing during synchronization of slow cortical rhythms.
- The RAS receives input from all afferent sensory systems in parallel to primary afferent sensory projections. That is, the "nonspecific" projection system to the RAS relays "arousal" information through the intralaminar thalamus (ILT) to the cortex. This system functions in parallel to the shuttling of "specific" sensory information through the primary sensory thalamic nuclei to the cortex. It is the

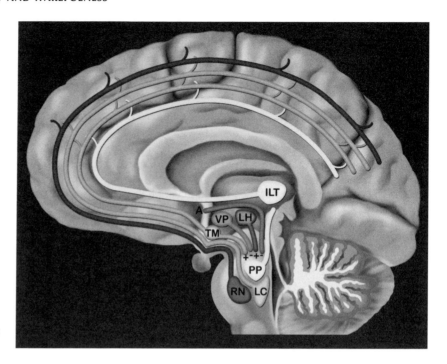

**Figure 4.1** Neural networks controlling sleep and wake states.

temporal summation of intralaminar nonspecific inputs (the context) with primary specific inputs (the content) at the level of the cortex that is thought to participate in "binding," that is, the conscious perception of a sensory event. Disturbances in RAS driving of the ILT and/or of thalamocortical reverberating activity thus can be expected to lead to disturbances in perception.

- The RAS also sends descending projections to postural and locomotion control systems. Such connectivity allows the RAS to act as the "fight-or-flight" control system, simultaneously activating higher centers while priming motor systems to respond appropriately to sudden stimuli. These descending projections modulate the following: (a) pontine inhibitory area (PIA) that is thought to control the atonia of REM sleep; (b) pontine neurons that generate the startle response, a flexor response that primes the motor system; and (c) reticulospinal systems that drive locomotion.

- Reticular activating system projections to the dorsal subceruleus region also modulate the generation of ponto–geniculo–occipital (PGO) waves during REM sleep. This region generates high-frequency bursts of activity (like those required for long-term potentiation) that have been proposed to promote consolidation of certain memories during REM sleep via its projections to the hippocampus. Recent evidence suggests that the subceruleus nucleus generates oscillatory activity by electrical coupling such that individual neurons capable of rhythmic activity are entrained into ensemble activity by the presence of electrical coupling via gap junctions. A similar process has been proposed for the PPN and may represent a novel mechanism for sleep–wake control.

These findings imply that agents that modulate electrical coupling may be expected to influence sleep–wake states.

- The hypothalamic sleep–wake modulatory system is composed mainly of: (a) tuberomammillary nucleus (TMN) with excitatory histaminergic projections; (b) lateral hypothalamus (LH) with excitatory orexinergic projections that project to many brain areas; and (c) ventrolateral preoptic (VLPO) region with mostly inhibitory gamma aminobutyric acid (GABA) ergic projections. These hypothalamic sleep–wake modulatory systems are thought to help stabilize sleep–wake states. On the one hand, the excitatory LH orexin projections were proposed to be an "on" switch promoting waking, partly through their activation of excitatory TMN histaminergic neurons, which are tonically active during waking (and significantly decrease firing during sleep), and of excitatory basal forebrain and RAS, especially cholinergic, neurons. Blockade of orexin receptors can be expected to decrease waking, whereas activation of these receptors can be expected to increase vigilance.

- The basal forebrain cholinergic projection system is especially active during waking and serves to raise the excitability of the cortex. Interestingly, acetylcholine release from the basal forebrain is greater during REM sleep than during waking. On the other hand, the inhibitory VLPO GABAergic projections can be thought of as an "off" switch promoting slow wave sleep through its inhibition of the RAS, LH, basal forebrain, and cortex.

- The dorsal ascending cholinergic (PP) and monoaminergic (LC, RN) projections from the RAS to the ILT serve to activate the cortex via thalamocortical projections. There is also a massive set of ventral projection systems that bypass the thalamus to terminate diffusely throughout the cortex. These originate in the RAS (noradrenergic LC and serotonergic RN) and are joined by ascending projections from the TM (histaminergic TM), LH (orexinergic), and VP (GABAergic VLPO), as well as from the basal forebrain (acetylcholine, not shown). In turn, the TMN, LH, and VP send descending projections to the RAS that may act reciprocally to stabilize sleep–wake states.

- In addition to these transmitters, adenosine is a ubiquitous homeostatic factor thought to be involved in sleep–wake regulation. Conditions of high metabolic activity or prolonged wakefulness lead to a buildup of adenosine, which decreases subsequent to sleep. Therefore, adenosine also may modulate sleep-wake states via its inhibitory actions on most cells, but particularly on excitatory cholinergic RAS and basal forebrain neurons. Adenosine injections into the RAS are known to decrease waking, while adenosine levels in the basal forebrain (but not in the thalamus) progressively increase during prolonged wakefulness and decrease during subsequent recovery of sleep.

- The close relationship between sleep–wake regulation and other homeostatic control functions should be remembered. These systems, especially hypothalamic sleep–wake modulatory regions, interact with the regulation of food intake, metabolism, hormone release, and temperature. This means that disorders of hypothalamic sleep–wake modulatory regions, or psychoactive agents that modulate them, can be expected to also affect homeostatic control systems. For example, Kleine–Levin syndrome is a postpubertal onset disorder characterized by episodes of hypersomnia, mood disturbances (especially depression), compulsive hyperphagia (especially carbohydrates), hypersexuality, and signs of dysautonomia. This disorder points to a pathologic locus bridging sleep–wake control, mood control, and homeostatic control systems.

## BLOOD FLOW DURING SLEEP AND WAKING

The state of slow-wave sleep is marked by decreases in regional cerebral blood flow throughout the brain, but more significantly in the RAS, thalamus, hypothalamus, and basal forebrain. This state is characterized by decreased activity of cholinergic RAS and basal forebrain neurons, of LH orexinergic cells, and of TMN histaminergic cells. That is, the major excitatory projection systems decrease their outputs during slow-wave sleep.

- Rapid eye movement sleep is characterized by increased blood flow in the RAS, the thalamus, and anterior cingulate cortex, among others, with decreases in blood flow in the dorsolateral prefrontal cortex. It has been proposed that the unregulated activity of RAS cholinergic neurons is responsible for REM sleep and, via unknown mechanisms, for decreased frontal lobe blood flow, or "hypofrontality." The hypofrontality of REM sleep is thought to account for the lack of critical judgment during dreaming (and during hallucinations). This state is also characterized by the generation of PGO waves (triggered by descending cholinergic PPN projections to the pons), now thought to be involved in sleep-dependent plasticity. Unlike sleep, the process of awakening entails two stages, a rapid (5-min) reestablishment of consciousness that is marked by increases in cerebral blood flow in the RAS and thalamus, followed by a slower (15-min) increase in cerebral blood flow, primarily in anterior cortical regions.

- Psychoactive agents that affect blood flow can be expected to alter sleep–wake states. It should also be noted that cholinergic RAS neurons have some of the highest concentrations of nitric oxide in the brain. Therefore, wherever the PPN projects, a corollary effect may include vasodilation.

## NEUROPHARMACOLOGY

Psychoactive agents that affect the function of sleep–wake regulating systems can also have profound effects on a host of processes, including higher cognitive performance, attention, learning and memory, homeostatic regulation, and more.

### Alcohol

Alcohol appears to preferentially affect small neurons, particularly granule cells throughout the cerebral and cerebellar cortices, and the hippocampus, perhaps by enhancing GABAergic transmission. Direct effects on sleep–wake control regions appear to also involve potentiation of GABAergic transmission.

- At high doses, its effects are neurotoxic, mainly on basal forebrain neurons, and thus may impair diffuse cholinergic input to the cortex. Significant impairment in motor performance, such as driving, occurs at very low blood alcohol concentrations, an effect potentiated by sleep deprivation or sleep loss. Most alcoholic patients suffer from insomnia, which is clinically important since alcoholism can exacerbate the adverse consequences of insomnia, such as mood changes and anxiety, and because insomnia has been associated with alcohol relapse. In general, sleep loss has greater sedative effects than low doses of alcohol, but similar effects on psychomotor performance. Alcohol produces greater memory impairment than sleep loss, probably because of its marked effects on the hippocampus.

- Alcohol, aside from its recreational uses, is the prototypical anxiolytic, having a calming effect on the stressed, or overstressed, organism. It is evident that alcohol intake is a form of self-medication used as an anxiolytic by patients suffering from psychiatric disorders that involve hypervigilance, for example, schizophrenia, anxiety disorders, and depression. Because alcohol ingestion can lead to decreased frontal lobe blood flow, the ultimate effect will be to exacerbate the "hypofrontality" already evident in these psychiatric patients, further impairing decision-making capacity and lowering the threshold for uncritical action.

### Anesthetics and Sedatives

The proposed mechanisms of action of anesthetics have typically involved a myriad of cellular effects at different sites by disparate drugs. The primary site of action of most anesthetics may be the sleep–wake control system. The parallel manifestations between sleep and anesthesia suggest that anesthetics basically "hijack" the sleep–wake control system to induce anesthesia.

- Most anesthetics, including barbiturates, etomide, propofol, neuroactive steroids, and volatile anesthetics, act on GABAa receptors among other receptors. Sedation and natural sleep occur greatly as a result of enhanced GABAergic transmission, which in turn affects the release of a number of excitatory transmitters such as acetylcholine, excitatory amino acids, and histamine. These actions may take place specifically in such regions as the RAS, TMN, and basal forebrain (all of which have local circuit GABAergic neurons, and receive GABAergic input from VLPO), thereby regulating the level of arousal.

- *Barbiturates* are dangerous drugs with a narrow therapeutic index between the dose required for sedation and the dose that will cause coma and death. These agents typically decrease cerebral blood flow, although regional differences between agents are evident.

- *Volatile and steroid anesthetics* are also known to reduce cerebral blood flow along with cerebral oxygen metabolism, an effect that maintains the coupling between metabolism and flow. Halothane and propofol appear to block gap junctions. Oleamide, which promotes sleep, is also known to block electrical coupling. Anandamide, which enhances adenosine levels to promote sleep, can block gap junctions. Carbenoxolone, a putative gap junction blocker, is known to decrease gamma-band oscillations [high-frequency electroencephalogram (EEG)], while connexin 36 (the neuronal gap junction protein) knockout mice exhibit low gamma-band power. These findings support a role for electrical coupling via gap junctions in the control of sleep–wake states and their modulation by anesthetic agents.

- *Benzodiazepines* act by binding to a site that modulates GABA receptors, especially, GABAa receptors. These agents produce sedative, hypnotic, anxiolytic, and anticonvulsant activities. They act generally by amplifying GABAergic transmission, such that short-acting agents have been used to promote sleep in insomnia patients, although more recently, effective nonbenzodiazepine hypnotics

have been developed. These agents (e.g., eszoplicone, zolpidem, and zaleplon) also act to facilitate GABAa receptor function.

- *Gammahydroxybyrate* (GHB) is a naturally occurring metabolite of GABA, is a potent central nervous system (CNS) depressant, and acute intoxication with GHB or its analogs can lead to respiratory depression and even death. Like most hypnotics, GHB can induce tolerance and produce dependency. In pharmacologic doses, it is used as a sedative/anesthetic, in alcohol/opiate detoxification, and for the treatment of cataplexy in narcolepsy. How does GHB act to decrease cataplexy? The cellular mechanisms are unknown, but one possible mechanism may be through direct or indirect activation of GABAb receptors, which can inhibit PPN neurons (which induce REM sleep) and elicit slow-wave activity, including spike and wave activity via the thalamus, a form of nonconvulsive epilepsy; this agent, when administered before bedtime appears to induce the symptoms of narcolepsy and contain them at night. High doses of GHB can decrease glucose metabolism but, surprisingly, do not significantly alter global blood flow.

### Antihistamines

Pathology and lesions of the TMN cause hypersomnia. Histaminergic inputs to the RAS suppress slow-wave sleep and promote waking, although they do not affect REM sleep significantly. Administration of antihistamines (histamine receptor blockers) results in sedation. Such an effect may result from blockade of histaminergic inputs to the RAS, basal forebrain, and/or LH.

- The cortex has the highest concentration of histamine receptors, so that widespread changes in cortical excitability are also possible through that mechanism. Antihistamines reduce blood flow in frontal cortex and midbrain, which could also account for the cognitive impairments and decrement in psychomotor function observed. Some tolerance can develop over time that can decrease such impairments. In children, first- and second-generation antihistamine intoxication can induce coma, although the newer (third-generation) pediatric formulations (e.g., fexofenadine, loratadine, cetirizine, etc.) appear to be safer.

### Caffeine

The popularity of caffeine is related to its stimulant properties, which are mediated by its ability to reduce adenosine release in the brain. Caffeine appears to block adenosine A1 and A2a receptors, producing a psychomotor stimulant effect. Because of the high levels of A2a receptors in the striatum, the potential use of caffeine for the treatment of Parkinson's disease has been advanced. Since adenosine A2a receptor blockade appears to protect dopaminergic neurons from toxic agents, a neuroprotective role has been proposed for caffeine in the treatment of Parkinson's disease. Caffeine intake has also been associated with a decreased risk of Alzheimer disease, again presumably acting as a neuroprotective agent.

- Caffeine is known to lower cerebral blood flow while simultaneously inducing an increase in metabolism through inhibition of adenosine receptors, leading to a state of relative hypoperfusion for prolonged periods of time. However, its alerting effects are obviously mediated by inhibition of adenosinergic inputs to RAS and basal forebrain cholinergic neurons.

## Nicotine

Inhaled nicotine in cigarette smoke is known to permeate the lungs where >80% of the available nicotine is absorbed into the bloodstream. The short delivery time and elimination half-lives (8 min and 2 h, respectively) assure that, within a short time, smoking another cigarette can reproduce the effect. After absorption into the blood, nicotine readily crosses the blood–brain barrier and appears to be rapidly partitioned into brain tissue. Concentrations of nicotine in the brain have been reported to be 5–7 times higher than blood concentrations. Smokers assert that, in addition to its positive effects on concentration and attention, the primary positive effect of smoking is that it calms and relaxes.

- One of the sites of action of nicotine may be in the RAS, specifically, on PPN neurons. Systemic administration of nicotine, or localized injection of a nicotinic receptor agonist into the PPN, leads to a dose-dependent decrease in the amplitude of the P13 potential in the rat, the rodent equivalent of the sleep-state-dependent P50 potential in the human, suggesting that nicotinic agonists, at least initially, may reduce the level of arousal.
- The calming effects of nicotine, via stimulation of presynaptic inhibition of cholinergic RAS neurons, appears to differ from the role of smoking in reducing the incidence of Parkinson disease, which is a neuroprotective action on dopaminergic neurons.
- Cerebral vasodilation is seen immediately after smoking, but chronic smokers show global reductions in cerebral blood flow ("hypofrontality"). The initial beneficial, calming effects of nicotine may be followed by deleterious consequences on cortical blood flow. Such an effect may drive craving for the next cigarette, creating a vicious cycle of continuous self-administration.

## Stimulants

The most common stimulant, amphetamine, induces release of monoamines, especially dopamine, but also blocks reuptake and may have neurotoxic effects on nigral neurons, and, more recently, is suspected of inducing degeneration of certain striatal neurons.

- *Amphetamine* is abused for recreational purposes and continues to be prescribed for the treatment of attention deficit hyperactivity disorder. Methylphenidate does not appear to have such neurotoxic effects. The difference between these agents appears to be that methylphenidate is mainly a dopamine uptake inhibitor without major influence on release. While any psychotropic agent can have deleterious effects on brain cells, particularly if abused, great care is required when using amphetamine, especially in the young. Amphetamine psychosis occurs in two forms, acute intoxication after a single large dose (characterized by confusion and disorientation), and chronic abuse after repeated use that produces a schizophrenia-like syndrome. The increased release of dopamine by amphetamine is considered a model for schizophrenia and contributes to the "dopamine theory" of schizophrenia.
- *Methamphetamine* is a popular street drug similar to amphetamine, has become widely abused, and probably has severe neurotoxic effects. One potential mechanism via which these agents promote hypervigilance is through activation of the striatum and disinhibition of cholinergic RAS neurons. A more direct effect would be induced release of dopamine and noradrenaline at the level of the cortex. These effects are accompanied by transient increases in cerebral blood flow (midbrain, thalamus, and frontal cortex), but abstinent abusers are known to have decreased blood flow in basal ganglia and certain cortical areas, that is, long-term effects on blood flow may be deleterious.
- *MDMA* (3,4-methylenedioxymethamphetamine) or "ecstasy" is another recreational abused amphetamine that is even more neurotoxic, has hallucinogenic properties at high doses, and has been linked to a number of deaths.
- *Modafinil* is a newer stimulant that does not appear to act through dopaminergic mechanisms, like amphetamine. Modafinil does seem to affect structures involved in the regulation of sleep–wake states and to affect a number of transmitter systems, including decreased GABAergic and increased noradrenergic, histaminergic, and orexinergic, as well as excitatory amino acid and serotonin, release. Modafinil has been found to be effective in the treatment of daytime sleepiness in patients with narcolepsy. Modafinil's mode of action on cortical, reticular thalamic, and inferior olivary neurons is to increase electrical coupling, an effect reduced by gap junction blockers. Modafinil may also facilitate electrical coupling in RAS nuclei such as the PPN and subceruleus. The membrane resistance of these neurons is decreased by modafinil in the presence of fast synaptic blockers, an effect reversed by a gap junction blocker. Modafinil also affects the pedunculopontine neuron whose input resistance is decreased by the superfusion of modafinil in the presence of fast synaptic blockers, with a decrease in resistance that occurs in electrically coupled neurons. There is a decrease in resistance

over time with modafinil that is partially blocked by the gap junction blocker mefloquine.

- The P50 midlatency auditory evoked potential is a sleep-state-dependent potential thought to be generated by the RAS, specifically the PPN. Oral modafinil increased the amplitude of the P50 potential in subjects with daytime sleepiness, suggesting that the amplitude of this waveform can be used as a measure of arousal level. The same effect is observed on the midlatency P13 potential (the rodent equivalent of the human P50 potential) amplitude via a local action within the RAS.

- Modafinil has recently been reported to alleviate spatial neglect from cortical stroke and to increase the amplitude of the P50 potential in stroke patients. This suggests that sensory neglect arising from stroke (right hemisphere strokes typically lead to persistent spatial neglect of the left spatial field, whereas left hemisphere strokes lead to only transient spatial neglect of the contralateral spatial field) can be treated successfully by "waking up" the involved cortex, implying that the consequences of stroke may be to decrease activity, blood flow, or metabolism, one or more of which modafinil may counteract.

- The wake-promoting property of modafinil may make it beneficial for the treatment of other disorders involving decreased activity, blood flow, or metabolism. For example, the hypofrontality in various psychiatric disorders may be amenable to such therapy, as long as the hypervigilance present in these conditions is not exacerbated. Cocaine abusers show reduced frontal cortex blood flow, a mechanism thought to promote risky or erroneous decision making. The RAS is thought to be damaged in about 85% of cases of coma, with the rest accounted for by hypothalamic damage. While the use of amphetamine or methylphenidate has been advocated in patients with coma, a better alternative that does not induce significant cardiovascular effects could be modafinil. While the mechanism of action of modafinil is unknown, recent studies show that it may increase electrical coupling, thereby promoting ensemble activity at higher frequencies, thus promoting waking.

**Schizophrenia, Anxiety Disorder, and Depression**   The serotonergic RN is known to inhibit the PPN and LC, with the cholinergic PPN exciting the LC and the noradrenergic LC inhibiting, via alpha-2 adrenergic receptors, the PPN. The PPN sends excitatory cholinergic projections to the substantia nigra (SN), which, in turn, sends dopaminergic projections to the striatum.

- The treatment of depression previously included tricyclic antidepressants such as amitryptiline, imipramine, and clomipramine, agents that mainly blocked reuptake of noradrenaline and serotonin, and blocked histamine and acetylcholine release, thus accounting for increased sleepiness. The selective serotonin reuptake inhibitors (SSRIs) more selectively affect the RAS, thus downregulating arousal levels, especially through promoting inhibition of the PPN and LC. It is not clear if the etiology of depression is related to disinhibition of the PPN and LC by a decrement in serotonergic tone, although this would seem a likely origin for the sleep–wake symptomatology of depression.

- The treatment of anxiety disorder has involved the use of benzodiazepine amplification of GABAergic inhibition. In addition, the use of the alpha-2 receptor agonist clonidine produces anxiolytic effects, probably by inhibiting autoreceptors in the LC and postsynaptic receptors in the PPN, thus downregulating vigilance. Because of the peripheral cardiovascular effects of clonidine, alpha-2 adrenergic receptor agonists without such actions would be more desirable (e.g., the use of the alpha-2 adrenergic receptor agonist dexmedetomidine as an anxiolytic for the treatment of anxiety disorders such as posttraumatic stress disorder, panic attacks, and general anxiety disorder. The etiology of anxiety disorder has been proposed to include downregulation or degeneration of LC outputs (possibly induced by stress hormones), which would act to release, or disinhibit, PPN neurons.

- The treatment of schizophrenia previously involved the use of the dopaminergic receptor blocker haloperidol, which induced tardive dyskinesia, among other serious side effects. Newer antipsychotics such as risperidone and quetiapine appear to block dopaminergic, noradrenergic, and serotonergic receptors. More striking antipsychotic effects were provided by the use of clozapine, which was designed as a muscarinic cholinergic blocker for the treatment of Parkinson's disease. The serious but rare side effect of agranulocytosis made this a dangerous agent; one later-generation agent that has maintained anticholinergic activity without this side effect is olanzapine. These agents appear to have partial penetrance at serotonergic, cholinergic, and dopaminergic receptors, basically reducing muscarinic cholinergic activation of the SN, as well as partially blocking dopaminergic actions in the striatum. The etiology of schizophrenia has been suggested to include increased PPN output, accounting for marked hypervigilance and hallucinations. Excessive PPN output would overactivate the SN and, in turn, increase striatal release of dopamine, that is, complying with the "dopamine theory" of schizophrenia.

### Development

The human newborn sleeps 16 h per day, half of these in REM sleep and half in slow-wave sleep. Between birth and after puberty, there is a developmental decrease in REM sleep such that the adult has 1 h of REM sleep and 6–7 h of slow-wave sleep per day. Therefore, the developmental decrease in REM sleep is mostly replaced by a postpubertal increase in waking. It has been suggested that REM sleep has the biological function of serving to direct the course of brain maturation, such that REM sleep could provide endogenous stimulation at a time when the brain has little or no exogenous input. However, REM sleep does not appear to be essential for survival in the adult. When the stressful components of REM sleep deprivation are removed, REM sleep suppression does not lead to death or disease. It has been proposed that the increased vigilance and REM sleep drive seen in such disorders as schizophrenia, depression, and anxiety disorder represent a regression to a neonatal state with abundant REM sleep. Recent evidence suggests that a number of transmitter systems change during the developmental decrease in REM sleep and may modulate the decrease, and that agents that affect electrical coupling, for example, halothane, propofol, and modafinil, may have much greater effects during the developmental decrease in REM sleep, which in the human is not over until well after puberty, than in the adult.

### Additional Considerations

Particular attention to hormonal conditions is warranted. After all, the first sign of puberty is pulsatile hormone (LH) release during sleep. For example, narcolepsy is tightly linked with certain human leukocyte antigen (HLA) haplotypes, suggesting that it is an autoimmune disorder. Kleine–Levin syndrome is linked to similar haplotypes, which suggests an autoimmune etiology. Interestingly, in most cases of narcolepsy, Kleine–Levin syndrome, as well as schizophrenia, panic attacks, and obsessive–compulsive disorder, the age of onset is soon after puberty. It has been suggested that developmental dysregulation, either pre- or perinatally (initial insult), becomes pathologically manifest after exposure to puberty and its hormonal onslaught. These considerations point to complex interactions between development, environment, and hormonal status, all of which seem to affect sleep–wake regulation in as yet unknown ways. These findings suggest that the effects of hormones, either prescribed or taken as dietary supplements, or abused, need to be more closely studied and considered in the design of therapeutic interventions.

### KEY POINTS

1. At least some anesthetics may act by "highjacking" the sleep–wake control system. One example is the blockade of gap junctions by agents such as halothane and propofol, and the increased coupling induced by the stimulant modafinil.

2. The control of sleep–wake states is a phylogenetically conserved system such that dysregulation of this system may indicate a drastic alteration of homeostasis. Such dysregulation may also presage the onset of other neurologic and psychiatric disorders, for example, many REM behavior disorder patients will go on to develop more widespread neurodegenerative changes while many Parkinson's disease patients suffered from sleep dysregulation years before the onset of parkinsonian signs.

3. One of the first signs of puberty is during the nighttime release of leutenizing hormone, and gonadal steroids dramatically affect sleep–wake states, suggesting that these two homeostatic systems are highly interdependent.

### ACKNOWLEDGMENT

This work was supported by USPHS awards NS20246, RR20146 and NS39384.

### BIBLIOGRAPHY

Garcia-Rill E. Disorders of the reticular activating system. *Med Hypoth* 1997; 49:379–387.

Garcia-Rill E, et al. Electrical coupling: Novel mechanism for sleep-wake control. *Sleep* 2002; 30:1405–1414.

Garcia-Rill E, et al. Magnetic sources of the M50 response are localized to frontal cortex. *Clin Neurophysiol* 2008; 119:388–398.

Heister DS, et al. Evidence for electrical coupling in the SubCoeruleus (SubC) nucleus. *J Neurophysiol* 2007; 97:3142–3147.

Mamiya N, et al. Nicotine suppresses the P13 auditory evoked potential by acting on the pedunculopontine nucleus in the rat. *Exp Brain Res* 2004; 164:109–119.

Maquet P, et al. Functional neuroanatomy of human slow wave sleep. *J Neurosci* 1997; 17:2807–2812.

Saper SB, et al. The sleep switch: Hypothalamic control of sleep and wakefulness. *Trends Neurosci* 2001; 24:726–731.

Schenck CH, et al. Delayed emergence of a parkinsonian disorder in 38% of 29 older men initially diagnosed with idiopathic rapid eye movement sleep behavior disorder. *Neurology* 1996; 46:388–393.

Seiden LS, et al. Neurotoxicity of methamphetamine and methylenedioxymethamphetamine. *Neurotox Res* 2001; 3:101–116.

Woods AJ, et al. Bias in magnitude estimation following left hemisphere injury. *Neuropsychologia* 2006; 44:1406–1412.

# 5

## INSOMNIA: PREVALENCE AND DAYTIME CONSEQUENCES

W. David Brown
Sleep Diagnostics of Texas, The Woodlands, Texas

### INTRODUCTION

Insomnia is a common, though varied complaint, and includes difficulty falling asleep, maintaining sleep for a sufficient duration, or a sense of nonrestorative sleep. The term has been used to describe a symptom of another medical or psychiatric disorder, or it may be considered a distinct diagnostic entity.

### PREVALENCE OF INSOMNIA

#### General Population

Most studies assessing the prevalence of insomnia in the general population report that 30–35% of individuals experienced some difficulty sleeping in the previous year. In addition, roughly 10–20% of the population describes their sleep complaints as severe (i.e., disrupted sleep every night or almost every night for at least 2 weeks and generally includes daytime symptoms).

- The 1991 National Sleep Foundation Survey found that 36% of U.S. respondents reported a current sleep problem; of this group, 27% had occasional insomnia and 9% had chronic sleep disturbance. This is consistent with a 1989 survey that found that 10.2% of the U.S. population had chronic insomnia.

#### Primary Care

Insomnia is more prevalent in primary care populations. In one study, the prevalence of insomnia was 69% (50% with occasional insomnia and 19% with chronic insomnia). The higher rate in a medical population would be expected due to concomitant psychiatric and medical illness.

- While many primary care patients have significant sleep problems, few are actually being treated. In a large survey of five managed-care organizations, insomnia with daytime dysfunction was reported by 32.5% of the respondents. However, only 0.9% was seeing a physician specifically for sleep, 11.6% of those with daytime dysfunction group were taking a prescription medication for sleep, and 21.4% were taking an over-the-counter medication for sleep.

#### Gender

Insomnia prevalence is higher in women than in men. The prevalence of insomnia in women is about 1.3 times that of men.

- The gender differences are strongly influenced by age. Before the age of 30 years, the prevalence rates are very similar.
- There are three factors that distinguish women from men, namely the menstrual cycle, childbirth, and menopause. About 15% of women experience sleep disturbance premenstrually. During pregnancy, sleep worsens progressively, with 13–60% of women reporting sleep disturbance during the first trimester, and 66–97% by the third trimester. Estimates of insomnia among peri- and postmenopausal women range from 36 to 50% and are attributed to hot flashes, mood disorders, and sleep-disordered breathing.
- Although women clearly report more subjective sleep problems, objective disturbances in sleep have been difficult to demonstrate apart from insomnia related to pregnancy.

#### Age

The prevalence of insomnia increases with age for a variety of reasons, including retirement, loss of a spouse or close friend, illness, or side effects from medications.

- In one survey of 9000 elderly persons (> 65 years old), 57% reported at least one chronic sleep complaint, and 29% had chronic difficulty falling asleep or waking too early; only 12% had no sleep complaints.

*Sleep Medicine Essentials*, edited by Teofilo L. Lee-Chiong

• In another study involving older population, the prevalence of insomnia in African Americans was significantly lower than among Caucasians.

## Psychiatric Patients

In patient samples, over 60% of those with major depressive disorder report sleep disturbances, and between 30–50% of patient's with chronic insomnia have a psychiatric disorder, typically a mood disorder.

• Alcoholics have high rates of insomnia. One study documented that 61% of alcoholics had insomnia during the 6 months prior to treatment, and the insomnia may persist for weeks to months after initiating abstinence. Compared to patient's without insomnia, patient's with insomnia were about twice more likely to report frequent alcohol use for sleep, had worse polysomnographic measures of sleep continuity, and had more severe alcohol dependence and depression. Both severity of alcohol dependency and level of depression are significantly associated with insomnia. Insomnia is a robust predictor of alcohol relapse.

## CONSEQUENCES OF INSOMNIA

### Quality of Life

Quality of life (QOL) is a concept used to describe an individual's ability to function and to derive satisfaction from doing so. QOL is impaired in insomnia patients.

• In a 1991 Gallup survey found that 72% of insomnia subjects woke up feeling drowsy or tired. Thirty percent of chronic insomnia subjects reported that their quality of life was fair or poor compared to 19% of occasional insomniacs and only 4% of no-insomnia subjects. Fewer of the insomnia group reported enjoying relationships, and they had more problems with their spouse as well as friends. They reported feeling physically worse than a no-insomnia group, mood was worse, and they reported difficulty handling minor irritations.

• In a survey of a German population, quality of life was rated as "bad" in 22% of severe insomniacs compared to only 3% of subjects without a sleep complaint. QOL was rated as "good" in only 28% of severe insomniacs versus 68% of subjects without sleep problems. Despite this finding, only 55% of the severe group had ever discussed their sleep with a doctor and only 27% were taking medication for sleep.

• Quality of life scores were measured in three matched groups of severe insomnia, mild insomnia, and good sleepers. QOL scores were progressively worse from good sleepers to severe insomnia. Insomnia patients report poorer cognitive ability including decreased attention, concentration, mental acuity, reasoning, and problem-solving ability. Even when individuals with psychiatric illness are excluded, insomnia patients produce higher scores on depression, anxiety, and health status scales. In general, insomnia can have a negative impact on home life and recreational functioning. Insomnia patients report decreased enjoyment of interpersonal relationships, are more likely to feel irritated by their children, are less likely to help them with their homework, and tend to watch TV more than read or exercise.

### Use of Medical Services

Insomnia is associated with poorer health, although the cause-and-effect relationship has not been established. Insomnia patients use more medical services, both directly for treatment of the sleep complaint and secondarily for increased medical complaints.

• Moderate to severe insomnia sufferers have up to two times as many doctor visits and hospital stays as do good sleepers. This increased usage is not accounted for by direct treatment for insomnia alone. Only a small percentage of insomnia patients seek treatment specifically for their sleep complaint, and only a minority of insomnia patients take prescription medications for sleep. Insomnia patients take more medications for other medical problems, including cardiovascular, genitourinary, and gastrointestinal drugs. After controlling for demographic variables and comorbid conditions, the negative association of insomnia remained significant on emergency room visits, calls to physician, and over-the-counter drug use.

• Nursing home care for the elderly is the largest source of direct costs attributable to insomnia. Between 40 and 51% of caregivers who institutionalize an elderly person cite sleep disruption as a major factor.

### Work Performance

Absenteeism from work is far more prevalent in severe insomniacs than in good sleepers. A severe insomnia complaint may be one of the best predictors of absenteeism from work. In addition, insomnia patients experience fewer promotions and pay raises, remain in lower pay grades, are less optimistic about their future job opportunities, receive fewer positive recommendations, have more difficulty with concentration and finishing their work, have more work-related accidents, and have higher attrition rates.

### Accidents

In a 1991 Gallup survey, 5% of insomnia subjects reported having an automobile accident due to sleepiness compared to only 2% of the occasional or no-insomnia groups.

• Middle-aged drivers dissatisfied with their sleep were three times as likely to have had an auto accident in the previous year compared to other drivers.

- In a French study, severe insomnia patients had seven times as many industrial accidents as did good sleepers.

## Cognitive Functioning

Insomnia patients report poorer cognitive ability, including poorer attention, concentration, mental acuity, reasoning, problem-solving ability, and mental reactivity. Although there is no consistent evidence of cognitive dysfunction for any neuropsychological functions in insomnia patients, the areas that are most likely to show reduced performance are attention span and vigilance performance.

## Risk for Depression

Insomnia patients have higher rates of depression. Although often perceived as a symptom of depression, insomnia can also be a precursor of depression. Insomnia complaints tend to precede or occur with a mood disorder (first episode or relapse) but tend to appear at the same time or to follow an anxiety disorder episode.

- Both insomnia and hypersomnia are associated with suicidal behavior in patients with major depression. Sleep disturbance is associated with suicidality in patients with major depression and is a significant independent predictor of completed suicide in psychiatric patients. Insomnia may be a better predictor of suicidal behavior than a specific plan or suicide note.

## Cost

Chronic insomnia can be associated with increased use of medical services, decrements in work performance, family problems, emotional problems, automobile and industrial accidents, and may lead to increased use of alcohol.

- In the United States based on a prevalence of 10% there would be 25 million people with insomnia. Direct costs have been estimated at $13.9 billion with a large majority of the costs attributed to nursing home care. In addition to the direct cost of medical treatment and drugs, indirect costs may include reduced productivity, increased absenteeism, accidents, and hospitalization, as well as increased medical costs due to increased morbidity and mortality, depression due to insomnia, and increased alcohol consumption.
- Estimates of the total direct, indirect, and related costs of insomnia have been estimated to range from $30–35 billion to a high of $92.5–$107.5 billion.

## KEY POINTS

1. Insomnia is a common problem and the prevalence rates are similar in most surveys. The disorder is more common in a general medical practice, in women, and in the elderly.
2. Insomnia is associated with negative consequences including increased use of medical services, absenteeism from work, automobile and industrial accidents, poorer work performance, and greater risk for depression. It can have a negative impact on family life.
3. The direct and indirect costs associated with insomnia are estimated to be in the billions of dollars each year.

## BIBLIOGRAPHY

Agargun MY, et al. Sleep disturbances and suicidal behavior in patients with major depression. *J Clin Psychiatry* 1997; 58:249–251.

Althius MD, et al. The relationship between insomnia and mortality among community-dwelling older women. *J Am Geriatr Soc* 1998; 46:1270–3.

Ancoli-Israel S, et al. Characteristics of insomnia in the United States: Results of the 1991 National Sleep Foundation Survey. I. *Sleep* 1999; 22:S347–S353.

Brower KJ. Insomnia, alcoholism and relapse. *Sleep Med Rev* 2003; 7:523–539.

Brower KJ, et al. Insomnia, self-medication, and relapse to alcoholism. *Am J Psychiatry* 2001; 158:399–404.

Drake CL, et al. Insomnia causes, consequences, and therapeutics: An overview. *Depress Anxiety* 2003; 18:163–176.

Foley DJ, et al. Incidence and remission of insomnia among elderly adults: An epidemiologic study of 6800 persons over three years. *Sleep* 1999a; 22:S366–S372.

Foley DJ, et al. Incidence and remission of insomnia among elderly adults in a biracial cohort. *Sleep* 1999b; 22:S373–S378.

Fulda S, et al. Cognitive dysfunction in sleep disorders. *Sleep Med Rev* 2001; 5:423–445.

Hajak G. Epidemiology of severe insomnia and its consequences in Germany. *Eur Arch Psychiatry Clin Neurosci* 2001; 251:49–56.

Hall RC, et al. Suicide risk assessment: A review of risk factors for suicide in 100 patients who made severe suicide attempts. Evaluation of suicide risk in a time of managed care. *Psychosomatics* 1999; 40:18–27.

Hatoum HT, et al. Prevalence of insomnia: A survey of the enrollees at five managed care organizations. *Am J Manag Care* 1998a; 4:79–86.

Hatoum HT, et al. Insomnia, health-related quality of life and healthcare resource consumption. A study of managed-care organization enrollees. *Pharmacoeconomics* 1998b; 14:629–637.

Ishigooka J, et al. Epidemiological study on sleep habits and insomnia of new outpatients visiting general hospitals in Japan. *Psychiatry Clin Neurosci* 1999; 53:515–522.

Leger D, et al. Prevalence of insomnia in a survey of 12,778 adults in France. *J Sleep Res* 2000; 9:35–42.

Leger D, et al. SF-36: Evaluation of quality of life in severe and mild insomniacs compared with good sleepers. *Psychosom Med* 2001; 63:49–55.

Leger D, et al. Medical and socio-professional impact of insomnia. *Sleep* 2002; 25:625–629.

Leigh JP. Employee and job attributes as predictors of absenteeism in a national sample of workers: The importance of health and dangerous working conditions. *Soc Sci Med* 1991; 33: 127–137

Manber R, et al. Sex, steroids, and sleep: A review. *Sleep* 1999; 22:540–555.

Ohayon MM. Epidemiology of insomnia: What we know and what we still need to learn. *Sleep Med Rev* 2002; 6:97–111.

Ohayon MM, et al. Prevalence and consequences of insomnia disorders in the general population of Italy. *Sleep Med* 2002a; 3:115–120.

Ohayon MM, et al. Prevalence of insomnia and associated factors in South Korea. *J Psychosom Res* 2002b; 53:593–600.

Ohayon MM, et al. Place of chronic insomnia in the course of depressive and anxiety disorders. *J Psychiatr Res* 2003; 37:9–15.

Ohayon MM, et al. Daytime consequences of insomnia in the French general population. *Encephale* 2004; 30:222–227.

Roth T, et al. Daytime consequences and correlates of insomnia in the United States: results of the 1991 National Sleep Foundation survey. II. *Sleep* 1999; 22:S354–S358.

Shochat T, et al. Insomnia in primary care patients. *Sleep* 1999; 22: S359–S365.

Simon G, et al. Prevalence, burden, and treatment of insomnia in primary care. *Am J Psychiatry* 1997; 154:1417–1423.

Walsh JK, et al. The direct economic costs of insomnia in the U.S. for 1995. *Sleep* 1999; 22:S386–S393.

Walsh J, et al. Prevalence and health consequences of insomnia. *Sleep* 1999; 22:S427–S436.

Young T, et al. Objective and subjective sleep quality in premenopausal, perimenopausal, and postmenopausal women in the Wisconsin sleep cohort study. *Sleep* 2003; 26:667–672.

Zammit G, et al. Quality of life in people with insomnia. *Sleep* 1999; 22:S379–S385.

# 6

## CAUSES OF INSOMNIA

EDWARD J. STEPANSKI
Accelerated Community Oncology Research Network, Memphis, Tennessee

## INTRODUCTION

Insomnia is defined as self-reported difficulty falling asleep, difficulty staying asleep, or having nonrestorative sleep, usually in association with daytime impairment. There are many causes of insomnia, covering a broad range of medical, psychiatric, and behavioral factors. In many instances, insomnia is assumed to be secondary to another primary medical, psychiatric, or sleep disorder. However, specific cause-and-effect pathways have not yet been demonstrated, and a complete understanding of the causes of insomnia remains elusive. Several models are commonly used to explain causes of insomnia.

## PRIMARY VERSUS SECONDARY INSOMNIA

One model often used to understand causes of insomnia is to differentiate whether the insomnia is secondary to another primary disorder or is an independent disorder. This distinction is important since a diagnosis of secondary insomnia will lead to focusing treatment efforts on the primary disorder, rather than on the symptom.

- Psychiatric disorders, such as depression and anxiety, are examples of primary disorders commonly associated with secondary insomnia. The comorbidity between insomnia and depression is particularly strong, and patients with severe insomnia are eight times more likely to have depression than patients without insomnia.
- Patients with medical disorders also have high rates of insomnia.
- "Secondary insomnia" occurs much more frequently than primary insomnia. In one study involving patients who presented to sleep centers with reports of insomnia, 20% of cases were diagnosed with primary insomnia, 44% of cases with insomnia secondary to a mental disorder, and 8% of cases with insomnia secondary to a medical disorder or substance abuse disorder.
- Primary insomnia is diagnosed using criteria from the *Diagnostic and Statistical Manual of Mental Disorders—IV* when the insomnia appears to be an independent disorder. Various behavioral and cognitive factors are theorized as contributing to primary insomnia. This is reflected by the fact that the International Classification of Sleep Disorders-2 (ICSD) provides subtypes for primary insomnia that specifically implicate behavioral and cognitive factors as causes of the insomnia. Subtypes of primary insomnia categorized within the ICSD nosology include *psychophysiological insomnia*, *inadequate sleep hygiene*, *idiopathic insomnia*, and *paradoxical insomnia*.
- Inadequate sleep hygiene has been hypothesized to result from behavioral factors such as spending excessive time in bed, napping during the day, drinking caffeine near bedtime, and using the bed for work.
- Psychophysiological insomnia is thought to result from learned associations between the bed and increased tension and arousal. This category can also be thought of as "conditioned insomnia." This category is the most commonly diagnosed of the primary insomnia subtypes.
- Idiopathic insomnia begins in childhood and is thought to result from a neurophysiologic abnormality in the central nervous system.
- Paradoxical insomnia is diagnosed when the patient reports being awake most or all of the night, although there is evidence that the patient has been asleep. Polysomnography in these patients will show normal sleep time concurrent with the patient's report of having been awake much of the night.

*Sleep Medicine Essentials*, edited by Teofilo L. Lee-Chiong
Copyright © 2009 John Wiley & Sons, Inc.

## LIMITATIONS OF THE SECONDARY INSOMNIA MODEL

Research shows a strong association between insomnia and psychiatric and medical disorders, but it is not clear that insomnia is a direct consequence of these disorders. In many cases, the relation between insomnia and other presumed primary conditions does not follow a straightforward cause-and-effect model.

- An episode of insomnia predicts subsequent development of new depression; conversely, episodes of insomnia have been shown to predict a recurrence of depression in previously recovered individuals. Thus, insomnia, at least in some cases, can be a cause of depression rather than a consequence of depression. Alternatively, insomnia and depression may both result from a common vulnerability or other factor.
- Insomnia can also precede serious medical disorders; for instance, insomnia is a significant predictor of an incident coronary event.
- Definitive determination that insomnia is secondary to another primary disorder is often impossible in clinical practice. There must be contiguity between the origin and course of the insomnia, relative to the suspected primary disorder, before insomnia is considered as definitively secondary to the associated primary condition. If only either the origin or the course of the insomnia is associated with that of the primary disorder, the insomnia is only viewed as partially related to the primary condition.
- Another shortcoming of viewing insomnia as a consequence of another primary disorder is that not all patients with the primary disorders associated with insomnia actually develop insomnia. If insomnia is secondary to a medical condition, shouldn't all patients with the condition develop insomnia? This is clearly not the case. Other factors are at work in causing insomnia beyond the presence or absence of another "primary" disorder. A National Institutes of Health (2005) state-of-the-science conference addressed this issue and concluded that the concept of "comorbid insomnia" is more accurate than the notion of "secondary insomnia."

## THEORETICAL MODEL FOR CHRONIC INSOMNIA: PREDISPOSING, PRECIPITATING, AND PERPETUATING FACTORS

Determining a specific cause of chronic insomnia is often challenging because of multiple contributing factors. A model of chronic insomnia has been proposed that assumes a multifactorial etiology and categorizes causal factors according to their role in the formation of the insomnia as predisposing, precipitating, or perpetuating. This model helps to improve the understanding of how various factors interact together to produce insomnia and also illustrates how an episode of acute insomnia evolves into chronic insomnia.

- According to this model, all individuals have a certain level of predisposition to insomnia, and insomnia occurs when this predisposition interacts with exposure to a precipitating factor. Individuals who are highly predisposed will experience insomnia in response to minor precipitants, while others are robust sleepers with a low predisposition to insomnia and experience insomnia only in response to very significant precipitating events. Over time, the precipitating factor recedes or disappears entirely but is replaced by perpetuating factors that maintain the insomnia. The predisposing factors explain why only certain patients develop insomnia (highly predisposed) when experiencing pain or another condition that commonly precipitates insomnia, while others (with low predisposition) continue to sleep well in the presence of the same disorder.

### Causal Factors in Development of Insomnia

Predisposing factors
- Somatic hyperarousal
- Cognitive hyperarousal
- Decreased homeostatic sleep drive

Precipitating factors
- Medical disorders
- Psychiatric disorders
- Medication effects
- Substance abuse
- Circadian rhythm disorders
- Primary sleep disorders

Perpetuating factors
- Behavioral factors
- Cognitive factors

### Predisposing Factors

The presence of predisposing factors is inferred by the different thresholds observed across individuals for the development of insomnia. Specific mechanisms underlying a predisposition to insomnia have not been elucidated. Theories include:

- *Physiological Hyperarousal* Individuals with chronic insomnia, as compared to normal sleepers, have a faster increase in heart rate in response to stress, increased metabolic rate, increased heart rate variability, increased beta activity in the sleep electroencephalography (EEG), increased secretion of adrenocorticotropic hormone (ACTH), increased cerebral glucose metabolism during sleep and wake, and increased daytime alertness despite short sleep. Studies using positron emission tomography scans also showed less decrease in cerebral glucose metabolism between wake and sleep in those areas of the brain associated with arousal in subjects with insomnia as compared to normal sleepers. Nevertheless, it has not yet been shown whether hyperarousal itself is a cause or consequence of insomnia. In addition to these measures of physiologic hyperarousal, there is evidence that patients with chronic insomnia are prone to increased cognitive arousal or emotional arousal.

- *Decreased Homeostatic Drive for Sleep*  Sleep initiation, as well as overall regulation of a coherent sleep–wake schedule, has been shown to be related to homeostatic and circadian mechanisms. Patients with chronic insomnia do not show the same increase in slow-wave sleep following sleep deprivation that is observed in normal sleepers, consistent with decreased homeostatic drive. A reduced sleep drive would be expected to make it more difficult to initiate and maintain sleep under both baseline and sleep-deprived conditions. Decreased sleep drive could interact with precipitating factors to produce chronic insomnia.

## Precipitating Factors

Precipitating factors are those disorders or conditions typically hypothesized as causes of secondary insomnia. Common precipitating factors include medical disorders, psychiatric disorders, environmental factors, medication effects, primary sleep disorders, or circadian rhythm changes that negatively affect sleep.

- Precipitating factors can be acute stressful events, acute environmental changes (e.g., excessive noise or light in the bedroom, or sleeping in a new environment), or changes in the sleep–wake schedule (e.g., jet lag or shift work).
- *Chronic medical and psychiatric conditions* (e.g., pain, dyspnea, neurodegenerative disorders, renal failure, hyperthyroidism, and mood disorders) can also precipitate insomnia.
- *Medications* are also associated with insomnia, including stimulating antidepressants, steroids, beta blockers, bronchodilators, and decongestants.
- *Primary sleep disorders* causing insomnia include restless leg syndrome, periodic limb movement disorder, and sleep-disordered breathing. All of these primary sleep disorders become more prevalent with aging.

## Perpetuating Factors

Perpetuating factors are behavioral and cognitive changes that occur once an individual has been sleeping poorly for a period of time.

- Examples include keeping an irregular sleep–wake schedule, spending excessive amounts of time in bed attempting to gain more sleep time, taking daytime naps, and engaging in stimulating activities during the night. These are changes that people often make in response to insomnia in an effort in obtain additional sleep and rest. However, while such changes might help alleviate symptoms in the short term, they promote continued insomnia in the long term.
- Cognitive changes that occur with insomnia include an increased preoccupation with sleep during daytime hours, as well as a fear of not sleeping and of daytime impairment. These cognitive changes lead to increased tension at bedtime and upon awakening during the night.
- Patients may develop irrational fears regarding the effects of insomnia (e.g., inability to sleep will lead to loss of employment or even death) as well as unreasonable expectations regarding sleep (e.g., requiring 9 h of total sleep time, although optimal daytime performance is regularly achieved with only 7–8 h of sleep).
- The role of these behavioral and cognitive changes in maintaining chronic insomnia helps to explain another finding that conflicts with the presumed cause-and-effect relation between insomnia and primary disorders: The primary disorder can remit with treatment, but the insomnia continues on. If the insomnia is truly secondary to the primary condition, it should remit in conjunction with the primary disorder. A multifactorial model of chronic insomnia with predisposing, precipitating, and perpetuating factors shows that the primary disorder initially triggers the insomnia but is not needed for insomnia to continue.

## KEY POINTS

1. There are many possible causes of insomnia, covering a broad range of medical, psychiatric, and behavioral factors. Chronic insomnia can best be understood as resulting from a combination of predisposing, precipitating, and perpetuating factors.
2. A traditional model of insomnia distinguishes between secondary insomnia that occurs as a consequence of another primary disorder, and primary insomnia, which is an independent disorder. This model explains the high comorbidity between insomnia and psychiatric and medical disorders.
3. Chronic insomnia has also been shown to predict the subsequent development of psychiatric and medical disorders, and therefore is worthy of evaluation and treatment as an independent disorder.

## REFERENCES

National Institutes of Health State of the Science Conference statement on Manifestations and Management of Chronic Insomnia in Adults, June 13–15, 2005. *Sleep* 2005; 28:1049–1057.

## BIBLIOGRAPHY

Besset A, et al. Homeostatic process and sleep spindles in patients with sleep-maintenance insomnia: Effect of partial (21 h) sleep deprivation: *Electroencephal Clin Neurophys* 1998; 107:122–132.

Bonnet MH, et al. Hyperarousal and insomnia. *Sleep Med Rev* 1997; 1: 97–108.

Chang PP, et al. Insomnia in young men and subsequent depression. The Johns Hopkins precursors study. *Am J Epidemiol* 1997; 146:105–114.

Foley D, et al. Sleep disturbances and chronic disease in older adults. Results of the 2003 National Sleep Foundation Sleep in America survey. *J Psychosom Res* 2004; 56:497–502.

Glovinsky P, Spielman A. *The Insomnia Answer.* Berkeley Publishing Group, New York, 2007.

Harvey AG, et al. Catastrophic worry in primary insomnia. *J Behav Ther Exp Psychiatry* 2003; 34:11–23.

Jinda RD, et al. Electroencephalographic sleep profiles in single-episode and recurrent unipolar forms of major depression: II. Comparison during remission. *Biol Psychiatry* 2000; 51:230–236.

Katz DA, et al. Clinical correlates of insomnia in patients with chronic illness. *Arch Intern Med* 1998; 158:1099–1107.

Nofzinger EA, et al. Functional neuroimaging evidence for hyper-arousal in insomnia. *Am J Psychiatry* 2004; 161:2126–2128.

Perlis ML, et al. Self-reported sleep disturbance as a prodromal symptom in recurrent depression. *J Affect Disord* 1997; 42:209–212.

Perlis ML, et al. Beta EEG in insomnia. *Sleep Med Rev* 2001; 5:363–374.

Schwartz S, et al. Insomnia and heart disease: A review of epidiemologic studies. *J Psychosom Res* 1999; 47:313–333.

Stepanski E, et al. Effects of sleep deprivation on daytime sleepiness in primary insomnia. *Sleep* 2000; 23:215–219.

Stepanski EJ, et al. Emerging research on the treatment of secondary or comorbid insomnia. *Sleep Med Rev* 2006; 10:7–18

Tang NK, et al. Sleeping with the enemy: Clock monitoring in the maintenance of insomnia. *J Behav Ther Exp Psychiatry* 2007; 38:40–55.

Taylor DJ, et al. Comorbidity of chronic insomnia with medical problems. *Sleep* 2007; 30:213–218.

Vgontzas AN, et al. Chronic insomnia is associated with nyctohemeral activation of the hypothalamic-pituitary-adrenal axis: Clinical implications. *J Clin Endocrinol Metab* 2001; 86:3787–3794.

Zayfert C, et al. Residual insomnia following cognitive behavioral therapy for PTSD. *J Traumat Stress* 2004; 17:69–73.

# 7

## EVALUATION OF INSOMNIA

Douglas E. Moul and Daniel J. Buysse
Sleep and Chronobiology Center, Department of Psychiatry, University of Pittsburgh, Pittsburgh, Pennsylvania

## INTRODUCTION

Insomnia is a complaint of inability to obtain enough sleep or restorative sleep despite enough time given for sleep. It may be present even if a person has daytime complaints of subjective sleepiness, provided that they are not objectively sleepy.

- The evaluation of insomnia is an ongoing process that may extend throughout a patient's medical, psychiatric, or psychological treatment course. Classification of the patient's insomnia syndrome provides a medical context, but the patient's style of presentation and life choices also provide data that guide the choice of treatment strategies. The intervention(s) chosen for the patient is(are) guided by how insomnia is classified.

## PRIMARY INSOMNIA

The *Diagnostic and Statistical Manual* (DSM-IV) defines *primary insomnia* as chronic insomnia in which insomnia and its consequences are the central and only features. This diagnosis requires the absence of other psychiatric, medical, or primary sleep disorders that can cause poor sleep. Difficulty initiating or maintaining sleep, or poor sleep quality, lasting for one month or more is required, along with the presence of daytime impairment (e.g., difficulty concentrating, moodiness, irritability, or fatigue) attributed to the sleep difficulty. Daytime consequences separate patients with *primary insomnia* from those with simple dissatisfaction with their sleep.

- The International Classification of Sleep Disorders (ICSD-2) includes the following disorders as primary insomnias: Psychophysiological Insomnia, Idiopathic Insomnia, and Paradoxical Insomnia. *Psychophysio-*

*logical insomnia* occurs when psychological conditioning factors have made bed or bedroom conditions discriminant stimuli for wakefulness, so that they evoke arousal responses that impair sleep. *Idiopathic insomnia* is a childhood-onset insomnia that has continued into adulthood. *Paradoxical insomnia* refers to an insomnia complaint where polysomnographic (PSG) data indicate that the patient is sleeping much more than the patient reports, accompanied by daytime impairments that result from the reported sleep deficits.

- While it may seem logical for insomnia to be classified by separable difficulties with initiating or maintaining sleep, or with early morning awakening, longitudinal studies have not established that these are stable subtypes.

## COMORBID INSOMNIA

Comorbid insomnia occurs in many sleep, medical, or psychiatric disorders.

Taking a medical/psychiatric history and conducting physical and mental status examinations can identify many diagnoses.

- Polysomnography is unlikely to provide helpful diagnostic information unless the clinical history is suggestive of obstructive sleep apnea, periodic limb movement disorder, narcolepsy, or a parasomnia. PSG may also be useful if initial therapy is unsuccessful, or if there is considerable diagnostic uncertainty. For example, a short rapid eye movement (REM) sleep latency may suggest a diagnosis of major depression in a patient with severe insomnia.

- Actigraphy measurements can be useful in clarifying patterns of sleep and wakefulness.

## DEMOGRAPHICS

Epidemiological studies estimate that one-third of the population has insomnia during a one-year period, with 10% having chronic insomnia. In primary care settings, chronic insomnia (both primary and comorbid) may be present in more than 30% of patients.

- The prevalence of various insomnia-related disorders depends on the referral patterns of particular clinics. An insomnia complaint in a pulmonary sleep clinic is more likely to be due to sleep apnea, whereas it is more likely to be related to an affective, anxiety, or substance abuse disorder in a general psychiatric clinic.

- A number of sleep disorders related to insomnia are probably common across many clinics. Obstructive sleep apnea should be suspected with a clinical history of loud snoring and obesity, and a physical finding of a crowded upper airway. Restless legs syndrome can often be diagnosed by a characteristic history of an urge to move the legs during physical inactivity at night. Delayed sleep phase syndrome can resemble insomnia with difficulties in falling asleep at conventional bedtimes. Finally, shift work sleep disorder can usually be clearly established from the patient's occupational history.

## EVALUATION OF INSOMNIA

A clinical history should be obtained from both the patient and bed partner. A sleep-focused physical and mental status examination is essential.

- Sleep diaries recorded before the clinic evaluation is useful to assess sleep patterns across nights, as are data from questionnaires that focus on sleepiness, anxiety, depression, general psychopathology, sleep quality, and insomnia.

## ASSESSMENT OF CHRONIC INSOMNIA

*Identifying information and chief complaint*
    Demographic risk factors
    Initial stated complaint
*History of present illness*
    Predisposing and initiating factors
    Diagnostic studies
    Therapy trials (e.g., drugs, behaviors)
    Course of illness
    Complicating disorders
    Obvious life stressors
*Sleep habits*
    When sleep is attempted in 24 h
    When sleep occurs in 24 h (include nighttime awakenings)
    Review of sleep logs over weeks
    Sleep schedules on weekends
    Bedtime routines and cognitions
    Influences over sleep schedules (time-zone travel, shift work, etc.)
*Sleep disturbances*
    Adverse bed conditions
    Problems with bed partner
    Symptoms of other sleep disorder (e.g., snoring, restless legs)
*Daytime functioning*
    Daytime inability to nap
    Symptoms of lowered concentration, fatigue, irritability, or moodiness
*Health habits*
    Review of prescribed and over-the-counter medications
    Use of caffeine, alcohol, nicotine, and street drugs
    Diet patterns or restrictions
    Exercise regimen
*Past medical history*
    Sources of pain or discomfort
    Neurologic syndromes
    Relevant medical syndromes
*Past psychiatric history*
    Hospitalization and rehabilitation
    Suicidal or self-harm attempts
    Diagnoses and treatments
    Past and current impairments
*Family history*
    Sleep disorders
    Substance abuse disorders
    Psychiatric disorders
    Relevant medical disorders
*Social and occupational history*
    Level of schooling
    Past and present quality of primary relationships
    Occupational exposures and stresses
    Significant losses
    History of verbal, physical, or sexual abuse or trauma exposures
    Life aspirations
*Assessment of self-report questionnaire data*
    Sleepiness
    Depression
    Anxiety
    General psychopathology
    Sleep quality
    Insomnia-specific
*Brief physical examination*
    Risk factors for sleep apnea
    Signs of neurologic illness
    Lab tests (as needed)

*Mental status examination*
- Quality of alertness and concentration
- Daytime and nighttime symptoms of depression, anxiety, psychotic, or obsessive–compulsive disorders
- Report of blank spells or other loss of awareness
- Fear of the bed, of nighttime, or of sleep
- Presence of frequent nightmares
- Impaired insight into psychological aspects of problem

## INDIVIDUALIZED COMPONENTS OF EVALUATION

### Psychiatric Disorders

Since psychiatric conditions are often associated with an insomnia complaint, adopting a psychiatric perspective is prudent. For example, dramatic statements like, "Doctor, I haven't slept at all," may not be intended to be taken literally, but thought of as "My poor sleep *really* bothers me."

- Sometimes a complaint of insomnia should lead to inquiries about more stigmatized or feared diagnoses; this is especially relevant when thought distortions (e.g., negative thoughts in depressed patients, and fearful thoughts in anxiety patients), or gross deficits in reality testing (e.g., delusions in psychotic patients) are present.

### Comorbid Disorders

There is high prevalence of comorbid clinical symptoms and disorders in patients with insomnia. Comorbid problems, including psychiatric, neurologic, and other medical syndromes that may contribute to the maintenance or severity of insomnia should be reviewed. For instance, in a patient with acute or chronic pain, focusing solely on the complaint of insomnia and ignoring issues of pain control is inadequate.

### DIFFERENTIAL DIAGNOSIS OF A PRESENTING COMPLAINT OF INSOMNIA

| Classification | Specific Causes |
| --- | --- |
| Primary insomnia | Psychophysiological |
| | Paradoxical |
| | Idiopathic |
| Miscellaneous causes | Adjustment (acute) insomnia |
| | Inadequate sleep hygiene |
| | Behavioral insomnia of childhood |
| | Insomnia not due to substance or known |
| | Physiologic condition, unspecified |
| | Physiologic insomnia, unspecified |
| Primary sleep disorders | Advanced sleep phase disorder |
| | Delayed sleep phase disorder |
| | Jet lag syndrome |

| Classification | Specific Causes |
| --- | --- |
| | Nightmare disorder |
| | Periodic limb movement disorder |
| | Restless legs syndrome |
| | Shift work sleep disorder |
| | Sleep apnea syndrome |
| Psychiatric disorders | Adjustment disorder |
| | Alcohol dependence/abuse |
| | Caffeine-induced sleep disorder |
| | Generalized anxiety disorder |
| | Major depressive episode |
| | Manic episode (bipolar disorder) |
| | Nicotine dependency |
| | Opiate withdrawal |
| | Pain disorder |
| | Panic disorder |
| | Posttraumatic stress disorder |
| | Psychotic episode |
| | Sedative/hypnotic withdrawal |
| | Separation anxiety disorder |
| | Somatoform disorder |
| | Stimulant dependency/abuse |
| | Tourette disorder |
| Neurological disorders | Dementia |
| | Fatal familial insomnia |
| | Head trauma |
| | Headache disorders |
| | Parkinson's disease |
| | Seizure disorders |
| | Stroke |

### Medication and Substance Use

If excessive caffeine use is a potential cause of sleep disturbance, it may be important to minimize or eliminate caffeine intake for a few weeks to determine if this intervention is beneficial. Counseling about alcohol use is especially important in the abstinent alcoholic with insomnia.

### Behavioral Factors

Even when physical and medication factors may be modifiable, they may not be as powerful or as relevant for treating insomnia as the psychological factors that may be motivating poor sleep practices. These factors may be grouped into those pertaining to erroneous or distorted ideas about *sleep time management*, *sleep habit training*, *consequences of insomnia*, and *arousal management*.

- *Sleep time management* and *habit training practices* of insomnia patients can work against getting sleep. Continuous time spent awake and circadian sleep–wake timing jointly govern a person's propensity to sleep. Many individuals with robust sleep systems can, no doubt, violate these principles without subjective distress; however, in insomnia patients, the practices of daytime or "nighttime napping" work against obtaining good continuous nocturnal sleep. The time a person spends for sleep across 24 h should be consolidated into the nocturnal bout of sleep, and limited to the amount of time the patient's brain can sustain sleep. Irregularly timed awake periods tend to produce irregularly timed and unpredictable sleep.

- Under normal conditions, the circadian system has a forbidden zone for sleep in the early evening, and a high sleep propensity period from 3:00 AM until dawn; thus, attempting to sleep during the early evening will be frustrating, and the circadian advantages of predawn sleep will be diminished. Going to bed early to permit more sleep is actually counterproductive.
- Variability in sleep timing undercuts not only stable biological rhythm timing, it also undermines the capacity of the patient's behavioral habit system to regulate the normal, unconscious, biologically based scheduling of sleep and wakefulness.
- *Distorted ideas about the consequences* of insomnia involve exaggerations of perception or distortions of inference that a person has in relation to the exact truth of the matter about sleep. While it is true that there are real daytime consequences from chronic insomnia, these consequences are not like what insomniacs sometimes imagine them to be. Some insomniacs believe that if they don't get a good night's sleep, they will be a total failure at their jobs, when the reality is more likely that they will not be at their best, but they will still do their jobs satisfactorily. When one chronically rehearses the perceived consequences of impending failure resulting from less-than-perfect sleep, an intense sense of sleep worry coupled with an impulsive, impatient style of managing sleep can develop. Such worry degrades sleep.
- Evaluation should also explore how the patient generally handles ideas about his/her own performance self-evaluations. A "perfectionist" may have an "all-or-none" cognitive management style that generally works poorly for managing sleep. First, since no one is perfect, some aspect of life will remain imperfect and be a cause of performance anxiety at bedtime. Performance anxiety may be helpful during the daytime in improving daytime performances but can only keep one awake at bedtime. Second, while going to sleep is an occurrence, it is not a performance; performance anxiety specifically about sleep can only make sleep worse.

## HYPERAROUSAL IN INSOMNIA

There are numerous sleep–wake forms of "arousal," and there is no universally accepted physiologic definition of arousal. A variety of metrics [e.g., higher electroencephalogram (EEG) beta frequencies and lowered heart rate variability] suggest the presence of biological hyperarousal.

- Overarousal can be a key cause of sleep disturbance in patients who lead very time-pressured or conflict-laden lives, and it is important to appreciate the stresses and strains that patients may face that increase arousal.
- It is important to ask patients if they ruminate while in bed, with anxiety and worry about events,

demands, contingencies, or sleep. This overaroused state due to an unmodulated and anxious pattern of thinking may exist even in the absence of a depressive or anxiety disorder.
- Arousals may be linked to factors related to the bed, bedroom, or bedtime. It is useful to inquire if the bed is used for activities other than sleeping or sex, or if the patient sleeps better when away from home.

## EVALUATION IN RELATION TO TREATMENT PLANNING

Treatment actually begins at the start of evaluation, and evaluation continues during treatment.

- It is important to assess the patient's lifestyle (e.g., late social activities on weekends) and preferences regarding therapy. The patient's lifestyle is an important factor that needs to be considered when planning treatment. In addition, knowledge of the patient's preferences among the available treatment options will guide the selection of interventions that will be acceptable to the patient.
- The patient should be educated about the importance of monitoring therapeutic efficacy of the prescribed treatment objectively with daily sleep logs.

## KEY POINTS

1. The evaluation of insomnia is an ongoing process that may extend throughout a patient's medical, psychiatric, or psychological treatment course. Classification of the patient's insomnia syndrome provides a medical context, but the patient's style of presentation and life choices also provide data that guide the choice of treatment strategies.
2. Comorbid insomnia occurs in many sleep, medical, or psychiatric disorders. Taking a medical/psychiatric history, and conducting physical and mental status examinations can identify many diagnoses. Sleep diaries recorded before the clinic evaluation is useful to assess sleep patterns across nights, as are data from questionnaires that focus on sleepiness, anxiety, depression, general psychopathology, sleep quality, and insomnia.
3. Polysomnography is unlikely to provide helpful diagnostic information unless the clinical history is suggestive of obstructive sleep apnea, periodic limb movement disorder, narcolepsy, or a parasomnia. PSG may also be useful if initial therapy is unsuccessful, or if there is considerable diagnostic uncertainty.
4. Actigraphy measurements can be useful in clarifying patterns of sleep and wakefulness.
5. Psychological factors may be motivating poor sleep practices. These factors may be grouped into those pertaining to erroneous or distorted ideas about sleep time management, sleep habit training, consequences of insomnia, and arousal management.

## BIBLIOGRAPHY

Bonnet MH, et al. 24-Hour metabolic rate in insomniacs and matched normal sleepers. *Sleep* 1995; 18:581–588.

Borbély AA, et al. Sleep initiation and initial sleep intensity: Interactions of homeostatic and circadian mechanisms. *J Biol Rhythms* 1989; 4:149–160.

Chesson A, et al. Practice parameters for the evaluation of chronic insomnia. An American Academy of Sleep Medicine report. Standards of Practice Committee of the American Academy of Sleep Medicine. *Sleep* 2000; 23:237–241.

Lavie P. Ultrashort sleep-waking schedule. III. "Gates" and "forbidden zones" for sleep. *Electroencephalogr Clin Neurophysiol* 1986; 63:414–425.

Morin CM, et al. Patients' acceptance of psychological and pharmacological therapies for insomnia. *Sleep* 1992; 15:302–305.

Moul DE, et al. Self-report measures of insomnia in adults: rationales, choices, and needs. *Sleep Med Rev* 2004; 8(3): 177–198.

Ohayon MM. Epidemiology of insomnia: What we know and what we still need to learn. *Sleep Med Rev* 2002; 6:97–111.

Ribeiro S, et al. Long-lasting novelty-induced neuronal reverberation during slow-wave sleep in multiple forebrain areas. PLoS Biol 2004; 2:E24.

Spielman AJ, et al. Treatment of chronic insomnia by restriction of time in bed. *Sleep* 1987;10:45–56.

Vincent NK, et al. Perfectionism and chronic insomnia. *J Psychosom Res* 2000; 49:349–354.

# 8

## PHARMACOLOGIC THERAPY OF INSOMNIA

Teofilo Lee-Chiong
National Jewish, Health Denver, Colorado

Michael Sateia
Sleep Disorders Center, Dartmouth-Hitchcock Medical Center, Lebanon, New Hampshire

## INTRODUCTION

The goals of pharmacologic therapy of insomnia consist of alleviation of nighttime sleep disturbance and relief of its daytime consequences. Clinicians should correctly identify any underlying comorbid factors, such as sleep disordered breathing, restless legs syndrome, or mood disorders, and manage them accordingly. Incorporation of nonpharmacologic interventions, including proper sleep hygiene practices and cognitive behavioral therapy is recommended.

- Hypnotic agents are primarily indicated for the treatment of transient sleep disruption such as those caused by jet lag, shift work, or acute stress, but are also used in selected persons with chronic insomnia (e.g., for primary insomnia that failed to respond to behavioral therapy, or comorbid insomnia that did not improve with treatment of the underlying condition).
- Medications used in the treatment of insomnia include the benzodiazepine receptor agonists (BzRAs), melatonin agonists, antidepressants, and the nonprescription hypnotic agents, such as histamine antagonists, melatonin, and herbal compounds.

## HYPNOTIC MEDICATIONS

The selection of a particular hypnotic agent among the numerous available compounds should be done cautiously with consideration of its hypnotic efficacy, absorption and elimination profile, onset and duration of action, effect on sleep stages, risks of tolerance, dependency and withdrawal, abuse potential, possible drug interactions, and cost. It is advisable to select an agent with minimal risk of daytime residual effects. Specific characteristics of the patient, including the presence of medical or psychiatric illnesses,

age, pregnancy or lactation, and occupation, should also be taken into account.

- Duration of action differs among the various hypnotic preparations, and this distinction has been used to select the appropriate agent for the specific insomnia complaint. Short-acting agents are most appropriate for persons who have difficulty falling asleep. Patients with both sleep-onset and maintenance insomnia may be given agents with intermediate action. Finally, long-acting compounds, including flurazepam and quazepam, may be useful for some patients with both early morning awakenings and daytime anxiety, although their long duration of action is associated with accumulation and daytime performance impairments. Hence, caution is advised with such agents, particularly in the elderly.
- It is generally recommended that sedative-hypnotic therapy be limited to short-term use. Whenever these agents are used for longer periods, indications should be reassessed on a regular basis. Monitoring for effectiveness of the drug, adverse reactions, self-escalation of the medication dose, and alterations in medical or psychiatric status must occur.
- Older hypnotic agents, such as barbiturates and chloral hydrate, have been superseded by newer, more effective and safer agents. In addition to the danger of psychological and physical dependency, barbiturates can interact with numerous other medications via their induction of liver enzymes. Overdose is an ever-present danger with barbiturates. The popularity of chloral hydrate has waned primarily due to the rapid development of tolerance as well as the potential for development of rashes, gastric discomfort, and hepatic toxicity following its use.
- Benzodiazepines and the nonbenzodiazepine agonist agents act at the gamma-aminobutyric acid (GABA)–

benzodiazepine receptor complex. Benzodiazepines act nonselectively at two central receptor sites, omega-1 and omega-2. The sedative action of benzodiazepines is related primarily to omega-1 receptors, whereas omega-2 receptors are believed to be responsible for their effects on memory and cognitive functioning. The hypnosedative action of the nonbenzodiazepine agents, eszopiclone, zolpidem, and zaleplon, is comparable with that of benzodiazepines. These agents interact preferentially with omega-1 receptors. These newer agents are less likely than benzodiazepines to impair daytime performance and memory due to their relatively short duration of action and their low potential for residual effect. With some exceptions, most studies on benzodiazepines and nonbenzodiazepine receptor agonists are of relatively short duration and lack data regarding long-term follow-up.

## BENZODIAZEPINES

In general, benzodiazepines are effective and safe in the treatment of various types of insomnia. They typically increase total sleep time, reduce sleep latency, and decrease the frequency of awakenings in patients with insomnia. In addition to their hypnotic properties, benzodiazepines are potent anxiolytics, muscle relaxants, and anticonvulsants. Benzodiazepines can be classified into three groups with respect to duration of action: short half-life ($< 3$ h), medium half-life ($3–10$ h), and long half-life ($> 10$ h).

- Benzodiazepines, although typically well tolerated, may be associated with several adverse consequences. Short-acting agents may cause rebound daytime anxiety and greater withdrawal symptoms following cessation of their use. The effect of agents with long elimination half-lives may persist into the next day, producing sleepiness, incoordination, and cognitive impairment. Patients should be cautioned against operating motor vehicles or performing tasks that require vigilance and alertness when using these drugs. The residual effects of long-acting hypnotics are particularly of concern among the elderly. The presence of preexisting memory impairment, reduced clearance of the agent, and, possibly, increased central nervous system sensitivity may increase the risk for confusion among elderly patients. When prescribing hypnotic agents to elderly patients, one should start at a low dose and monitor its effects closely.
- Benzodiazepines should generally be avoided in pregnant women and in breast-feeding mothers. Due to the theoretical dangers of respiratory depression, benzodiazepines should be given cautiously, if at all, to patients with untreated sleep apnea and profound obstructive and restrictive ventilatory impairment, including emphysema and obesity-hypoventilation syndrome. Lethality with overdose of benzodiazepines, when ingested alone, is low, but rises with

co-ingestion of other compounds such as alcohol and other central nervous system depressants.

- Other potential disadvantages of benzodiazepines include the development of tolerance and risk for dependence and abuse, as well as withdrawal symptoms and rebound insomnia following cessation of chronic use, particularly with short-acting agents. However, the limited data on long-term usage precludes firm conclusions regarding the true prevalence of such complications.
- Abrupt discontinuation following long-term use of benzodiazepine use may result in withdrawal symptoms (agitation, anxiety, confusion, irritability, restlessness, tremulousness), relapse (recurrence of insomnia), or rebound (worsening of disturbed sleep compared to pretreatment baseline). The severity of benzodiazepine withdrawal syndrome is related to the medication dosage, duration of treatment, and the rapidity of tapering of drug use. In cases of severe withdrawal, significant morbidity or death can ensue. Relapse after benzodiazepine discontinuation is common, regardless of the type of intervention used to aid withdrawal.
- Rebound insomnia with deterioration of sleep quality and daytime well-being can occur among patients with insomnia following withdrawal of hypnotic agents, primarily short-acting medication. The duration of sleep deterioration can be protracted with marked internight variability. Although rebound insomnia can develop following short-term therapy with benzodiazepines, it is particularly prominent after chronic treatment with rapidly metabolized agents. Rebound insomnia can be minimized by intermittent use of hypnotic agents and by gradual reduction of the dose administered.

## NONBENZODIAZEPINE BENZODIAZEPINE RECEPTOR AGONISTS

*Zolpidem* is a nonbenzodiazepine imidazopyridine that binds preferentially to the omega-1 subtype of benzodiazepine receptors. In contrast to the benzodiazepines, it possesses no anticonvulsant or muscle relaxant activity. It has a quick onset of action and has a short half-life of approximately 2.4 h. The appeal of zolpidem as a hypnotic agent rests in its relative lack of any appreciable withdrawal symptoms, tolerance, rebound insomnia, or residual daytime cognitive and motor impairment. Compared to the benzodiazepines, it is less likely to disrupt normal sleep architecture. The dose of zolpidem is commonly 5–10 mg at bedtime. The lower dose is recommended for elderly patients and individuals that have underlying medical disorders. A sustained release form of the agent is also available and is given at a dose of 6.25–12.5 mg at bedtime.

*Zaleplon*, another NBBRA has minimal effects on sleep architecture, a rapid onset of action, and a short duration of action with half-life of only about 1 h. Zaleplon is administered at a dose of 5–10 mg at bedtime. Doses should start at 5 mg in elderly patients. It may also be given during prolonged middle-of-the-night awakenings as long as there are at least 4 h remaining prior to rising time.

*Eszopiclone* is a cyclopyrrolone, nonbenzodiazepine agent with intermediate duration of action of about 5–7 h. It is not restricted to short-term use in the pharmacologic treatment of chronic primary insomnia.

- Compared to conventional benzodiazepines, zolpidem, zaleplon, and eszopiclone are less likely to cause significant rebound insomnia or tolerance. However, risk of abuse remains a concern, particularly among patients with a history of abuse or dependence of alcohol or other drugs, and those with psychiatric disease.

## MELATONIN RECEPTOR AGONISTS

*Ramelteon* is a melatonin receptor agonist that is highly selective for ML1 receptors located mainly in cells of the suprachiasmatic nucleus. It is postulated to mediate the effects of melatonin on circadian rhythms. Ramelteon has clinically relevant sleep-promoting effects, including a decrease in sleep latency to persistent sleep, and minimal increases in sleep efficiency and total sleep time. Its very short half-life (~1 h) limits its use to sleep initiation problems.

## ANTIDEPRESSANTS

Antidepressants have been increasingly utilized over the past decade in the treatment of insomnia. However, despite their widespread use to aid sleep, there are limited data on their appropriate use among persons with insomnia, particularly in patients without mood disorders. Serotonin-specific antidepressants such as trazodone have fewer adverse effects than the older tricyclic agents, including doxepin and amitriptyline, and have surpassed the latter's popularity as hypnotic agents. The use of tricyclic antidepressants (e.g., amitriptyline, trimipramine, and doxepin) is associated with greater anticholinergic reactions, cardiotoxicity, and orthostatic hypotension.

*Trazodone* is a widely prescribed medication for insomnia. A 5-hydroxytryptamine (5-HT) (2) and alpha-1 receptor antagonist, it possesses both anxiolytic and sedative properties. Trazodone increases sleep efficiency, total sleep time, slow-wave sleep, and rapid eye movement (REM) sleep latency, and decreases REM sleep. Trazodone does not appear to possess any significant tolerance or dependence potential. Although widely prescribed for individuals with chronic primary insomnia, its effectiveness in this application has not been established. Limited data suggest improvement of sleep in depressed patients with insomnia when co-administered with other antidepressant medications. Side effects associated with the use of trazodone include atrial and ventricular arrhythmias and priapism. Serotonin syndrome can result with co-administration with similar serotonin-specific agents.

*Mirtazapine*, a noradrenergic and specific serotonergic antidepressant, acts by antagonizing central alpha-2-adrenergic and 5-HT (2) and 5-HT (3) receptors. Significant improvements in sleep latency, sleep efficiency, and wake after sleep onset have been noted during mirtazapine administration in patients with major depression and insomnia. Weight gain and daytime sedation may be problematic in some patients.

## OTHER PRESCRIPTION AGENTS

*Quetiapine* is an atypical antipsychotic with antihistaminergic, antidopaminergic, and antiadrenergic properties. It has been noted to increase total sleep time, sleep efficiency, stage 2 non-REM sleep, and subjective sleep quality when given to healthy subjects. It is commonly employed as a sleep aid for patients with psychiatric illness, although its effectiveness for this indication has not been established.

## NONPRESCRIPTION HYPNOTIC AGENTS

Patients with insomnia commonly self-administer nonprescription sleep agents, including alcohol, to manage their sleep disturbances. Frequently used nonprescription products include acetaminophen, diphenhydramine, melatonin, alcohol, and herbal products.

### Histamine Antagonists

A majority of over-the-counter hypnotic agents are composed of antihistamines. Aside from their actions on histamine H1 receptors, these agents may also act upon serotonergic, cholinergic, and central alpha-adrenergic receptors. The first-generation histamine H1-antagonists, such as diphenhydramine and chlorpheniramine, can induce sedation by virtue of their ability to cross the blood–brain barrier. In contrast, use of second-generation agents, including loratadine and fexofenadine, is less likely to result in sedation. There are few published data on the efficacy of nighttime administration of antihistamines as sleep aids for insomnia. In general, the effectiveness of antihistamines for treatment of chronic insomnia is not well demonstrated. Tolerance to the hypnotic effects of diphenhydramine may develop rapidly.

### Melatonin

The secretion of endogenous melatonin by the pineal gland is synchronized to the circadian rhythm with increased production at nighttime. Melatonin has been evaluated primarily for the therapy of insomnia secondary to circadian rhythm sleep disturbances. Studies on its use for primary insomnia are more limited. Some studies have demonstrated improvement in sleep following evening administration of melatonin in older individuals with reduced endogenous melatonin levels.

## Botanical Compounds

Self-medication with herbal preparations is common. Additional studies are required to better define the roles of these compounds in the management of both transient and chronic insomnia.

**Kava**    There has been little published data on the efficacy of kava (*Piper methysticum*), a psychoactive agent belonging to the pepper family, in the therapy of insomnia. Kavapyrones, the active constituents of kava, possess centrally acting skeletal muscle relaxant and anticonvulsant properties, and might possibly have an effect on GABA receptors as well. Adverse effects include dizziness, mild gastrointestinal disturbances, and allergic skin reactions. Kava has been removed from the market in a number of countries as a result of concern about numerous reported cases of hepatotoxicity. A scaly dermatitis known as kava dermopathy can follow chronic use of kava in supratherapeutic dosages.

**Valerian**    Valerian is a popular botanical sleep remedy and is often found as one of the ingredients for herbal compounds marketed for the therapy of insomnia. The sedative properties of valerian (*Valeriana officinalis*) have been ascribed to the possible interaction of its valepotriates and sesquiterpene constituents with GABA, adenosine, or barbiturate receptors. Evidence for the efficacy of valerian as a treatment for insomnia is inconclusive. Abdominal pain, chest tightness, tremor, lightheadedness, mydriasis, and fine hand tremors have been reported following overdoses with valerian.

**Other Botanical Agents**    Other natural products that have been used as mild sedatives include passionflower (*Passiflora incarnata*) and skullcap (*Scutellaria laterifolia*). These agents may be combined with valerian or kava in commercial botanical products. No clinical trials of the use of skullcap or passionflower for insomnia have been published in the medical literature.

## DISCONTINUING LONG-TERM USE OF HYPNOTIC AGENTS

The long-term use of hypnotic agents for chronic insomnia, although not recommended, is a clinical reality.

- Long-term use of hypnotics is common in both primary insomnia, when conservative and nonpharmacologic treatments have been unsuccessful, unavailable, or simply ignored, and in comorbid insomnia, as an adjunct to treatment of the primary condition, or when such treatment has failed to correct the insomnia. Patients receiving hypnotic agents chronically should be informed that this is an "off-label" use for some of medications.
- There is little literature that establishes the effectiveness of chronic benzodiazepine administration for insomnia. Some nonbenzodiazepines (eszopiclone and zolpidem) may maintain long-term effectiveness without significant safety problems.
- The usual clinical management for withdrawal from chronic benzodiazepine use is gradual tapering. A combination of cognitive-behavioral therapy and benzodiazepine tapering may be considered in the management of patients with insomnia and chronic benzodiazepine use.

## KEY POINTS

1. The management of insomnia should address not only the perceived difficulty with nighttime sleep but also its daytime consequences. The sleep disturbance related to insomnia may be due to many causes. One should, therefore, attempt to identify any factors that may precipitate or perpetuate these complaints and initiate appropriate corrective measures. It is of paramount importance to prevent the progression of transient complaints into chronic, unrelenting insomnia.

2. Most patients benefit from a combination of sleep hygiene counseling, cognitive behavior therapy, and the judicious administration of hypnotic agents.

3. Pharmacotherapeutic management is generally effective for transient insomnia due to jet lag or acute stressors. It may also be used intermittently in patients with more chronic complaints.

4. The selection of a particular hypnotic medication should be based on the characteristics of the patient, duration and timing of insomnia, and the pharmacologic profile of the agent. It is advisable to use the lowest effective dose and to monitor carefully both the therapeutic response as well as side effects.

## BIBLIOGRAPHY

Almeida Montes LG, et al. Treatment of primary insomnia with melatonin: A double-blind, placebo-controlled, crossover study. *J Psychiatry Neurosci* 2003; 28:191–196.

Baillargeon L, et al. Discontinuation of benzodiazepines among older insomniac adults treated with cognitive-behavioural therapy combined with gradual tapering: A randomized trial. *CMAJ* 2003; 169:1015–1020.

Bélanger L, et al. Benzodiazepine discontinuation in chronic insomnia: A survival analysis over a 24-month follow-up. *Sleep* 2003; 26:A308–A309.

Curran HV, et al. Older adults and withdrawal from benzodiazepine hypnotics in general practice: Effects on cognitive function, sleep, mood and quality of life. *Psychol Med* 2003; 33:1223–1237.

Donath F, et al. Critical evaluation of the effect of valerian extract on sleep structure and sleep quality. *Pharmacopsychiatry* 2000; 33:47–53.

Erman M, et al. Phase II study of the selective ML-1 receptor agonist TAK-375 in subjects with primary chronic insomnia. *Sleep* 2003; 26:A298.

Fugh-Berman A, et al. Dietary supplements and natural products as psychotherapeutic agents. *Psychosom Med* 1999; 61:712–728.

Hajak G, et al. Abuse and dependence potential for the non-benzodiazepine hypnotics zolpidem and zopiclone: A review of case reports and epidemiological data. *Addiction* 2003; 98:1371–1378.

Krystal AD, et al. Sustained efficacy of eszopiclone over 6 months of nightly treatment: Results of a randomized, double-blind, placebo-controlled study in adults with chronic insomnia. *Sleep* 2003; 26:793–799.

Lehrl S. Clinical efficacy of kava extract WS 1490 in sleep disturbances associated with anxiety disorders. Results of a multicenter, randomized, placebo-controlled, double-blind clinical trial. *J Affect Disord* 2004; 78:101–110.

Mendelson WB, et al. The treatment of chronic insomnia: Drug indications, chronic use and abuse liability. Summary of a 2001 New Clinical Drug Evaluation Unit Meeting Symposium. *Sleep Med Rev* 2004; 8:7–17.

Montplaisir J, et al. Zopiclone and zaleplon vs benzodiazepines in the treatment of insomnia: Canadian consensus statement. *Hum Psychopharmacol* 2003; 18:29–38.

Neubauer DN. Pharmacologic approaches for the treatment of chronic insomnia. *Clin Cornerstone* 2003; 5:16–27.

Noble S, et al. Zopiclone. An update of its pharmacology, clinical efficacy and tolerability in the treatment of insomnia. *Drugs* 1998; 55:277–302.

Roehrs T, et al. Hypnotics: An update. *Curr Neurol Neurosci Rep* 2003; 3:181–184.

Roth T, et al. Phase II study of the selective ML-1 receptor agonist TAK-375 in a first night effect model of transient insomnia. *Sleep* 2003; 26:A294.

Saletu-Zyhlarz GM, et al. Insomnia in depression: Differences in objective and subjective sleep and awakening quality to normal controls and acute effects of trazodone. *Prog Neuropsychopharmacol Biol Psychiatry* 2002; 26:249–260.

Schweizer E, et al. Benzodiazepine dependence and withdrawal: A review of the syndrome and its clinical management. *Acta Psychiatr Scand Suppl* 1998; 393:95–101.

Sproule BA, et al. The use of non-prescription sleep products in the elderly. *Int J Geriatr Psychiatry* 1999; 14:851–857.

Stevinson C, et al. Valerian for insomnia: A systematic review of randomized clinical trials. *Sleep Med* 2000; 1:91–99.

Terzano MG, et al. New drugs for insomnia: Comparative tolerability of zopiclone, zolpidem and zaleplon. *Drug Saf* 2003; 26:261–282.

Walsh JK, et al. A five week, polysomnographic assessment of zaleplon 10 mg for the treatment of primary insomnia. *Sleep Med* 2000; 1:41–49.

Walsh JK, et al. Efficacy and tolerability of four doses of indiplon (NBI-34060) modified-release in elderly patients with sleep maintenance insomnia. *Sleep* 2003; 26:A78.

Winokur A, et al. Comparative effects of mirtazapine and fluoxetine on sleep physiology measures in patients with major depression and insomnia. *J Clin Psychiatry* 2003; 64:1224–1229.

Zhdanova IV, et al. Melatonin treatment for age-related insomnia. *J Clin Endocrinol Metab* 2001; 86:4727–4730.

# 9

## NONPHARMACOLOGIC THERAPY OF INSOMNIA

MELANIE K. MEANS AND JACK D. EDINGER
Department of Veterans Affairs Medical Center, Durham, North Carolina, and Duke University Medical Center, Durham, North Carolina

### INTRODUCTION

Insomnia is a prevalent disorder characterized by diffi-culty initiating or maintaining sleep or by chronically poor sleep quality. Accompanying nocturnal sleep disrup-tion are daytime complaints (e.g., fatigue, poor concentra-tion, etc.) that can significantly compromise daily functioning, health status, and quality of life.

- Sleep difficulties may arise from a variety of events, conditions, or circumstances, such as stress, environ-mental factors, changes to the sleep–wake cycle, medical or psychiatric illnesses, or ingestion of sleep-disrupting substances. Regardless of the preci-pitating factors, insomnia may assume a chronic course perpetuated by psychologic and behavioral factors such as dysfunctional beliefs about sleep, heightened anxiety, and sleep-disruptive compensa-tory practices.

- Although sedative hypnotic medications are often prescribed for insomnia, such treatment is symptom focused and fails to address underlying behavioral and cognitive factors sustaining the sleep problems. In contrast, nonpharmacologic or behavioral insom-nia therapies specifically target behavioral and con-ditioning factors with the goals of eradicating these perpetuating mechanisms and restoring normal sleep–wake functioning. (Table 9.1)

### STIMULUS CONTROL

Stimulus control is a well-established insomnia therapy consisting of a structured behavioral regimen designed to disassociate a problem behavior or conditioned auto-nomic response from a specific environmental setting. This approach is based on the assumption that both the timing (bedtime) and setting (bed/bedroom) are associated

with repeated unsuccessful sleep attempts and over time become conditioned cues that perpetuate insomnia. As a result, the goal of this treatment is that of reassociating the bed and bedroom with successful sleep attempts. Sti-mulus control achieves this endpoint by curtailing sleep-incompatible activities in the bed and bedroom and by enforcing a consistent sleep–wake schedule.

- In practice, this therapy requires instructing the patient to: (a) go to bed only when sleepy; (b) estab-lish a standard wake-up time; (c) get out of bed whenever awake for > 15 – 20 min; (d) avoid reading, watching TV, eating, worrying, and other sleep-incompatible behaviors in the bed and bedroom; and (e) refrain from daytime napping.

- From a theoretical perspective, it is probable that strict adherence to this regimen not only corrects aberrant, sleep-disruptive conditioning, but it also likely reestablishes a normal sleep drive and sleep–wake rhythm. Because the treatment recommenda-tions may appear counterintuitive, it is important that the insomnia patient understand the therapeu-tic rationale.

- Stimulus control instructions usually can be admi-nistered in one visit; however, follow-up visits are beneficial to facilitate compliance and achieve opti-mal success.

### SLEEP RESTRICTION

Sleep restriction therapy reduces nocturnal sleep distur-bance primarily by restricting the time allotted for sleep each night so that the time spent in bed closely matches the individual's actual sleep requirement. Some insomnia sufferers attempt to alleviate their sleep difficulties by spending excessive time in bed. However, allotting too much time for sleep fragments the sleep pattern and

*Sleep Medicine Essentials*, edited by Teofilo L. Lee-Chiong
Copyright © 2009 John Wiley & Sons, Inc.

Table 9.1  Common Behavioral Therapies for Insomnia

| | |
|---|---|
| **Stimulus control** | A structured behavioral regimen designed to establish the bedroom as a stimulus for sleep by eliminating behaviors that are incompatible with sleep. |
| **Sleep restriction** | A behavioral strategy in which time in bed at night is restricted in order to encourage a more consolidated sleep pattern. |
| **Cognitive–behavioral insomnia therapy** | A multifaceted treatment approach designed to reduce dysfunctional beliefs about sleep and correct sleep-disruptive habits. |
| **Progressive muscle relaxation** | A relaxation strategy where the patient alternately tenses and relaxes muscle groups in order to reduce muscle tension. Typically, muscles are tensed and relaxed in a systematic order during a 15- to 20-min session. |

creates excessive time awake each night. By restricting time in bed, mild sleep deprivation may be induced. As a result, sleep drive is increased, wakefulness is reduced, and the sleep pattern is consolidated.

- This treatment typically begins by calculating the individual's average total sleep time (ATST) from a sleep log that is kept for at least 2 weeks. An initial time-in-bed (TIB) prescription may either be set at the ATST or at a value equal to the ATST plus an amount of time that is deemed to represent normal nocturnal wakefulness (e.g., ATST + 30 min). However, unless persuasive evidence suggests the individual has an unusually low sleep requirement, the initial TIB prescription is seldom set below 6 h per night. On subsequent visits, the TIB prescription is increased by 15- to 20-min increments following weeks the patient, on average, is sleeping > 85 or 90% of the TIB and continues to report daytime sleepiness. Conversely TIB is usually reduced by similar increments following weeks wherein the patient, on average, sleeps less that 80% of the time spent in bed. Since TIB adjustments often are necessary, sleep restriction typically entails an initial visit to introduce treatment instructions and follow-up visits to alter TIB prescriptions.
- Sleep compression therapy shares the same therapeutic goal and rationale as sleep restriction therapy but achieves this through an alternate methodology. Instead of immediately restricting TIB to an amount close to ATST, the therapist gradually reduces TIB over a number of weeks until this value approximates ATST.

## SLEEP HYGIENE

Sleep hygiene connotes a loosely defined set of recommendations targeting lifestyle and environmental factors. Patients are educated about healthy sleep behaviors and sleep-conducive environmental conditions. For example, insomnia patients may be encouraged to exercise daily, eliminate the use of caffeine, alcohol, and nicotine, eat a light snack at bedtime, and ensure that the sleeping environment is quiet, dark, and comfortable.

- Sleep hygiene is seldom used as a primary intervention but is often included with other interventions such as stimulus control or sleep restriction.

## RELAXATION THERAPIES

A variety of relaxation strategies, including progressive muscle relaxation, passive relaxation, autogenic training, biofeedback, imagery training, meditation, and hypnosis have been used to treat insomnia. Common to these approaches is their focus on factors such as performance anxiety and bedtime arousal, which often perpetuate sleep difficulties. Accordingly, the goal of these therapies is to reduce or eliminate the physiologic (e.g., muscle tension) and/or cognitive (e.g., racing thoughts) arousal that disrupts sleep.

- Regardless of the specific relaxation strategy employed, treatment typically entails conducting specific treatment exercises and teaching relaxation skills over multiple treatment sessions. The patient is encouraged to practice at home in order to gain mastery and facility with self-relaxation. Once the patient achieves sufficient relaxation skills, these can be applied to facilitate sleep initiation by reducing sleep-related anxiety and bedtime arousal.

## PARADOXICAL INTENTION

Designed mainly to address the excessive performance anxiety that contributes to sleep onset difficulties, paradoxical intention requires the insomnia patient to remain awake as long as possible after retiring to bed. The patient is instructed to purposefully engage in the feared activity (staying awake) in order to reduce performance anxiety that confounds associated goal-directed behavior (falling asleep). This method alleviates both the patient's excessive focus on sleep and anxiety over not sleeping; as a result, sleep becomes less difficult to initiate.

- Paradoxical intention is seldom used albeit seemingly effective. Like the other treatments, an initial visit to provide treatment instructions and follow-up sessions to support the patient and assure compliance are usually recommended when administering this intervention.

## COGNITIVE THERAPY

Cognitive therapy is a psychotherapeutic approach that alters cognitions contributing to emotional arousal and maladaptive behaviors. During the therapeutic process, unhelpful beliefs are first identified and monitored. The utility of these beliefs are challenged and then replaced with more adaptive and helpful substitutes.

- When applied specifically to insomnia patients, cognitive therapy targets unrealistic expectations about sleep as well as misconceptions or misattributions regarding the causes of insomnia, the consequences of insomnia, the ability to control and predict sleep, and sleep behaviors. The goal of this therapy is to reduce the cognitive arousal and anxiety contributing to insomnia by helping the patient adopt a more adaptive "mental set."

- Whether provided through formalized patient education modules or via the cognitive restructuring method similar to that commonly used in cognitive therapy with clinically depressed individuals, cognitive therapy involves multiple treatment sessions with a skilled therapist.

## COGNITIVE–BEHAVIORAL THERAPY

Cognitive–behavioral therapy (CBT) is a multicomponent treatment approach consisting of cognitive therapy strategies used in combination with behavioral therapies such as stimulus control, sleep restriction, and sleep hygiene. One presumed advantage of this treatment is that it includes treatment components addressing the range of cognitive and behavioral mechanisms that perpetuate insomnia. Although CBT is a seemingly more complex treatment than those previously described, in practice, this intervention usually requires no more therapist or patient treatment time than do the other treatments.

- CBT models have utilized two to up to eight treatment session protocols in their clinical applications. As with the other therapeutic approaches, multiple treatment sessions to provide patients with sufficient support and follow-up are recommended.

## OTHER APPROACHES

In efforts to maximize treatment response, the effects of combining pharmacotherapy with behavioral treatments have been investigated. These preliminary studies indicate that combination treatment equals or slightly outperforms medication-only and behavioral treatment-only conditions. At long-term assessments, however, sleep improvements are sustained in behavioral treatment but not combination treatment. Clearly, more research is needed to ascertain the potential benefits of combining behavioral interventions with hypnotic medications.

- When insomnia is caused by a desyncronization of the patient's sleep schedule with his or her biological circadian rhythm, therapeutic approaches such as chronotherapy or bright-light therapy may be indicated.

- Acupuncture is presumed to promote sleep by stimulating the release of neurotransmitters involved in the sleep–wake system. Although sufficient evidence does not exist to recommend acupuncture as a primary treatment for insomnia, some recent studies have shown this technique improves sleep patterns.

## EFFECTIVENESS OF NONPHARMACOLOGIC THERAPIES

Nonpharmacologic insomnia treatments produce significant improvements in sleep patterns that are durable over time. The magnitude of sleep improvements obtained with behavioral treatments equals or surpasses those obtained from medication alone, and patients generally prefer these behavioral treatments to pharmacologic approaches.

- Practice parameters issued by the American Academy of Sleep Medicine recognize stimulus control, sleep restriction, progressive muscle relaxation, biofeedback, paradoxical intention, and CBT as effective therapies for treating insomnia, whereas sleep hygiene, imagery training, and cognitive therapy lack sufficient evidence for recommending these approaches as a stand-alone therapy.

- Compared to other nonpharmacologic approaches, stimulus control and sleep restriction therapies demonstrate the most robust and sustained effects on sleep outcomes. Because most multicomponent CBT treatments include stimulus control and sleep restriction interventions, CBT is highly effective as well.

## KEY POINTS

1. Chronic insomnia often is perpetuated by dysfunctional beliefs about sleep, heightened anxiety, and sleep-disruptive compensatory practices.
2. Medications frequently prescribed to treat insomnia are symptom focused and fail to address these psychological and behavioral problems.
3. Nonpharmacologic behavioral insomnia therapies such as relaxation therapy, stimulus control, sleep restriction therapy, and cognitive–behavioral therapy target behavioral and psychological factors that maintain and exacerbate sleep difficulties.
4. The effectiveness of nonpharmacologic insomnia therapies is well established, and such therapies represent a first-line approach for the treatment of chronic insomnia.

## BIBLIOGRAPHY

Chesson AL, et al. Practice parameters for the nonpharmacologic treatment of chronic insomnia. An American Academy of Sleep Medicine report. Standards of Practice Committee of the American Academy of Sleep Medicine. *Sleep* 1999; 22:1128–1133.

Edinger JD, et al. A primary care "friendly" cognitive behavioral insomnia therapy. *Sleep* 2003; 26:177–182.

Harvey L, et al. Insomniacs' reported use of CBT components and relationship to long-term clinical outcome. *Behav Res Ther* 2002; 40:75–83.

Larzelere MM, et al. Anxiety, depression, and insomnia. *Primary Care Clin Office Pract* 2002; 29:339–360, vii.

McCrae CS, et al. Secondary insomnia: A heuristic model and behavioral approaches to assessment, treatment, and prevention. *Appl Prevent Psychol* 2001; 10:107–123.

Means MK, et al. Behavioral treatment of insomnia *Expert Rev Neurother* 2002; 2:127–137.

Morin CM, et al. Psychological and behavioral treatment of insomnia: Update of the recent evidence (1998–2004). *Sleep* 2006; 29:1398–1414.

Smith MT, et al. Comparative meta-analysis of pharmacotherapy and behavior therapy for persistent insomnia. *Am J Psychiatry* 2002; 159:5–11.

# 10

## NARCOLEPSY

Rafael Pelayo and Maria Cecilia Lopes
Stanford Sleep Disorders Clinic, Stanford University, Stanford, California

### INTRODUCTION

Narcolepsy is a chronic neurologic disorder of excessive daytime sleepiness (EDS), which characteristically has a childhood onset and is associated with hypocretin deficiency.

- Historically, the word "narcolepsy" was first coined by Gélineau in 1880 to designate a pathologic condition characterized by irresistible episodes of sleep of short duration recurring at close intervals. The symptoms of narcolepsy can be conceptualized as a blurring of the boundaries between the awake, sleeping, and dreaming brain. The awake narcoleptic may feel sleepy. The sleeping narcoleptic may have disturbed sleep due to arousals. Dreaming phenomenon may occur while the patient is awake.
- The onset of narcolepsy is typically in the second decade of life but may begin at a younger age or as an adult. Narcolepsy may have an abrupt or insidious onset. In the latter situation, the full syndrome may take up to 12 years to develop. During this time, patients may be misdiagnosed as simply lazy or depressed. It may not be until after the child becomes an adult that the correct diagnosis is made. It is therefore important for health care providers to consider narcolepsy as a possibility in any person with unexplained EDS.

### CLINICAL SYMPTOMS

The cardinal features of narcolepsy are daytime somnolence, cataplexy, sleep paralysis, and hypnagogic hallucinations, referred to as the "tetrad" of narcolepsy. The discovery of abnormal sleep onset rapid eye movement (REM) sleep periods in narcolepsy allowed for objective physiologic measurements. Disturbed nocturnal sleep has been described as an important complaint and may compose a fifth symptom associated with narcoleptic syndrome. The mnemonic aide *CHESS* may help the reader remember the five symptoms of narcolepsy: *C*ataplexy, *H*ypnagogic hallucinations, *E*xcessive daytime sleepiness, *S*leep paralysis, and *S*leep disruption.

*Cataplexy* is characterized by a sudden loss of muscle tone while awake, typically triggered by a strong positive emotion, such as laughter or surprise. It can also be triggered less commonly by anger or fear.

- Cataplexy is virtually a pathognomonic symptom of narcolepsy. When an experienced clinician witnesses a cataleptic attack, confirmatory sleep laboratory testing for narcolepsy might not be necessary.
- Narcoleptic patients remain conscious during the attack and are able to remember the details of the event afterwards. The episodes are typically brief and may only last a few seconds. Some patients can have other narcoleptic symptoms manifest during an episode of cataplexy, such as hypnagogic hallucinations or sleep paralysis, or may simply fall asleep.
- Cataplexy may involve only certain muscles or affect the entire voluntary musculature. Most typically, the jaw sags, the head falls forward, the arms drop to the side, and the knees buckle. The severity and extent of cataplexy can range from a state of absolute powerlessness, which seems to involve the entire body, to no more than a fleeting sensation of weakness. Although the extraocular muscles are supposedly not involved, the patient may complain of blurred vision. Respiration may become irregular during an attack, which may be related to weakness of the abdominal or intercostal muscles. Complete loss of muscle tone, which results in a fall with risk of serious injuries, might occur during a cataplectic attack. The attacks may also be subtle and not noticed by nearby individuals. An attack may consist only of a slight buckling of the knees, in which the patient may simply sit or stand against a wall. Speech may be slurred. If it involves the upper limbs, the individual may be described as clumsy

*Sleep Medicine Essentials*, edited by Teofilo L. Lee-Chiong
Copyright © 2009 John Wiley & Sons, Inc.

due to dropping cups or spilling liquids whenever surprised or laughing. A patient may present with repetitive falls that cannot be easily explained, and this may result in a misdiagnosis of atonic seizures.

- The duration of each cataplectic attack, partial or total, is highly variable. They usually range from a few seconds to 2 min, and rarely up to 30 min. The term *status cataplecticus* is applied to prolonged attacks.

- Attacks can be elicited by emotion, stress, fatigue, or heavy meals. Laughter and anger seem to be the most common triggers, but a feeling of elation while listening to music, reading a book, or watching a movie can also induce the attacks. Merely remembering a funny situation may induce cataplexy, and it may also occur without obvious precipitating acts or emotions. In children it often occurs while playing with others. Thus, the potential emotional impact of cataplexy cannot be overstated. Indeed, individuals may be misdiagnosed with a psychiatric disorder before recognition of narcolepsy.

*Hypnagogic hallucinations* are fragments of auditory or dreamlike imagery that occur at sleep onset. Similar episodes upon awakening are called hypnopompic hallucinations. This is a nonspecific symptom of narcolepsy and probably occurs clinically more frequently in any sleep-deprived individual. Hypnagogic hallucinations should not be confused with psychosis. Auditory hallucinations are common. The patient may be frightened by the imagery.

*Sleep paralysis* is a self-descriptive term that can be a terrifying experience. It is a transient inability to move usually upon awakening. Patients find themselves suddenly unable to move the limbs, to speak, or even to breathe deeply. This state is frequently accompanied by hallucinations. During episodes of sleep paralysis, particularly at the first occurrence, the patient may have extreme anxiety associated with a fear of dying. This anxiety is often greatly intensified by hallucinations, sometimes terrifying, which may accompany the sleep paralysis. Patients may be reluctant to talk about these events; or these experiences can be so frightful that the patient may resist going to bed to sleep.

- Sleep paralysis, like hypnagogic hallucinations, may occur in any sleep-deprived individual in the absence of narcolepsy. They do not occur in all narcoleptics and may be transitory. Patients with narcolepsy may, with time, learn to recognize hypnagogic hallucinations and sleep paralysis as frightening, but otherwise essentially benign, phenomena and be better able to tolerate them.

*Daytime sleepiness* or an inability to maintain wakefulness during the daytime is the most common complaint in narcoleptic patients. In young children, this may not be quickly recognized as abnormal. The parents may not complain if their children sleep more than usual or may view the sleepiness as a normal phase of development. Certainly, most adolescents falling asleep in the classroom

do not have narcolepsy. Delays in diagnosis are usually related to an absence of clinical suspicion for narcolepsy.

- In the 24-h cycle, established narcolepsy patients do not sleep more than average. The increase daytime sleep is countered by impaired nighttime sleep.

*Academic impairment* is not unusual in children with narcolepsy. Children and adolescents with narcolepsy may report embarrassment, academic decline, and loss of self-esteem. Patients may be misdiagnosed with an attention deficit disorder. Psychosocial problems are not uncommon.

## DIFFERENCES IN CLINICAL FEATURES BETWEEN ADULTS AND CHILDREN WITH NARCOLEPSY

The differences in clinical manifestations between children and adults are summarized in Table 10.1. It can be difficult to recognize daytime sleepiness in very young children, but cataplexy is a more obvious symptom in the young.

## EPIDEMIOLOGY

Narcolepsy is not a rare disorder. A survey in the United States found an incidence rate of 1.37 per 100,000 persons per year. The prevalence was estimated at 56.3 per 100,000 persons.

- The incidence rate was highest in the second decade, followed in descending order by the third, fourth and first decades. Approximately 36% of prevalence cases did not have cataplexy. Onset as young as age 2 years has been reported.

## PATHOPHYSIOLOGY

An animal model of narcolepsy has been developed using dogs. Using positional cloning, an autosomal recessive mutation responsible for narcolepsy was discovered in this canine model. Independent work using a gene knock-out mice model confirmed the role of hypocretin in narcolepsy.

- The hypocretins, which are also called orexins, are neuropeptides. Two novel neuropeptides have been described, namely Hcrt-1 and Hcrt-2, which are derived from the same precursor genes synthesized by neurons located exclusively in the lateral, posterior, and perifornical hypothalamus. Hypocretin-containing neurons have widespread projections throughout the central nervous system (CNS) with particularly dense excitatory projections to monoaminergic centers, such as the noradrenergic locus ceruleus, histaminergic tuberomammillary nucleus, serotoninergic raphe nucleus, and dopaminergic ventral tegmental area. The hypocretins were originally believed to be primarily important in the regulation of appetite; however, a major function

**Table 10.1   Clinical Features of Narcolepsy between Children and Adults**

| Symptom | Children | Adults |
|---|---|---|
| Cataplexy | Seen in most narcoleptic children because it is easy to recognize.<br>Often occurs while playing with other children.<br>Frequently the first symptom to be recognized.<br>Differential diagnosis includes other causes of drop attacks. | Present in about 70% of narcoleptic patients.<br>Usually associated with laugher.<br>It is the first symptom of narcolepsy in 5–8% of patients.<br>Can be clinically similar to drop attacks.<br>It may appear on average 6 years after the onset of excessive daytime sleepiness. |
| Hypnagogic hallucination | Symptoms such as nightmares and hypnagogic hallucinations may be considered as part of normal childhood development.<br>An accurate description may be difficult to elicit. | Present in 30% of adults.<br>Visual hallucinations usually consist of simple forms or shapes.<br>Auditory hallucinations are also common. |
| Excessive daytime sleepiness | May sometimes be difficult to recognize.<br>More usual symptom is falling asleep during class.<br>Sleepiness can be masked by other abnormal behavior such as hyperactivity. | Easier to recognize in adults than in children.<br>May present as difficulty with concentrating during slow activities.<br>May lead to problems at work because of the occurrence of sleep episodes during monotonous situations. |
| Sleep paralysis | Frequently accompanied by hallucinations.<br>Children dislike talking about these events. | Can sometimes be a terrifying experience.<br>May occur in healthy subjects.<br>Symptom decreases with age. |
| Disturbed nocturnal sleep | This symptom may not affect children.<br>Sometimes is a transitory complaint. | Worse during adulthood. |

emerging from research on these neuropeptides is the regulation of sleep and wakefulness. Deficiency in hypocretin neurotransmission results in narcolepsy in mice, dogs, and humans.

- Canine narcolepsy is an autosomal recessive disease caused by disruption of the hypocretin receptor 2 gene (Hcrtr2). In most humans with narcolepsy, the Hcrtr receptor is intact, but the actual peptide may be deficient or absent. Hypocretin levels can be measured in the cerebrospinal fluid (CSF) and has been found to be either very low or absent in most narcoleptics. This difference may account for differences in genetic transmission between the canine model and humans. In the canine model, narcolepsy can be predicted through breeding, whereas this is not the case in humans. Although, familial studies indicate a 20–40 times increased risk of narcolepsy among first-degree relatives, only 25–31% of monozygotic twins are concordant for narcolepsy.

- Since most identical human twins are discordant for narcolepsy, an additional pathophysiologic mechanism has been sought to explain the development of narcolepsy. The possibility that an autoimmune mechanism is damaging the hypocretin-producing cells in the hypothalamus has been raised. This is supported by the tight linkage of a subtype of human leukocyte antigen (HLA) DQ1 with humans with narcolepsy with cataplexy. Similar linkages have been found in other autoimmune disorders such as multiple sclerosis. However, extensive searches for physical evidence of an autoimmune process have been inconclusive or negative.

- The mechanisms through which hypocretin deficiency results in narcolepsy are unknown. A cholinergic/monoaminergic imbalance underlying the symptomatology of narcolepsy has been established and is most likely caused by an absence of hypocretin signaling; however, the widespread projections of hypocretin neurons make it difficult to elucidate its exact functional importance.

- The hypocretin system is consistently involved in the vast majority of patients with primary narcolepsy with cataplexy. There have been reports of secondary narcolepsy, particularly associated with head injuries or neoplasm.

## DIAGNOSIS

Within the context of an appropriate clinical history, an overnight polysomnography (PSG) with a short REM sleep latency, followed by a Multiple Sleep Latency Test (MSLT) with a maximum average sleep latency of 8 min and two or more sleep-onset REM periods (SOREMPs) has been considered diagnostic for narcolepsy. A urine toxicology screen is typically performed on the morning of the MSLT.

- If an experienced clinician observes unequivocal cataplexy, overnight PSG and MSLT are not required to establish the diagnosis. During an unequivocal bout of cataplexy, the deep tendon reflexes would be expected to be absent when elicited with a reflex hammer.

- The current diagnostic criteria for narcolepsy in children are the same as in adults. However, the established diagnostic criteria may not always be applicable to children since the MSLT was not validated for children younger than 8 years of age.

- If a person is taking a medication that suppresses REM sleep, such as with most antidepressants, the MSLT results may not be reliable. If a patient abruptly stops taking antidepressants, REM sleep rebound may occur giving a false-positive result. A similar situation can occur if the MSLT is started at a time in the morning that a person usually sleeps, a scenario that occurs in an adolescent with a delayed sleep phase pattern. Finally, a false-positive result for narcolepsy can occur if the subject is suffering from jet lag, is sleep deprived, or has subtle sleep disordered breathing.

- Direct assays of hypocretin levels are more specific for the diagnosis of narcolepsy. Hypocretin can be measured in the CSF, and its absence in the CSF is diagnostic of narcolepsy. CSF hypocretin level measurements may be particularly useful in complex or ambiguous clinical situations. However, a normal CSF level of hypocretin does not exclude the possibility of narcolepsy. A reliable blood serum equivalent test is not yet available.

## TREATMENT

Successful treatment of narcolepsy needs to include both behavioral and pharmacologic treatments. Behavioral treatment begins with the patient having as thorough an understanding of their condition as possible. Having the patient and family members meet other people with narcolepsy may be helpful. Volunteer support organizations such as the Narcolepsy Network have been established. Patients need to understand that developing healthy sleep habits are important for the rest of their lives. Two brief naps a day of about 20 min each should be strongly encouraged. For school-aged children, the health care provider should serve as an advocate on behalf of the patient to encourage the school to allow the child to nap in a safe and comfortable environment. Failure to consider or properly apply nondrug treatments as part of the comprehensive management may lead to unsatisfactory results for the patient and the family. These factors can result in patients with narcolepsy that are not properly managed due to either underdosing or overdosing of medication or incorrect medication selection.

- Drug therapy must take into account possible side effects since narcolepsy is a lifelong illness and patients will have to receive medications for years. Tolerance or addiction may be seen with some compounds. Treatment of narcolepsy, thus, balances avoidance of side effects, including tolerance, with maintenance of an active life. There are no double-blind placebo-controlled trials of medication specifically for children with narcolepsy, and the medications that are commonly prescribed are not specifically approved by the Food and Drug Administration (FDA) for narcolepsy in children.

- The drugs most widely used to treat excessive daytime sleepiness are the central nervous system stimulants. A number of side effects, including irritability, anxiety, nervousness, headache, psychosis, tachycardia, hypertension, nocturnal sleep disturbances, tolerance, and drug dependence, may arise with their use.

- There are two drugs with different modes of action that can be used for patients with narcolepsy. The first one, modafinil, is considered more as a "somnolytic" than a nonspecific stimulant. Headaches are the most common side effect of modafinil and may be avoided or minimized by starting at low doses and gradually increasing the dose. Modafinil should be considered the initial pharmacologic agent used to treat the EDS of narcolepsy. The second drug is gamma-hydroxybutyrate (GHB, or sodium oxybate), which is the first substance ever approved specifically for cataplexy. Nighttime use of GHB has also been approved for the excessive daytime sleepiness of narcoplepsy patients. Important CNS adverse events associated with abuse of GHB include seizures, respiratory depression, and profound decreases in level of consciousness, with instances of coma and death. GHB has powerful CNS depressant effects and can increase slow-wave sleep. This medication when given at bedtime may be of value to reduce cataplexy. Patients may prefer this medication over other medications used for cataplexy, particularly if insomnia is also present. Dosing guidelines for patients younger than 16 years old are not established.

- Cataplexy seems to respond best to medications with noradrenergic reuptake blocking properties. There are no systematic trials of anticataplexy drugs on children. Postpubertal teenagers are usually treated as young adults. In this group, two medications have been more commonly used, namely clomipramine and fluoxetine. Both of these drugs have active noradrenergic reuptake blocking metabolites (desmethylclomipramine and norfluoxetine), and it is through these metabolites that the therapeutic effect may be mediated.

## KEY POINTS

1. Narcolepsy is a chronic neurologic disorder of excessive daytime sleepiness (EDS), which characteristically has a childhood onset and is associated with hypocretin deficiency. Other key clinical features include EDS, sleep paralysis, hypnagogic hallucinations, and sleep disturbance.

2. Within the context of an appropriate clinical history, an overnight polysomnography (PSG) with a short REM sleep latency, followed by a Multiple Sleep Latency Test (MSLT) with a maximum average sleep latency of 8 min and two or more

sleep-onset REM periods (SOREMPs) has been considered diagnostic for narcolepsy. If an experienced clinician observes unequivocal cataplexy, overnight PSG and MSLT are not required to establish the diagnosis.

3. Successful treatment of narcolepsy needs to include both behavioral and pharmacologic treatments.

## BIBLIOGRAPHY

Boehmer LN, et al. Treatment with immunosuppressive and anti-inflammatory agents delays onset of canine genetic narcolepsy and reduces symptom severity. *Exp Neurol* 2004; 188:292–299.

Borgen LA, et al. Sodium oxybate (GHB) for treatment of cataplexy. *Pharmacotherapy* 2002; 22:798–799.

Dauvilliers Y, et al. A monozygotic twin pair discordant for narcolepsy and CSF hypocretin-1. *Neurology* 2004; 62:2137–2138.

Ebrahim IO, et al. Hypocretin (orexin) deficiency in narcolepsy and primary hypersomnia. *J Neurol Neurosurg Psychiatry* 2003; 74:127–130.

Fujiki N, et al. Analysis of onset location, laterality and propagation of cataplexy in canine narcolepsy. *Psychiatry Clin Neurosci* 2002; 56:275–276.

Guilleminault C, et al. Narcolepsy in prepubertal children. *Ann Neurol* 1998; 43:135–142.

Guilleminault C, et al. Narcolepsy in children: A practical guide to its diagnosis, treatment and follow-up. *Paediatr Drugs* 2000; 2:1–9.

Hecht M, et al. Report of a case of immunosuppression with prednisone in an 8-year-old boy with an acute onset of hypocretin-deficiency narcolepsy. *Sleep* 2003; 26:809–810.

Khatami R, et al. Monozygotic twins concordant for narcolepsy-cataplexy without any detectable abnormality in the hypocretin (orexin) pathway. *Lancet* 2004; 363:1199–1200.

Kilduff TS, et al. The hypocretin/orexin ligand-receptor system: Implications for sleep and sleep disorders. *Trends Neurosci* 2000; 23:359–365.

Krahn LE, et al. Hypocretin (orexin) levels in cerebrospinal fluid of patients with narcolepsy: Relationship to cataplexy and HLA DQB1*0602 status. *Sleep* 2002; 25:733–736.

Lin L, et al. The sleep disorder canine narcolepsy is caused by a mutation in the hypocretin (orexin) receptor 2 gene. *Cell* 1999; 98:365–376.

Littner M, et al. Practice parameters for the treatment of narcolepsy: An update for 2000. *Sleep* 2001; 24:451–466.

Marcus CL, et al. Secondary narcolepsy in children with brain tumors. *Sleep* 2002; 25:435–439.

Melberg A, et al. Hypocretin deficiency in familial symptomatic narcolepsy. *Ann Neurol* 2001; 49:136–137.

Mignot E. An update on the pharmacotherapy of excessive daytime sleepiness and cataplexy. *Sleep Med Rev* 2004; 8:333–338.

Mignot E, et al. The role of cerebrospinal fluid hypocretin measurement in the diagnosis of narcolepsy and other hypersomnias. *Arch Neurol* 2002; 59:1553–1562.

Mignot E, et al. On the value of measuring CSF hypocretin-1 in diagnosing narcolepsy. *Sleep* 2003; 26:646–649.

Overeem S, et al. Voxel-based morphometry in hypocretin-deficient narcolepsy. *Sleep* 2003; 26:44–46.

Pelayo R, et al. Pediatric sleep pharmacology: You want to give my kid sleeping pills? *Pediatr Clin North Am* 2004; 51:117–134.

Ripley B, et al. CSF hypocretin/orexin levels in narcolepsy and other neurological conditions. *Neurology* 2001; 57:2253–2258.

Rosen GM, et al. Sleep in children with neoplasms of the central nervous system: Case review of 14 children. *Pediatrics* 2003; 112:e46–54.

Schatzberg SJ, et al. The effect of hypocretin replacement therapy in a 3-year-old Weimaraner with narcolepsy. *J Vet Intern Med* 2004; 18:586–588.

Silber MH, et al. The epidemiology of narcolepsy in Olmsted County, Minnesota: A population-based study. *Sleep* 2002; 25:197–202.

Tafti M, et al. Pharmacogenomics in the treatment of narcolepsy. *Pharmacogenomics* 2003; 4:23–33.

Taheri S, et al. The role of hypocretins (orexins) in sleep regulation and narcolepsy. *Annu Rev Neurosci* 2002; 25:283–313.

# 11

## IDIOPATHIC HYPERSOMNIA

STEPHEN N. BROOKS
Austin, Texas

### INTRODUCTION

The term *idiopathic hypersomnia* (IH) is used to categorize individuals with prominent excessive daytime sleepiness (EDS) but who lack the classic features of narcolepsy or evidence of another disorder known to cause EDS [such as obstructive sleep apnea (OSA)].

- The imprecise definition of IH has led to diagnostic difficulties. Without doubt, many patients have been diagnosed with IH, when, in fact, they suffered from other disorders, such as narcolepsy without cataplexy, narcolepsy prior to the onset of cataplexy, delayed sleep phase syndrome, or upper airway resistance syndrome. Absence of specific biologic markers or animal models of IH adds to the challenge.

### EPIDEMIOLOGY

Idiopathic Hypersomnia is believed to be less common than narcolepsy, but estimates of prevalence are elusive because strict diagnostic criteria are lacking, and no specific biological marker(s) has been identified. It has been estimated that IH occurs in 2–5/100,000 in Caucasians and is even less common in African Americans. IH occurs equally in males and females.

- The etiology of the disorder is not known, but viral illnesses, including Guillain–Barré syndrome, hepatitis, mononucleosis and atypical viral pneumonia may herald the onset of sleepiness in a subset of patients. EDS may occur as part of the acute illness, but it persists after the other symptoms subside.
- A significant increase in HLA-DQß1*0602 in subjects with IH (52 vs. 17% in controls) has been described.
- Familial cases are known to occur, with an increased frequency of HLA-Cw2 and HLA-DR11. Neverthe-

less, most cases of IH are not associated with either a positive family history or an obvious viral illness.

### CLINICAL FEATURES

Patients present with complaints of excessive sleepiness or excessively deep sleep that is present for at least 6 months. Nocturnal sleep period can either be prolonged or normal in duration. *The International Classification of Sleep Disorders* (American Academy of Sleep Medicines, 2005) distinguishes IH with long sleep time (more than 10 h) from IH without long sleep time. There are often frequent daily sleep episodes. Onset is insidious and typically occurs before age 25 years. By definition, there is no history of head trauma within 18 months of presentation, no medical or mental disorder is present that could account for EDS, and symptoms do not meet the diagnostic criteria of any other sleep disorder that can cause EDS (e.g., narcolepsy, OSA, or posttraumatic hypersomnia).

- The onset of EDS is usually insidious over a period of weeks or months, beginning in adolescence or early adulthood. In some cases, the onset of hypersomnia follows a period of insomnia. Daytime sleepiness is prominent and continuous but is not irresistible in contrast to the "sleep attacks" that may occur in narcolepsy. No amount of sleep ameliorates the daytime sleepiness.
- Naps are usually more than an hour in duration and, in contrast to narcolepsy, are nonrefreshing. "Microsleeps," with or without automatic behavior, may occur throughout the day.
- Nocturnal sleep is prolonged and uninterrupted. There is difficulty awakening from sleep, which may assume the characteristics of "sleep drunkenness."
- Psychiatric symptoms, especially depression, are prevalent in patients suffering from IH. It remains

to be determined whether these symptoms constitute essential features of IH or represent responses to the chronic, debilitating disorder.

- Hypnagogic hallucinations and sleep paralysis are reported to occur in approximately 40% of patients with IH, a proportion similar to what has been found in narcolepsy without cataplexy.

- Some patients experience symptoms suggesting autonomic nervous system dysfunction, including orthostatic hypotension, syncope, vascular-type headaches, and Raynaud-like phenomena.

- There is a subgroup of patients with IH who complain of only EDS (monosymptomatic type). Restless sleep with frequent awakenings is common. A few patients may have irresistible sleep episodes similar to narcolepsy.

- Symptoms of IH are generally severe enough to cause significant problems with work, school, and social functioning. Almost all patients have difficulties with driving because of sleepiness.

- Some patients describe increased hypersomnia with excessive physical activity, heavy meals, alcohol, psychological stress, or menses. Many, however, report no obvious aggravating factors.

- Although IH is typically a lifelong disorder with a stable course after the progressive onset of symptoms, spontaneous improvement or even complete resolution of EDS has occurred in some patients.

## POLYSOMNOGRAPHIC FEATURES

Nocturnal polysomnography (PSG) demonstrates shortened initial sleep latency (less than 10 min); normal or increased total sleep time; normal sleep architecture; and normal rapid eye movement (REM) sleep latency. In contrast, narcoleptic patients exhibit significant sleep fragmentation.

- Ideally, prolonged PSG monitoring across 24-h period(s) would be more useful in characterizing the sleep–wake patterns in these patients. However, this is not practical in clinical practice, and even in research settings, methodological and standardization issues need to be addressed.

- Mean sleep latency on Multiple Sleep Latency Test (MSLT) is usually reduced (i.e., often 8–10 min), and there are fewer than two sleep-onset REM periods (SOREMPs).

- Spectral analysis has demonstrated a decrease in slow-wave activity during the first two nonrapid eye movement (NREM) episodes of nocturnal sleep; increased REM density (in patients with polysymptomatic IH); and increased sleep spindle density (especially during the second half of the night), suggesting excessive thalamic blockade occurring at the end of the night. A prolonged visual P300 latency, longer auditory P300 latency, and reduced auditory P300 amplitude have been described.

## PATHOPHYSIOLOGY

Little is known about the pathophysiology of idiopathic hypersomnia. No animal model is available for study, and no specific biologic markers have been identified. Neurochemical studies using cerebrospinal fluid (CSF) have suggested that individuals with idiopathic hypersomnia may have a derangement in the noradrenergic system.

- A phase delay in the circadian rhythm of melatonin compared to controls, with a shift in elevated nocturnal melatonin levels to morning hours as well as a (nonsignificant) prolongation of the melatonin signal in IH subjects, perhaps contributing to difficulty with awakening, has been described.

## DIFFERENTIAL DIAGNOSIS

Other disorders producing EDS (such as sleep disordered breathing, periodic limb movement disorder, psychiatric illness, insufficient sleep syndrome, or circadian rhythm sleep–wake disorders) must be ruled out before a diagnosis of IH is made. EDS may have multiple causes in an individual patient, and IH may still be a consideration in cases when EDS persists despite what appears to be adequate treatment of other identified disorders.

- *Upper airway resistance syndrome* may present with EDS. Snoring may or may not occur with this disorder. Anatomic features of upper airway crowding and multiple cortical arousals during nocturnal PSG are important clues to the diagnosis. Monitoring of esophageal pressure during PSG, demonstrating increased respiratory effort leading to cortical arousals, provides definitive diagnosis. If this technique is not available, the use of nasal cannulae may be helpful to demonstrate the presence of flow limitation associated with cortical arousals.

- *Narcolepsy without cataplexy* (or prior to the onset of cataplexy) may present a difficult diagnostic challenge. Several clinical features are useful in distinguishing narcolepsy without cataplexy from IH. Patients suffering from narcolepsy without cataplexy tend to have disrupted nocturnal sleep with multiple awakenings. Daytime sleepiness tends to be more compelling and naps tend to be briefer and more refreshing than in IH. The presence of SOREMP during the MSLT in patients with narcolepsy without cataplexy is very helpful in making the distinction. Total sleep time across the 24-h period is generally normal in narcolepsy, but this may also be the case in some patients with IH. Since symptoms of sleep paralysis and/or hypnagogic hallucinations may occur in either disorder, their presence is not a distinguishing feature. HLA typing is not helpful. The association with HLA-DQß1*0602 is less robust in narcoleptic patients without cataplexy than in those with cataplexy. This allele may also be found in a significant number of patients with IH and in up to 25% of the general population. The measurement of CSF Hcrt-1 is useful if the peptide is decreased or undetectable, but this occurs in only a minority (10–20%) of patients with narcolepsy without cataplexy.

- *Psychiatric disorders* (particularly depression) are often associated with hypersomnia. In such cases, the severity of daytime sleepiness tends to vary more from one day to the next than in patients with IH. Nocturnal sleep is often poor. Longer mean sleep latency on MSLT and shorter total nocturnal sleep time in patients with mood disorders compared to those with IH has been reported. Patients with psychiatric hypersomnia may also have longer sleep latency, longer wake time after sleep onset, and shorter total sleep time during nocturnal PSH.

- *Delayed sleep phase disorder* (DSPD) may be mistaken for IH because of similar age of onset and some shared features. Patients with DSPD may be profoundly sleepy during the day and difficult to arouse from sleep. In pure form, however, there should also be times during the 24-h period when alertness is normal. Total sleep time, sleep latency, sleep architecture, and ease of awakening should be normal in DSPD if the affected individual is allowed to follow the dictates of his circadian clock. Diagnosis becomes problematic when school or work schedules mandate variance from the individual's ideal circadian sleep–wake rhythm. Furthermore, insufficient sleep is common during adolescence and early adulthood, leading to marked variations in sleep time (especially during weekends), need for naps, and some degree of sleepiness throughout the day. Nocturnal PSG and MSLT may be misleading if performed at inappropriate (i.e., phase advanced) times. In such situations, prolonged sleep latency may occur on the nocturnal PSG, and MSLT may demonstrate decreased mean sleep latency (and even SOREMPs). Sleep diaries, with actigraphy in difficult cases, may be helpful in demonstrating changes in sleep patterns and daytime symptoms during weekends or vacations. Measurement of dim light melatonin onset is useful in defining the individuals underlying circadian rhythm.

- "*Long sleepers*" are individuals who require more sleep (10 or more hours per 24-h period) than what is typically considered normal, but whose sleep is otherwise normal in architecture and physiology. They may develop EDS if they are unable to obtain their biologic quota of sleep time. Basically, this amounts to insufficient sleep syndrome at one end of the spectrum of sleep need. It has been suggested that the symptoms of IH are a consequence of chronic sleep deprivation in very long sleepers. Questioning the patient about sleep schedules and daytime symptoms during periods during which they are able to sleep *ad lib* may yield useful information. Adjustment of schedules to allow increased total sleep time should be sufficient to reduce EDS and clarify the diagnosis.

## TREATMENT

Treatment of IH is often less than satisfactory. Lifestyle and behavioral modifications, including good sleep hygiene, are appropriate, but treatment with stimulant medication or modafinil is usually necessary.

- The administration of melatonin at night has been reported to be useful in treating some patients with features of IH.

## KEY POINTS

1. The definition of IH has evolved over time and will continue to do so as understanding of the neurologic underpinnings of sleep and wakefulness deepens.
2. IH is believed to be less common than narcolepsy (perhaps by a factor of 10).
3. The differential diagnosis of IH can be challenging even to experienced clinicians. Currently, no specific marker is available to confirm the diagnosis. Whether IH represents a collection of distinct disorders with overlapping features but different neurological mechanisms or a single pathophysiologic entity with variable manifestations among affected individuals remains to be determined. More refined characterization of subgroups of IH patients will likely broaden treatment options.

## REFERENCE

American Academy of Sleep Medicine (AASM). *The International Classification of Sleep Disorders* 2nd ed. AASM, Westchester, IL, 2005: 98–103.

## BIBLIOGRAPHY

Bassetti C, et al. Idiopathic hypersomnia. A series of 42 patients. *Brain* 1997; 120:1423–1435.

Billiard M, et al. Idiopathic hypersomnia. *Psychiatry Clin Neurosci* 1998; 52:125–129.

Billiard M, et al. Idiopathic hypersomnia. *Sleep Med Rev* 2001; 5:351–360.

Billiard M, et al. Physiopathology of idiopathic hypersomnia. Current studies and new orientations. *Rev Neurol* 2001; 157: S101–106.

Dauvilliers Y, et al. CSF hypocretin-1 levels in narcolepsy, Kleine-Levin syndrome, and other hypersomnias and neurological conditions. *J Neurol Neurosurg Psychiatry* 2003; 74:1667–1673.

Ebrahim IO, et al. Hypocretin (orexin) deficiency in narcolepsy and primary hypersomnia. *J Neurol Neurosurg Psychiatry* 2003; 74:127–130.

Kanbayashi T, et al. CSF hypocretin-1 (orexin-A) concentrations in narcolepsy with and without cataplexy and idiopathic hypersomnia. *J Sleep Res* 2002; 11:91–93.

Lesperance P, et al. Effect of exogenous melatonin on excessive daytime somnolence associated with disturbed sleep: An open clinical trial. *Sleep Res* 1997; 26:111.

Mignot E, et al. The role of cerebrospinal fluid hypocretin measurements in the diagnosis of narcolepsy and other hypersomnias. *Arch Neurol* 2002; 59:1553–1562.

Montplaisir J, et al. Idiopathic hypersomnia: A diagnostic dilemma. *Sleep Med Rev* 2001; 5:361–362.

Nevsimalova S, et al. A contribution to pathophysiology of idiopathic hypersomnia. *Suppl Clin Neurophysiol* 2002; 53:366–370.

Sforza E, et al. Homeostatic sleep regulation in patients with idiopathic hypersomnia. *Clin Neurophysiol* 2000; 111(2):277–282.

Vankova J, et al. Increased REM density in narcolepsy-cataplexy and the polysymptomatic form of idiopathic hypersomnia. *Sleep* 2001; 24(6):707–711.

Vgontzas AN, et al. Differences in nocturnal and daytime sleep between primary and psychiatric hypersomnia: Diagnostic and treatment implications. *Psychosom Med* 2000; 62:220–226.

# 12

## POSTTRAUMATIC AND RECURRENT HYPERSOMNIA

CAROLYN M. D'AMBROSIO
Tufts-New England Medical Center, Boston, Massachusetts

JOSHUA BARON
Department of Pediatric Neurology, Tufts-New England Medical Center, Boston, Massachusetts

## POSTTRAUMATIC HYPERSOMNIA

Head trauma is a major cause of morbidity and mortality in the United States. The sequelae of head trauma span the neuropsychological spectrum, ranging from headaches and poor concentration to significant disability and coma.

- Commonly, patients who have suffered even minor head trauma complain of sleep disturbances, including hypersomnia and insomnia. While sleep complaints are nonspecific, several studies have shown an association between traumatic brain injury (TBI) and obstructive sleep apnea (OSA), upper airway resistance syndrome (UARS), and narcolepsy.

- Posttraumatic hypersomnia has also been described. This is defined as subjective sleepiness, objective proof of sleepiness on an Multiple Sleep Latency Test (MSLT) [i.e., latency of ≤ 10 min with fewer than two rapid eye movement (REM)-onset naps], and an unremarkable polysomnogram (PSG), all occurring after a traumatic brain injury. In one study of patients with a history of head and neck trauma, factors that predicted an MSLT mean sleep latency of ≤ 5 min included the presence of coma of at least 24 h and skull fracture.

- The development of delayed sleep phase disorder (DSPD) after trauma has been described, including adolescents and adults who, after sustaining traumatic brain injury, were unable to fall asleep until the early morning hours. While the pathophysiology of posttraumatic DSPD has yet to be elucidated, it is postulated to be secondary to damage to the suprachiasmatic nucleus and its connections. One such study demonstrated a 12-h delay in peak melatonin concentration, which could be phase advanced to its normal time with the use of 5 mg of endogenous melatonin. Chronotherapy, which is useful for idiopathic DSPD, has also been attempted, but compliance to this treatment is poor.

## HYPERSOMNIA ASSOCIATED WITH MOOD DISORDERS

- Hypersomnia is one of the "atypical" symptoms of depression and is present in a minority of patients with unipolar depression. Hypersomnia is thought to be more common in patients with bipolar disorder and in childhood depression.

- The prevalence of hypersomnia in patients with unipolar and bipolar depression is higher among men compared to women and in those under the age of 30 years than in older patients.

- Patients who complain of hypersomnia may not necessarily be hypersomnolent on objective measures. Depressed patients complaining of hypersomnia tend to have significantly longer sleep latencies on MSLT and to sleep for a significantly shorter period of time when given the opportunity to do so compared to patients with idiopathic hypersomnia. Similarly, patients with bipolar disease have been found to have longer mean sleep latencies (exceeding 10 min) on MSLT compared to patients with narcolepsy. These finding suggest that the degree of hypersomnia may be overreported in patients with unipolar and bipolar depression, possibly due to misperception of extended time in bed as evidence of increased sleep.

- In a study of patients with hypersomnia in seasonal affective disorder, analysis of sleep logs of those patients complaining of increased sleep during the winter months compared to the summer months (9.9 vs. 7.4 h) revealed that only 6% of patients truly slept more than 9 h during the winter months. Likewise, although light box treatment has been reported to reduce hypersomnia on subjective measures, there is no effect of treatment on sleep duration when sleep diaries were examined.

## POSTINFECTIOUS HYPERSOMNIA

In 1931, von Economo described the syndrome of encephalitis lethargica, which was thought to have an infectious or postinfectious etiology. The key symptoms consisted of drowsiness progressing to coma, along with ophthalmoplegia, oculogyric crises, and basal ganglia or cerebellar signs. Patients also presented with disorders of psychiatric disturbances and akinetic mutism. This syndrome is now quite rare.

- Although there is no definitive treatment for encephalitis lethargica, one study showed improvement with methylprednisolone treatment.

## KLEINE–LEVIN SYNDROME

In 1925, Kleine first described two adolescent boys with periodic hypersomnia, accompanied by confusion and excessive food consumption. Levin added a third case in 1929.

- The Kleine–Levin syndrome (KLS) is a rare disorder that occurs most commonly in adolescent boys with a male to female ratio of 3:1. It is characterized by the triad of hypersomnia, hyperphagia, and hypersexuality, all co-occurring periodically. Patients may develop delusions or hallucinations, behavioral disinhibition, confusion, and amnesia for the episodes. Autonomic symptoms, such as facial flushing and bradycardia, may also occur. Each episode lasts from 3 days to 2 weeks at a time; the interval between episodes lasts from several weeks to months. Cognitive function and sleep are normal between attacks.
- Patients are often unable to identify factors that had provoked their initial Kleine–Levin attack; however, patients have described febrile illnesses, extremes of ambient temperature, alcohol use, head trauma, and emotional stress preceding some of the attacks.
- Polysomnography features of patients with KLS are variable. While there is an increase in total sleep time and decrease in sleep efficiency during an attack, the architecture of sleep both during and between attacks is discrepant among studies. One study noted an increase in REM sleep and a decrease in nonrapid eye movement (NREM) stages 1, 3, and 4 sleep during an attack; however, a more recent study reported a decrease in REM and slow-wave sleep, and an increase in NREM stage 1 sleep. PSGs obtained between attacks typically show a similar decrease in sleep efficiency and mild decreases in REM and slow-wave sleep. Electroencephalography (EEG) is usually normal between attacks and may show generalized slowing during an attack. Imaging studies, including head computed tomography (CT) and magnetic resonance imaging (MRI), and lumbar puncture are normal in patients.
- The etiology of KLS is unknown. Suggestions of a genetic basis arise from an association with the

HLA-DQB1 haplotype and description of a pair of siblings with KLS, each with the HLA-DR2, DQ1, and DR5 haplotypes. Nonetheless, familial groupings of KLS are few. A single-photon-emission computed tomography (SPECT) scan of one patient showed hypoperfusion of the frontal and temporal lobes during, and between, attacks. Inflammatory microglia in the thalamus and a small locus ceruleus with decreased substantia nigra pigmentation have also been demonstrated.

- A more probable etiology is a primary neuroendocrinologic disturbance, as patients with KLS have symptoms similar to individuals with hypothalamic-pituitary masses or damage. Six patients have been found to have diminished cortisol responses to insulin-induced hypoglycemia during attacks.
- Treatment for KLS has included light therapy, stimulants (e.g., methylphenidate or ephedrine), and anticonvulsants (e.g., valproic acid or carbamazepine) with variable success. Lithium, in doses of 300 mg per day, is the current mainstay of treatment.

## IDIOPATHIC RECURRING STUPOR

Several cases of periodic stupor or periodic coma have been described. These episodes are similar to KLS attacks in their characteristic periodicity, presence of hypersomnia, and increased frequency in males. However, while KLS tends to occur in adolescent males, the mean age of onset of idiopathic recurring stupor (IRS) attacks is the middle- to upper-40s, and only two cases with adolescent onset have been described.

- In almost all reported instances of IRS, the onset of an episode is heralded by dysarthria, ataxia (i.e., "staggering about as if drunk"), and sensation of malaise or fatigue, which precede each episode by hours to a few days. Patients then descend into a state of obtundation, lasting from 2 h to 5 days, from which they can be aroused only by noxious stimuli. Once aroused, patients may be able to perform simple cognitive tasks before returning to a stuporous state. Recollection is poor when the episode ends, and patients may confabulate about the preceding days' events. They may also remain "stunned" for hours after the episode ends.
- Frequency of episodes ranges from every 3 days to one event annually; in many cases, there are no precipitating events.
- During episodes, patients demonstrate diffuse hypotonia with diminished reflexes. The characteristic EEG during an IRS attack is a slow beta activity (14–16 Hz) that is most prevalent anteriorly. EEG is normal between episodes. PSG between episodes is also normal; however, some patients may have sleep fragmentation, reduced sleep efficiency of sleep, and decreased slow-wave and REM sleep.
- Analysis of cerebrospinal fluid (CSF) collected during an IRS attack yielded significantly increased

concentrations of a benzodiazepine-like substance, endozepine-4, compared to CSF collected between attacks or from normal controls. The cause(s) of the elevated endozepine-4 levels remains unclear.

## MENSTRUAL-RELATED HYPERSOMNIA

Menstruation-linked hypersomnia, another type of recurrent hypersomnia, was first described in 1975 by Billiard, Guilleminault, and Dement.

- Periodic hypersomnia precedes the menses by 2–3 days and continues until spontaneous recovery several days after the cessation of menstruation. During each episode, patients may awaken only to void, and intake of food and fluids can be decreased significantly. The onset of hypersomnia may be preceded by hostility and withdrawal.

- Onset of symptoms occurs from early adolescence to the early fifth decade.

- During periods of hypersomnia EEG reveals low-amplitude theta activity, with interictal EEGs showing poorly organized posterior rhythm or less prominent theta rhythms. PSG performed between episodes is generally normal. During an event, PSG may demonstrate an increase in total sleep time with no significant alteration in sleep architecture in most cases.

- Abnormalities in monoamine metabolites have been described, including abnormally elevated levels of 5-HIAA and homovanillic acid during specific periods of the menstrual cycle.

- Estrogen, which blocks progesterone release and inhibits ovulation, has been used successfully to prevent menstrual-related hypersomnia, with symptoms recurring upon return of ovulatory cycles. This has led to the hypothesis that progesterone precipitates hypersomnia in patients prone to menstrual-related hypersomnia. Methylphenidate may be considered for patients who fail to respond to conjugated estrogen therapy.

## KEY POINTS

1. Posttraumatic hypersomnia is characterized by the development of sleep disturbances, including hypersomnia and insomnia, following head trauma. Some of the sleep complaints may be associated with obstructive sleep apnea, upper airway resistance syndrome, narcolepsy, or delayed sleep phase disorder.

2. Certain mood disorders, including bipolar disorder, childhood depression, and seasonal affective disorder, may present as hypersomnia.

3. The Kleine–Levin syndrome (KLS) is a rare disorder that occurs most commonly in adolescent boys and is characterized by the triad of periodic hypersomnia, hyperphagia, and hypersexuality.

4. Periodic hypersomnia can precede menses by several days and continue until spontaneous recovery several days after the cessation of menstruation.

5. In idiopathic recurring stupor, onset of an episode of hypersomnolence is heralded by dysarthria, ataxia, and sensation of malaise or fatigue, which evolves into a state of obtundation, lasting from 2 h to 5 days.

## BIBLIOGRAPHY

Castriotta RJ, et al. Sleep disorders associated with traumatic brain injury. *Arch Phys Med Rehabil* 2001; 82:1403–1406.

Crumley FE. Valproic acid for Kleine-Levin syndrome. *J Am Acad Child Adolesc Psychiatry* 1997; 36:868–869.

Crumley FE. Light therapy for Kleine-Levin syndrome. *J Am Acad Child Adolesc Psychiatry* 1998; 37:1245.

Dauvilliers Y, et al. Kleine-Levin syndrome: An autoimmune hypothesis based on clinical and genetic analyses. *Neurology* 2002; 59:1738–1745.

Gadoth N, et al. Clinical and polysomnographic characteristics of 34 patients with Kleine-Levin syndrome. *J Sleep Res* 2001; 10:337–341.

Guilleminault CG, et al. Hypersomnia after head-neck trauma: A medicolegal dilemma. *Neurology* 2000; 54:653–659.

## DISORDERS CAUSING EXCESSIVE SLEEPINESS

| Disorder | Age of Onset/Sex | Interictal EEG | Ictal EEG | PSG | Treatment |
|---|---|---|---|---|---|
| Kleine–Levin syndrome | Adolescence, M>F | Normal | Generalized slowing | Increased TST and decreased sleep efficiency during attack | Lithium Anticonvulsants Stimulants |
| Idiopathic recurring stupor | Fifth decade, M>F | Normal | 14–16 Hz background | 14–16 Hz background during attack | Flumazenil |
| Menstrual-related hypersomnia | Variable: early adolescence to fifth decade | Poorly organized posterior rhythm | Low-amplitude theta | Increase in TST during attack | Conjugated estrogens |

Katz JD, et al. Familial Kleine-Levin syndrome: Two siblings with unusually long hypersomnic spells. *Arch Neurol* 2002; 59:1959–1961.

Lam RW, et al. Hypersomnia and morning light therapy for winter depression. *Biol Psychiatry* 2002; 31:1062–1064.

Landtblom A-M, et al. A case of Kleine-Levin syndrome examined with SPECT and neuropsychological testing. *Acta Neurol Scand* 2002; 105:318–321.

Lugaresi E, et al. Endozepine stupor: Recurring stupor linked to endozepine-4-accumulation. *Brain* 1998; 121:127–133.

Malhotra S, et al. A clinical study of Kleine-Levin syndrome with evidence for hypothalamic-pituitary axis dysfunction. *Biol Psychiatry* 1997; 42:299–301.

Mukkades NM, et al. Carbamazepine for Kleine-Levin syndrome. *J Am Acad Child Adolesc Psychiatry* 1999; 38:791–792.

Nagtegaak JE, et al. Traumatic brain injury-associated delayed sleep phase syndrome. *Functional Neurol* 1997; 12:345–348.

Papacostas SS, et al. The Kleine-Levin syndrome. Report of a case and review of the literature. *Eur Psychiatry* 2000; 15:231–235.

Posternak MA, et al. Symptoms of atypical depression. *Psychiatry Res* 2001; 104:175–181.

Quinto C, et al. Posttraumatic delayed sleep phase syndrome. *Neurology* 2000; 54:250–252.

Soriani S, et al. Endozepine stupor in children. *Cephalalgia* 1997; 17:658–661.

# 13

## EVALUATION OF EXCESSIVE SLEEPINESS

MERRILL S. WISE
Methodist Healthcare Sleep Disorders Center, Memphis, Tennessee

### INTRODUCTION

Characterization of excessive daytime sleepiness (EDS) is one of the most important challenges faced by the sleep medicine specialist. Pathological sleepiness occurs in association with a variety of sleep disorders, medical and psychiatric diseases, inadequate sleep, and medication side effects. Excessive sleepiness is defined as sleepiness that occurs in a situation when an individual would usually be expected to be awake and alert.

- Excessive daytime sleepiness is a chronic problem for approximately 5% of the general population, and is associated with significant morbidity and increased mortality risk to the individual and others.
- The identification of pathological sleepiness begins the process of establishing a proper diagnosis and allows initiation of treatment and follow-up of the individual's response. The diagnostic process begins with, and is based primarily on, a thorough sleep and general medical history. Since some patients are not fully aware of the extent of their excessive sleepiness, the sleep specialist may need to query the patient's spouse, co-workers, or others who are in daily contact with the patient.
- Questionnaires such as the Epworth Sleepiness Scale (ESS) provide information about the individual's subjective perception of sleepiness on a daily basis (see Tables 13.1 and 13.2). Sleep diaries provide documentation of the individual's typical sleep–wake schedule. Selective use of nocturnal polysomnography (PSG) provides useful objective data regarding sleep architecture and continuity, respiratory disturbance, limb movements or abnormal behaviors in sleep, and other intrinsic sleep pathology.
- The Multiple Sleep Latency Test (MSLT) is performed during the day to quantify the degree of

sleepiness and to identify sleep-onset rapid eye movement (REM) periods as part of the evaluation of individuals with possible narcolepsy.

- Several other techniques have been used to characterize daytime sleepiness such as pupillography and continuous electroencephalography (EEG)/video monitoring, but these tools are not widely used in routine clinical practice.

### CLINICAL HISTORY AND EXAMINATION

During the patient encounter, the examiner may observe clinical features of sleepiness such as ptosis, yawning, blank facial expression, loss of postural tone, or overt sleep.

- Patients with pathologic sleepiness are notorious for overestimating or underestimating their degree of sleepiness. A helpful approach involves having the patient review the frequency and severity of sleepiness in a variety of circumstances. Individuals with *mild* excessive sleepiness tend to fall asleep primarily in sedentary situations, such as riding in an automobile or during long lectures. Individuals with *moderate to severe* sleepiness fall asleep in more active situations, such as while sitting and talking with another person or while driving. Those with severe *pathologic* sleepiness may fall asleep suddenly in the midst of an active conversation, while standing up, while taking a shower, or while eating.
- The sleep history should include a detailed review of the patient's usual sleep–wake schedule in order to identify problems with inadequate nocturnal sleep or circadian problems. Individuals who perform shift work, college students, and those with medical or

**Table 13.1   The Epworth Sleepiness Scale**

How likely are you to doze off or fall asleep in the following situations, in contrast to feeling just tired? This refers to your usual way of life in recent times. Even if you have not done some of these things recently, try to work out how they would have affected you. Use the following scale to choose the *most appropriate number* for each situation:

0 = would never doze
1 = slight chance of dozing
2 = moderate chance of dozing
3 = high chance of dozing

*Situation*
Sitting and reading
Watching TV
Sitting, inactive in a public place (e.g., a theater or a meeting)
As a passenger in a car for an hour without a break
Lying down to rest in the afternoon when circumstances permit
Sitting and talking to someone
Sitting quietly after a lunch without alcohol
In a car, while stopped for a few minutes in traffic

The numbers in the eight situations are added together to give a global score between 0 and 24.

MW Johns, A new method for measuring daytime sleepiness: The Epworth sleepiness scale. *Sleep* 14:540–545, 1991. Used with permission.

military professions are especially prone to irregular sleep patterns and inadequate sleep. For the patient with inadequate nocturnal sleep, having the patient increase the duration of sleep on a consistent basis can be diagnostically helpful. The patient who continues to experience pathologic sleepiness despite improved sleep hygiene and adequate sleep duration is likely to have a primary sleep disorder or medical disorder.

## CONDITIONS ASSOCIATED WITH EXCESSIVE SLEEPINESS

Extrinsic causes
    Insufficient sleep syndrome
    Inadequate sleep hygiene
    Environmental sleep disorder
    Circadian rhythm problems: jet lag syndrome, shift work syndrome
    Medication-related hypersomnia
Intrinsic causes
    Obstructive sleep apnea
    Narcolepsy
    Idiopathic hypersomnia
    Periodic limb movement disorder
    Restless legs syndrome
    Periodic hypersomnia
    Circadian rhythm sleep disorders
        Delayed sleep phase syndrome
        Irregular sleep–wake pattern
        Non-24-h sleep–wake disorder
    Structural central nervous system (CNS) lesions
        Obstructive hydrocephalus
        Hypothalamic and diencephalic lesions

- A thorough review of the patient's medication history will sometimes uncover a sedating medication or evidence of medication toxicity. Medications that may be associated with excessive sleepiness include barbiturates, benzodiazepines, trazodone, tricyclic antidepressants, antipsychotic medications, lithium, clonidine, propranolol, and traditional antihistamines, such as diphenhydramine. Exposure to toxins such as heavy metals may produce an encephalopathy that includes somnolence.

- The terms used by patients to describe their symptoms may require clarification. The patient who complains of fatigue or tiredness is generally describing a feeling of listlessness, loss of energy, or weakness, and not overt sleepiness. Fatigue should be differentiated from excessive sleepiness, which is characterized by lapses in awareness, impaired cognitive and motor function, and a propensity for transition into overt sleep. This latter history is suggestive of a sleep disorder, whereas chronic fatigue or "feeling tired" generally indicates a medical or psychiatric disorder.

**Table 13.2   Groups of Experimental Subjects, Ages, and Epworth Sleepiness Scale Scores**

| Subjects/Diagnoses | Number (M/F) | Age in Years (Mean ± SD) | ESS Scores (Mean ± SD) |
|---|---|---|---|
| Normal controls | 30 (14/16) | 36.4 ± 9.9 | 5.9 ± 2.2 |
| Primary snoring | 32 (29/3) | 45.7 ± 10.7 | 6.5 ± 3.0 |
| Obstructive sleep apnea syndrome | 55 (53/2) | 48.4 ± 10.7 | 11.7 ± 4.6 |
| Narcolepsy | 13 (8/5) | 46.6 ± 12.0 | 17.5 ± 3.5 |
| Idiopathic hypersomnia | 14 (8/6) | 41.4 ± 14.0 | 17.9 ± 3.1 |
| Insomnia | 16 (6/12) | 40.3 ± 14.6 | 2.2 ± 2.0 |
| Periodic limb movement disorder | 18 (16/2) | 52.5 ± 10.3 | 9.2 ± 4.0 |

MW Johns, A new method for measuring daytime sleepiness: The Epworth sleepiness scale. *Sleep* 14:540–545, 1991. Used with permission.

## CONDITIONS ASSOCIATED WITH CHRONIC FATIGUE

Psychiatric conditions
> Depression
> Anxiety with or without insomnia
> Personality disorders

Medical conditions
> Chronic infection
> Malignancy
> Autoimmune disorders
> Hypothyroidism

Neurological conditions
> Myasthenia gravis
> Multiple sclerosis
> Parkinson's disease
> Myopathies and neuropathies

Chronic fatigue syndrome
Pregnancy

- Excessive sleepiness should be differentiated from lethargy or stupor, problems that generally indicate a neurologic disturbance due to a medical disorder or a structural central nervous system lesion. This distinction may be difficult in patients with severe respiratory disturbance during sleep or the patient in an intensive care unit (ICU) setting with chronic severe sleep deprivation.

- Individuals with excessive sleepiness should be questioned carefully about respiratory problems during sleep. Sleepiness with persistent loud snoring, especially snoring in all sleeping positions, is strongly suggestive of obstructive sleep apnea. Bed partner reports of gasping or choking sounds or observed apnea are also features that strongly suggest obstructive sleep apnea. These symptoms indicate the need for overnight PSG to assess respiratory function during sleep.

- The patient with narcolepsy reports chronic daily sleepiness regardless of the quantity of nocturnal sleep obtained. Narcolepsy is generally associated with moderate to severe daily sleepiness that consists of periodic overwhelming sleep attacks superimposed on a background of chronic sleepiness across the day. If the narcolepsy patient is allowed to sleep, he or she generally reports feeling refreshed for one to several hours, followed by the return of overwhelming sleepiness. The history should incorporate questions regarding auxiliary symptoms of narcolepsy, including cataplexy, sleep paralysis, and hypnagogic hallucinations. The individual with narcolepsy often experiences fragmented nocturnal sleep, and narcolepsy patients are not spared from the possibility of coexisting obstructive sleep apnea, periodic limb movement disorder, or other sleep disorders.

- A special challenge exists with regard to individuals with structural brain lesions leading to somnolence. Patients with obstructive hydrocephalus generally experience progressive deterioration in their level of consciousness, headache, nausea, and, possibly, vomiting. The patient with intracranial hemorrhage, such as subdural hematoma or expanding epidural hematoma, may complain of headache and may manifest focal neurologic deficits. Occasionally, sleepiness may be confused with the lapse in awareness that can occur with seizures, including complex partial or absence seizures, or the fugue state associated with nonconvulsive status epilepticus. An EEG or prolonged EEG/video monitoring study may be helpful in identifying and characterizing seizures.

- The sleep history should include questions about the patient's work and social habits, including shifts in circadian rhythm. The individual with late work hours is predisposed to the delayed sleep phase syndrome or inadequate nocturnal sleep. Pilots and flight attendants who travel frequently across multiple time zones are at risk for jet lag and other circadian problems. Shift workers often struggle to obtain adequate sleep, and the health effects of frequently changing shifts is significant.

- A history of excessive alcohol use or drug abuse is important, and, in certain cases, performance of urine drug screening may be indicated to identify illicit drug abuse as the cause of sleepiness.

- Regardless of the eventual diagnosis, patients with excessive sleepiness should be counseled regarding the potential risks associated with sleepiness, including motor vehicle accidents, work-related accidents, and loss of productivity. Individuals with excessive sleepiness may struggle with emotional and cognitive problems, including problems with attention and concentration, distractability, memory difficulties, depressed mood, and interpersonal problems due to irritability and poor coping skills.

- Excessive sleepiness may present in unique ways in children and adolescents. Because children are often teased or disciplined for sleepiness in the classroom, they may deny having sleepiness, or they may attempt to conceal sleepiness through a variety of strategies. Young children often manifest a paradoxical overactivity during drowsiness, possibly in an effort to self-stimulate. Excessive sleepiness may be associated with a variety of behavior problems including irritability and emotional lability, acting out behaviors, attention deficit/hyperactivity disorder symptoms, and learning problems. Children with excessive sleepiness may miss key social or athletic opportunities, and they often show a tendency to become socially isolated or withdrawn.

## POLYSOMNOGRAPHY

Nocturnal polysomnography is indicated in the evaluation of patients with suspected respiratory disturbances during sleep, narcolepsy, idiopathic hypersomnia, and those in whom an adequate explanation of excessive sleepiness is not reached following a thorough sleep history. PSG should be initiated within 30 min of the patient's usual sleep time.

## MULTIPLE SLEEP LATENCY TEST

The Multiple Sleep Latency Test is a validated, objective measure of the ability or tendency to fall asleep under standardized conditions. For proper interpretation, the MSLT must be preceded by overnight polysomnography to document the patient's total sleep time and sleep stage distribution.

- An MSLT is indicated for evaluation of suspected narcolepsy and possibly for suspected idiopathic hypersomnia. The MSLT is not routinely indicated for patients with excessive sleepiness due to other sleep disorders or medical or psychiatric disorders, for evaluation of sleepiness associated with obstructive sleep apnea, or for documenting response to nasal continuous positive airway pressure (CPAP) therapy. If there is clinical suspicion of narcolepsy in the patient with documented obstructive sleep apnea, the patient should first undergo appropriate treatment of sleep apnea followed by repeat PSG (with CPAP if being used to treat sleep apnea), then an MSLT.

- The rationale for the MSLT is based on the premise that the speed at which an individual falls asleep is an indication of the severity of sleepiness. The MSLT consists of a series of five nap opportunities at 2-h intervals during the patient's usual period of wakefulness. Nap opportunities begin 1.5–3 h after the patient's usual rise time, and the patient is observed and not allowed to sleep between nap opportunities. The patient is placed in a dimly lit, quiet room in a reclining position and instructed to "Please lie quietly, assume a comfortable position, keep your eyes closed, and try to fall asleep." The patient is given a 20-min opportunity to sleep.

- Sleep latency is measured from the time of "lights out" until the first epoch of any stage of sleep. If the patient falls asleep, he or she is allowed to sleep for an additional 15 min to provide an opportunity for entry into REM sleep (sleep-onset REM period). If the patient does not sleep during a 20-min nap opportunity, sleep latency is scored as 20 min. Because sleep latency is influenced by the quantity and quality of sleep the previous night, the patient must be studied with an overnight PSG for proper interpretation.

- The clinical usefulness of the MSLT in diagnosing narcolepsy is based on two physiological parameters measured by the test. The mean sleep latency value (the arithmetic mean of sleep latencies from all nap opportunities) provides objective documentation of pathological sleepiness under standardized condi-

tions. Analysis of data from four papers that were reasonably free of inclusion bias (39 subjects with narcolepsy) indicates that the weighted mean sleep latency among narcolepsy subjects was $3.0 \pm 3.1$ min. Control subjects without evidence of sleep disorders demonstrated a weighted mean sleep latency of $10.5 \pm 4.6$ min. These findings indicate that most patients with narcolepsy have objective evidence of hypersomnia as determined by a mean sleep latency of less than 5 min on the MSLT.

- The second useful parameter for the diagnosis of narcolepsy using the MSLT involves identification of sleep-onset REM periods (SOREMPs). The presence of two or more SOREMPs was associated with a sensitivity of 0.78 and a specificity of 0.93 for narcolepsy. SOREMPs do not occur exclusively in patients with narcolepsy and can be observed in patients with obstructive sleep apnea, or any condition associated with reduced nocturnal REM sleep leading to a "REM rebound" during the day. Recent withdrawal of REM suppressing medications such as selective serotonin reuptake inhibitors (SSRIs) may lead to REM rebound during the day as well.

- Diagnostic sensitivity and specificity of the MSLT are optimal when standardized procedures are followed and when interpretation is meticulous. Occasionally, for various reasons, patients with suspected narcolepsy do not meet polygraphic diagnostic criteria. Repeat MSLT testing may be indicated when the initial test is affected by extraneous circumstances, when appropriate study conditions were not present during initial testing, when ambiguous or uninterpretable findings are present, or when the patient is suspected to have narcolepsy on clinical grounds but earlier MSLT evaluation did not provide polygraphic confirmation. Patients with evolving narcolepsy may not meet MSLT diagnostic criteria initially, but criteria may be met on repeat testing 6–12 months later. Narcolepsy may also be diagnosed on clinical grounds when unequivocal cataplexy is present in addition to chronic pathological sleepiness. However, in North America and Europe, most sleep centers utilize routine polygraphic evaluation to provide objective confirmation of SOREMPs. Since narcolepsy is a serious and lifelong disorder with a major impact on the patient and others, the routine use of the MSLT for confirmation seems justified. In addition, MSLT diagnostic criteria for narcolepsy must be met when the patient has no history of cataplexy.

- Establishing normative mean sleep latency values for the MSLT is complicated by several factors. Mean sleep latency values are influenced by physiologic, psychologic, and test protocol variables. The quantity and continuity of nocturnal sleep prior to the MSLT clearly influence mean sleep latency values. At least 6 h of sleep the preceding night is required for a valid MSLT. There is no large systematically collected repository of normative data for the MSLT, and methodological variations may exist from center to center, and deviation from the standard protocol has the potential to alter sleep latencies significantly. Normative studies vary with regard to how rigorously control subjects are screened, how carefully subjects maintained a consistent sleep–wake pattern prior to the MSLT, whether subjects were allowed to use caffeine or medications, and whether urine drug screens were performed. Delineation of normative ranges is limited by the large standard deviation in mean sleep latency values, as well as ceiling and floor effects that indicate that mean sleep latency values are not normally distributed. These latter factors result in overlap between values among healthy controls and individuals with excessive sleepiness.

- Pooled data from normal subjects across all ages on the MSLT give a mean sleep latency of $10.4 \pm 4.3$ min when using the four-nap protocol and $11.6 \pm 5.2$ minutes when using the five nap protocol. Based on the traditional 2 standard deviations from the mean approach, 95% of the values from control populations on the four-nap test would fall between 1.8 and 19 min, and for the five-nap test, the mean sleep latency value would fall between 1.2 and 20 min. Thus, the MSLT does not discriminate well between clinical and control populations. However, within the clinical population, MSLT is useful for diagnostic purposes. Mean sleep latency values on MSLT are as follows:

| Test Protocol | Mean $\pm$SD (min) |
|---|---|
| MSLT (4-nap protocol) | $10.4 \pm 4.3$ |
| MSLT (5-nap protocol) | $11.6 \pm 5.2$ |
| MSLT in patients with narcolepsy | $3.1 \pm 2.9$ |

- Based on these data, the mean sleep latency should not be the sole criterion for determining the presence or severity of excessive sleepiness, certifying a diagnosis, or monitoring response to treatment. Global assessment should integrate the clinical history, objective test results, and other medical information.

## MAINTENANCE OF WAKEFULNESS TEST

The Maintenance of Wakefulness Test (MWT) is an objective, laboratory-based measure of a patient's ability to remain awake under standardized conditions for a defined period of time. The MWT is potentially useful in assessing response to treatment of disorders associated with excessive sleepiness. The test is not used to diagnose a condition.

## COMPARISON OF MSLT AND MWT

| | MSLT | MWT |
|---|---|---|
| Objective | To measure an individual's ability or tendency to fall asleep and propensity for entry into REM sleep | To measure an individual's ability to remain awake (usually after treatment of an underlying sleep disorder) |
| Time of test | During usual period of wakefulness | During usual period of wakefulness |
| Protocol | 4 or 5 nap opportunities at 2-h intervals beginning 1.5–3 h after waking; 20-min opportunity to nap | 4 tests at 2-h intervals; 20- or 40-min tests |
| Instructions to patient | "Please lie quietly, assume a comfortable position, keep your eyes closed, and try to fall asleep." | "Please sit still and remain awake for as long as possible." |
| Rule for termination | End nap opportunity after 20 min if no sleep occurs; end nap 15 min after sleep onset if sleep occurs | End test at first epoch of any stage of sleep, or after 20 or 40 min of wakefulness |
| Rule for determination of sleep latency | Arithmetic mean of all nap opportunities | Arithmetic mean of all four tests |
| Reporting results | Mean sleep latency (minutes); number of SOREMPs | Mean sleep latency (minutes) |
| Recommendations regarding CNS active medications | Optimal: Patient tapered off all CNS active medications for at least 14 days before test<br>Suboptimal: Patient continues on usual medications without change<br>Unacceptable: Patient tapered abruptly off CNS active medication just before test (may lead to REM rebound) | Patient on usual dosage of medication or CPAP at the time of the test |

- The MSLT and MWT measure different aspects of sleepiness and wakefulness during the day, and, as a consequence, mean sleep latency values do not correlate well between the two tests.

- The MWT is performed during the day after a typical night of sleep and when the individual is treated for a condition causing excessive sleepiness. The MWT consists of four tests at 2-h intervals. With each test, the subject is placed in a dimly lit, quiet room with a 7.5-W lamp positioned 3 ft lateral to the patient's head and 1 ft off the floor. The subject is given instructions to ``Please sit still and remain awake for as long as possible. Look directly ahead of you, and do not look directly at the light.''

- Sleep onset is defined as the first epoch of greater than 15 s of cumulative sleep in a 30-s epoch. There are two protocols for the MWT based on the duration of each test. Twenty- and 40-min protocols can be used, but the 40-min protocol is recommended.

- As with the MSLT, establishing normative mean sleep latency values for the MWT has been difficult. Whereas the MSLT shows a "floor effect" in subjects with severe sleepiness, the MWT shows a "ceiling effect" in subjects with normal levels of wakefulness, with many subjects remaining awake during each trial. The MWT data for a (40-min protocol) are as follows:

  Mean sleep latency (using latency to first epoch of any sleep stage): $30.4 \pm 11.2$ min

  Upper limit of 95% confidence interval: 40.0 min

## KEY POINTS

1. Characterization of excessive sleepiness begins with, and is based primarily on, a carefully taken clinical history. Questionnaires such as the Epworth Sleepiness Scale and sleep–wake diaries may provide additional data.

2. Overnight polysomnography is indicated as part of the evaluation of respiratory disturbances in sleep, narcolepsy, and for characterization of certain abnormal movements or behaviors in sleep.

3. The MSLT is indicated for evaluation of suspected narcolepsy in order to quantify the degree of excessive sleepiness and to document sleep-onset REM periods. The MSLT is not routinely indicated for evaluation of all patients with sleepiness.

4. The MWT is used selectively when objective data are necessary to document response to treatment for conditions that cause excessive sleepiness. The determination of a patient's response to treatment is especially important when the person's work involves public safety. Examples include pilots, air traffic controllers, bus, train, or subway drivers, and military and medical professionals.

## BIBLIOGRAPHY

Arand D, et al. Clinical use of the MSLT and MWT. *Sleep* 2005; 28:123–144.

Chesson AL, et al. The indications for polysomnography and related procedures. *Sleep* 1997; 20:423–487.

Doghramji K, et al. A normative study of the maintenance of wakefulness test (MWT). *Electroencephal Clin Neurophysiol* 1997; 103:554–562.

Littner MR, et al. Practice parameters for clinical use of the Multiple Sleep Latency Test and the Maintenance of Wakefulness Test. An American Academy of Sleep Medicine Report: Standards of Practice Committee of the American Academy of Sleep Medicine. *Sleep* 2005; 28:113–121.

Wise MS. Childhood narcolepsy. *Neurology* 1998; 1:S37–S42.

# 14

## THERAPY FOR EXCESSIVE SLEEPINESS

MAX HIRSHKOWITZ
Baylor College of Medicine, Houston, Texas, and Department of Medicine and Department of Psychiatry,
Michael E. DeBakey VAMC Sleep Center, Houston, Texas

### INTRODUCTION

Sleepiness can occur naturally or be induced. It may be defined in terms of self-report, physiologic response, or observation. Clinically significant sleepiness interferes with activities of daily living and is associated with a struggle to remain awake, inappropriate lapses into sleep, or both.

- In general, sleepiness may be viewed as a serious, noncontiguous, potentially life-threatening condition, that affects not only the afflicted individual but also his or her family, friends, co-workers, and society at large. Innumerable traffic and industrial accidents are either directly caused by, or are contributed to, by sleepiness.

### SLEEPINESS IN THE GENERAL POPULATION

Treating sleepiness can be easy or difficult, depending on the cause, the cooperation of the patient, or both. Sleep deprivation represents the leading cause of sleepiness. The internal sleep homeostatic mechanism accrues sleep debt in response to sleep loss. Sleepiness can be conceptualized as the alerting message that your account is overdrawn.

- When schedule permits, the individual naps or extends his or her sleep time (e.g., sleeping-in on weekends). If daytime alertness improves and sleepiness is reduced with these simple behavioral interventions, then the problem is likely nonmedical. Further lifestyle advice, sleep hygiene improvements, and avoidance of soporific substances or intoxicants is recommended.

### ADENOSINE ANTAGONISM

The judicious use of caffeinated substances may provide acute relief because methylxanthine stimulants counteract sleepiness. Caffeine and theobromine, usually consumed as coffee or chocolate, are widely traded commodities used the world over. In this country, major sources of caffeine also include tea, cola, and other sodas.

- Adenosine is an inhibitory neurotransmitter in the central nervous system (CNS). Caffeine is a CNS stimulant that inhibits adenosine, thereby producing activation. It is an alkaloid with the formula $C_8H_{10}N_4O_2$ with a mean half-life of 5 h (ranging widely from 1.5 to 9.5 h). Caffeine is rapidly absorbed (99% within 1 h). A typical 10-ounce mug of drip-brewed coffee will contain approximately 200–250 mg of caffeine. A typical can of cola soda (12-ounce) will have 40 mg caffeine, while 4- ounces of chocolate ranges from an average of 24 (milk), to 80 (dark), to 140 (Baker's) mg of theobromine.
- Caffeine can produce acute blood pressure elevations (5–15 mm Hg systolic, 5–10 mm Hg diastolic) with even more exaggerated increases in people experiencing stress. Caffeine is thought to account for as many as 14% of coronary heart disease and 20% of stroke-related deaths. The pharmacologically lethal oral dose in humans is estimated at 10–15 g.

### SLEEPINESS IN THE PATIENT POPULATION

While caffeine is the stimulant of choice of sleep-deprived individuals who self-medicate for sleepiness, it is also used by many individuals suffering from disorders of excessive sleepiness. These disorders include obstructive

*Sleep Medicine Essentials*, edited by Teofilo L. Lee-Chiong
Copyright © 2009 John Wiley & Sons, Inc.

sleep apnea, narcolepsy, idiopathic hypersomnia, circadian rhythm disorders, and sleepiness secondary to medical, neurologic, and psychiatric conditions. Sleepiness can also be iatrogenic.

- Sleepiness is sometimes treated with specifically targeted therapeutics designed to ameliorate the underlying cause (e.g., positive airway pressure for obstructive sleep apnea). In such cases, the goal is to correct the sleep-disrupting pathophysiology. By contrast, in sleep disorders where the sleepiness is presumably related to an underlying core neurological deficit, focused treatments are unavailable and therapy tends to be palliative.

- Currently, positive airway pressure is the preferred and most widely used therapy; it comes in three varieties, continuous, bi-level, and automatically self-adjusting. Continuous positive airway pressure (CPAP) is the most common modality. In general, it works by delivering a fan or turbine-generated flow at a set pressure to the nares. This positive pressure creates a "pneumatic splint" that maintains airway patency. It is highly effective in most patients; however, it requires nightly use. Patients who are sleepier before treatment tend to be more adherent to therapy. Normalization of sleep can be immediate and impressive. Sleep in a patient with SDB is marked by frequent brief arousals. These arousals are needed

## SLEEP DISORDERS ASSOCIATED WITH EXCESSIVE SLEEPINESS

| Type of Condition | Sleep Disorder | Comments |
|---|---|---|
| Primary sleep disorder | Obstructive sleep-disordered breathing | Sleepiness arises from sleep loss and fragmentation produced by frequent awakenings and arousals. |
| | Narcolepsy and idiopathic hypersomnia | Sleepiness is thought to relate to dysfunction in the basic CNS sleep-control mechanisms. |
| | Circadian rhythm sleep disorders | Sleepiness results from a mismatch of the circadian sleep–wake mechanisms and the behavioral schedule. |
| Secondary sleep disorder | Dyssomnias associated with medical conditions | Sleepiness can arise from sleep disturbances associated with pain, gastroesophageal reflux, fever, metabolic conditions, cardiopulmonary diseases, and endocrine disorders. |
| | Dyssomnias associated with neurological conditions | Sleepiness is associated with focal CNS lesions, myotonic dystrophy, encephalitis, cerebral palsy, Parkinson's disease, multiple sclerosis, head injuries, Prader–Willi syndrome, Kleine–Levin syndrome. |
| | Dyssomnias associated with psychiatric conditions | Sleepiness is associated with atypical depression, seasonal affective disorder, schizophrenia, or bipolar disorder (depressed phase). |

## TREATING SLEEPINESS IN OBSTRUCTIVE FORMS OF SLEEP-DISORDERED BREATHING

Obstructive forms of sleep-disordered breathing (SDB) include disorders ranging from upper airway resistance syndrome to severe obstructive sleep apnea. These sleep-related breathing impairments are caused by airway obstruction. During obstructive events, respiratory efforts continue but airflow decreases due to reduced or loss of airway patency.

- Many treatments are available for SDB, including weight loss, positive airway pressure therapy, oral appliances, and surgery. Weight loss is difficult to achieve and maintain; therefore, it is recommended but seldom relied upon.

to return ventilatory control to the voluntary system so that the airway can be dilated and airway patency restored. Pressures are titrated in an ascending fashion while the patient sleeps, and once an appropriate pressure is reached, the constant sleep disruptions disappear, permitting the patient to sleep uninterrupted, possibly for the first time in decades.

## TREATING SLEEPINESS IN NARCOLEPSY AND IDIOPATHIC HYPERSOMNIA

Stimulant medications are the mainstay of therapy for sleepiness associated with narcolepsy or idiopathic hypersomnia.

- Modafinil is effective for treating daytime sleepiness related to narcolepsy. The drug has a favorable benefit-to-risk ratio. Modafinil has a Food and Drug Administration indication for use for treating narcolepsy. Additionally, the Academy of Sleep Medicine Standards of Practice Guideline recommends modafinil as a first-line treatment for narcolepsy. It is generally effective and well tolerated. Side effects at therapeutic doses include headache, nervousness, nausea, insomnia, irritability, and, rarely, a serious life-threatening skin disease. High doses (greater than 800 mg) may cause tachycardia and hypertension. Modafinil does not appear to induce euphoria until doses exceeding 800–1000 mg are reached. Extended clinical trials report little or no loss of efficacy due to tolerance.

- Amphetamine, methamphetamine, dextroamphetamine, and methylphenidate are also recommended for treating sleepiness in narcolepsy, but their benefit-to-risk ratio is not well documented. Selegiline may also be considered for patients with narcolepsy and excessive sleepiness. Amphetamine and related stimulants increase activity and arousal level. Side effects include tremor, anorexia, insomnia, gastrointestinal complaints, irritability, and headaches. These medications directly activate the sympathetic nervous system and may adversely affect the cardiopulmonary system. Amphetamine psychosis, paranoia, and hallucinations can also occur. Amphetamines tend to produce euphoria and, therefore, have a high abuse potential; thus, they are Drug Enforcement Agency (DEA) Scheduled II substances. Tolerance may develop with chronic use and this, in turn, can lead to dose escalation. Tolerance and other side effects are reportedly less common with methylphenidate than other amphetamines. Abrupt discontinuation is discouraged, although little or no data are available concerning rapid withdrawal. Amphetamine discontinuation is characterized by profound excessive sleepiness and long episodes of recovery sleep.

- Other stimulants (pemoline and mazindol) were previously used to treat sleepiness in narcolepsy and idiopathic hypersomnia but due to limited efficacy and/or severe side effects, they are seldom used now.

- No practice guidelines are available for treating sleepiness in idiopathic insomnia; however, most clinicians use a similar approach to that used for narcolepsy.

## DRUGS USED TO TREAT EXCESSIVE SLEEPINESS

| Name | Therapeutic Dose | Comments |
|---|---|---|
| Modafinil | 100–400 mg | Wake-promoting substance with a 10- to 12-h half-life that is chemically different from amphetamines. Mechanism of action is not known but thought to work via histamine and gamma-aminobutyric acid (GABA) pathways. |
| Methylphenidate | 10–80 mg | Structurally similar to amphetamine and is rapidly absorbed. As with amphetamines, it works through dopamine release and reuptake blockade. Has a half-life of 2–4 h and is usually taken three or four times daily in divided doses. |
| Amphetamine Methamphetamine | 5–60 mg | This is the classic form of amphetamine. It is a racemic mixture of levo- and dextro- amphetamine isomers. It has less central and more peripheral action than dextroamphetamine and is usually taken three or four times daily in divided doses. |
| Dextroamphetamine | 20–60 mg | D-isomer of amphetamine. Moderately long half-life of 8–12 h. Usually taken in divided doses, twice or three times daily. |
| Levoamphetamine | 20–60 mg | L-isomer of amphetamine. Not available in the U.S. and does not appear to have any advantages over the D-isomer form. |
| Selegiline | 10 mg | Monoamine oxidase type B inhibitor that increases dopamine levels. Catabolizes to levo-amphetamine and methamphetamine. Can provoke hallucinations and contraindicated for concurrent administration with 5-HT reuptake inhibitors. |
| Mazindol | 2–12 mg | Chemically different from amphetamines. Mixed reports on efficacy. Known tolerance and abuse potential. |

## TREATING SLEEPINESS IN CIRCADIAN RHYTHM DISORDERS

One of the principal mechanisms regulating the sleep–wake cycle involves an internal 24-h biological clock (circadian pacemaker). This clock is responsible for providing stimulation to counteract the increasing homeostatic drive for sleep that accrues as a function of wakefulness. When this clock is out of synch with our schedule due to rapid movement through time zones or reversing the sleep–wake schedule, sleepiness and/or insomnia may result.

- In *jet lag*, an individual rapidly relocates to a different time zone. If in the new time zone, the patient has a desired awake time that occurs during the sleepy phase of the circadian cycle, excessive sleepiness may result.
- In *advanced sleep phase disorder*, the circadian rhythm is shifted earlier; the sleep–wake cycle is advanced with respect to the environmental clock time, making the individual drowsy in the evening.
- *Delayed sleep phase disorder* results when the biological clock is shifted later than the desired schedule. Individuals with delayed sleep phase are more alert in the evening and early nighttime, stay up later, and are sleepy in the morning.
- In the past, chronotherapy was used to reentrain the circadian rhythm; however, it has largely been replaced by bright light therapy. Bright light appears to be the critical factor controlling the biological clock. With precise timing of bright light exposure, the biological clock can be phase advanced, phase delayed, or stopped and reset. Bright light in the evening will delay the sleep phase, whereas bright light in the morning will advance the sleep phase.
- It also appears that melatonin or melatonin receptor agonists may be effective chronobiotics. Melatonin serves as a signal of darkness to the brain, and will advance the sleep phase when administered in the evening, and delay the sleep phase when given in the morning.
- Individuals with *shift work sleep disorder* (SWSD) continually struggle to remain awake during their night shift and to sleep during the day. If their internal biological clock does not shift with their schedule, they remain in a perpetual state of circadian misalignment. Shift workers face unique challenges to their sleep integrity. The sleep environment must be optimized. Sleep time must be given priority and not violated by intrusions by family and friends. Regularity is critical, and the patient should strive to arise at the same time daily and get an adequate amount of sleep. Low dose of pharmaceutical-grade melatonin or a melatonin agonist may promote sleep. Randomized clinical trials with modafinil have found improved alertness at night among patients with SWSD.

## TREATING SLEEPINESS IN MEDICAL, NEUROLOGIC, AND PSYCHIATRIC CONDITIONS

In cases where the sleepiness is due to an underlying medical, neurologic, or psychiatric condition, the standard approach is to treat the cause.

- In some cases, excessive sleepiness persists notwithstanding optimized treatment of the underlying condition(s). Some research indicates the efficacy of augmentation therapies with modafinil or stimulants. Augmentation studies have evaluated patients with depression, seasonal affective disorder, Parkinson's disease, pain-related fatigue, myotonic dystrophy, multiple sclerosis, and obstructive sleep apnea. Such an approach should be pursued with the utmost care, and only when the additional medication is not contraindicated by the patient's current drug regimen and/or comorbid conditions.

## TREATING IATROGENIC SLEEPINESS

The three major sources of iatrogenic sleepiness involve (a) soporific side effects of drug therapy; (b) direct sleep-promoting effects of a nondrug therapeutic intervention (e.g., radiation therapy), and (c) sleepiness produced by sleep disturbance resulting from a primary intervention (e.g., postsurgical pain).

- Drugs known to promote sleepiness as their primary effect include sedative-hypnotics and minor tranquilizers. Other agents may induce sleepiness as an unwanted side effect.
- Patients using sedative-hypnotics may experience sleepiness if a medication's duration of action extends beyond the scheduled sleep period (i.e., a "hang-over" effect). Switching to a shorter acting substance and/or lowering the dose may alleviate this problem.
- When the sleepiness is an unwanted side effect, the problem may be unavoidable; however, medication review often provides an opportunity to switch to less soporific substances with similar therapeutic efficacy.
- The following medications are associated with sleepiness: anxiolytics (diazepam, alprazolam), central-acting antihistamines (diphenhydramine), antidepressants (trazodone, amitriptyline, doxepin, sinequan, mirtazepine), antipsychotics (chlorpromazine, haloperidol, thioridazine, olanzapine, risperidone, quetiapine), antihypertensives (clonidine), anticonvulsants (carbamazepine, phenytoin, gabapentin), narcotics (meperidine, codeine, oxycododone, hydrocodone), and some steroids.

## KEY POINTS

1. Sleepiness can be associated with a wide variety of conditions. When improved alertness can be

attained by improved sleep hygiene and lifestyle interventions, these approaches are recommended.

2. Caffeine is widely used as a countermeasure for sleepiness arising from both behavioral and medical origins.

3. When sleepiness results from a primary sleep disorder affecting a presumed underlying sleep–wake mechanism (e.g., narcolepsy), wake-promoting substances and/or psychostimulants are generally used palliatively to manage the condition. These medications may have serious side effects and carry a potential for abuse. Therefore, they should be used properly and only under physician supervision.

4. If sleepiness is secondary to a medical, neurologic, or psychiatric condition, the underlying condition should be addressed first, and if residual sleepiness persists, augmentation therapy may be appropriate.

5. Medication review should be considered in patients being treated concurrently for other conditions in order to rule out iatrogenic factors.

## BIBLIOGRAPHY

Adler CH, et al. Randomized trial of modafinil for treating subjective daytime sleepiness in patients with Parkinson's disease. *Mov Disord* 2003; 18:287–293.

Billiard M, et al. Idiopathic hypersomnia. *Sleep Med Rev* 2001; 5:349–358.

Broughton RJ, et al. Randomized, double-blind, placebo-controlled crossover trial of modafinil in the treatment of excessive daytime sleepiness in narcolepsy. *Neurology* 1997; 49:444–451.

DeBattista C, et al. A prospective trial of modafinil as an adjunctive treatment of major depression. *J Clin Psychopharmacol* 2004; 24:87–90.

Fishbain DA, et al. Modafinil for the treatment of pain-associated fatigue: Review and case report. *Pain Palliat Care Pharmacother* 2004; 18:39–47.

Happe S. Excessive daytime sleepiness and sleep disturbances in patients with neurological diseases: Epidemiology and management. *Drugs* 2003; 63:2725–2737.

James JE. Critical review of dietary caffeine and blood pressure: A relationship that should be taken more seriously. *Psychosom Med* 2004; 66:63–71.

Littner M, et al. Practice parameters for the treatment of narcolepsy: An update for 2000. *Sleep* 2001; 24:451–466.

Lundt L. Modafinil treatment in patients with seasonal affective disorder/winter depression: An open-label pilot study. *J Affect Disord* 2004; 81:173–178.

MacDonald JR, et al. Modafinil reduces excessive somnolence and enhances mood in patients with myotonic dystrophy. *Neurology* 2002; 59:1876–1880.

Rammohan KW, et al. Efficacy and safety of modafinil (Provigil) for the treatment of fatigue in multiple sclerosis: A two centre phase 2 study. *J Neurol Neurosurg Psychiatry* 2002; 72:179–183.

Rye DB. Sleepiness and unintended sleep in Parkinson's disease. *Curr Treat Options Neurol* 2003; 5:231–239.

Schwartz JR, et al. Modafinil as adjct therapy for daytime sleepiness in obstructive sleep apnea: A 12-week, open-label study. *Chest* 2003; 124:2192–2199.

U.S. Modafinil in Narcolepsy Multicenter Study Group. Randomized trial of modafinil for the treatment of pathological somnolence in narcolepsy. *Ann Neurol* 1998; 43:88–97.

U.S. Modafinil in Narcolepsy Multicenter Study Group. Randomized trial of modafinil as a treatment for the excessive daytime somnolence of narcolepsy. *Neurology* 2000; 54: 1166–1175.

# 15

## ADULT SLEEP-DISORDERED BREATHING

Reena Mehra[1,2] and Kingman P. Strohl[1,2,3]
[1]Case School of Medicine, Cleveland, Ohio
[2] University Hospitals Case Medical Center, Cleveland, Ohio
[3] Department of Veterans Affairs Medical Center, Cleveland, Ohio

### INTRODUCTION

Sleep-disordered breathing (SDB) is a process characterized by repetitive partial or complete upper airway occlusion often associated with episodic, intermittent oxygen desaturation, hypercapnia, and arousals leading to sleep fragmentation. Several signs and symptoms adversely affecting quality of life and health status may accompany SDB. These include snoring, excessive daytime sleepiness (EDS), neurocognitive deficits, irritability, functional impairment, poor work performance, depression, automobile accidents due to drowsy driving, morning headaches, nocturnal enuresis, bed partner sleep disruption, and cardiovascular morbidity.

- Sleep-disordered breathing encompasses a spectrum of disorders including obstructive sleep apnea (OSA), central sleep apnea (CSA), upper airway resistance syndrome (UARS), and sleep hypoventilation syndrome. The prevalence of OSA [defined as an apnea–hypopnea index (AHI) of at least 5 events/hour], and excessive daytime somnolence has been estimated at 2% of women and 4% of men in a group of middle-aged adults, but there are pockets of higher prevalence in patients who are obese and have chronic cardiovascular disease.
- In addition, the cost of losses in work productivity and auto accidents must be considered. Failure to recognize SDB is costly both to the individual and to society; underdiagnosis is thought to cost the United States $3.4 billion in additional medical costs per year.

### CLINICAL FEATURES

Daytime symptoms include EDS, fatigue, morning headaches, poor concentration, reduced libido, personality changes, depression, and/or insomnia. Nocturnal symptoms include restlessness, snoring, witnessed apneas, nocturnal choking, nocturia, diaphoresis, reflux symptoms, dry mouth, drooling, and/or bed partner sleep disruption.

- Stratification of patients with suspected sleep apnea may be based on the following four symptoms: habitual snoring, excessive daytime somnolence, a body mass index (BMI) $>35 \, kg/m^2$, and observed/witnessed apneas. Each of these factors by itself has low sensitivity. On the other hand, patients with all 4 of the above symptoms may be placed in a high-risk group, and have an approximately 70% likelihood of having an apnea–hypopnea index $> 10$ events/hour.
- Other risk factors include male gender, postmenopausal women, age, race, obesity (BMI$=28$–$35 \, kg/m^2$), and craniofacial abnormalities. Figure 15.1 provides a reasonable symptom-based algorithm of polysomnography (PSG)-related decision making in the setting of suspected SDB.

Indications for PSG for SDB based on symptom presentation are shown in Fig 15.1.

### Snoring

This is strongly associated with SDB; this correlation is more pronounced in men than women. Snoring is also the most frequent symptom of sleep apnea, occurring in 70–95% of patients, but because it is so common in the general population, it is a poor predictor of sleep apnea. A study has shown that the absence of snoring makes SDB unlikely since only 6% of patients with SDB do not report snoring.

- Nearly all levels of snoring frequency were associated with a greater likelihood of sleep apnea, with

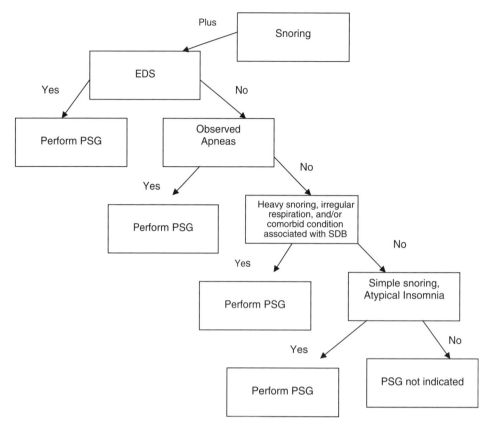

**Figure 15.1** PSD indications for SDB. (*Adapted from Chesson A, et al. Practice Parameters for the Indications for Polysomnography and Related Procedures, 1997.*)

sensitivities approximating 90% in men and specificities approximating 90% in women.

- Associations between snoring and sleep apnea are generally independent of age and sex.
- Parental-report questionnaires of children's snoring and other sleep and wake behaviors can be used as surrogate predictors of snoring or sleep-disordered breathing in children. In one study of preschool children and those between 5 and 7 years of age, parental report of frequent snoring was highly sensitive and specific in both age groups.
- Among older adults, men with SDB have two-fold higher odds of snoring compared to those without SDB even after adjustment for potential confounders; this association between snoring and SBD is likely attenuated compared to the middle-aged population.

### Witnessed Apneas

Witnessed or observed apneas are a common reason for referral to the sleep clinic. The patient may report waking up with acute panic and choking. Episodes usually only last for a few seconds but can cause considerable distress.

- Bed partners, however, often do not provide a reliable account of apneas during sleep, and even

trained medical staffs are suboptimal when diagnosing respiratory events in patients with SDB through clinical observation.

- Gender-related reporting bias may occur, as female patients with SDB are less likely to report nocturnal apneas.
- These events should be differentiated from other causes of nocturnal breathlessness such as paroxysmal nocturnal dyspnea in the patient with congestive heart failure, panic disorder, sleep-related asthma, sleep-related laryngospasm, and sleep-related choking syndrome.

### Excessive Daytime Sleepiness

Excessive daytime sleepiness is caused by fragmented sleep related to frequent arousals. Like snoring, sleepiness is common and by itself a poor discriminator, and 30–50% of the general population without sleep apnea report moderate to severe sleepiness.

- It is important to attempt to differentiate sleepiness (the urge or pressure to fall sleep) from reports of fatigue, lethargy, malaise, or exhaustion. Patients themselves may underreport their sleepiness, either because they are not aware of it or because there are social pressures to deny that it is a problem.

- Other common causes of EDS, such as insufficient sleep, poor sleep hygiene, drugs, shift work, should always be asked about in the history.
- Similar to snoring, the association between sleepiness and SDB in the elderly appears to be attenuated but present.

## PHYSICAL EXAMINATION

The physical examination of an individual with SDB may be normal. Specific physical examination findings in the setting of SDB may include obesity (BMI $>30\,kg/m^2$), neck circumference $> 40\,cm$, deviated nasal septum, narrow maxilla, narrow mandible, dental overjet/retrognathia, micrognathia, crossbite/dental malocclusion, high and narrow hard palate, elongated/low-lying uvula, prominent tonsillar pillars and, macroglossia.

## CLINICAL PREDICTION RULES

Several tools and symptom score clinical prediction rules have been developed to better identify those individuals with a high pretest probability of SDB prior to further evaluation with diagnostic PSG. A recent study examined four clinical prediction rules; however, sensitivities of these rules ranged from 33–39% and specificities ranged from 87–93% and are therefore not sufficiently accurate to discriminate between patients with and without SDB. Clinical prediction rules may be useful in prioritizing patients for split-night PSG.

- The Berlin questionnaire is a survey tool that has demonstrated efficacy in the setting of SDB. Survey items address the presence and frequency of snoring behavior, sleepiness or fatigue, and history of obesity or hypertension. Patients with persistent and frequent symptoms in any two of these three domains are considered to be at high risk for sleep apnea.
- Several tools are available for measuring sleepiness both subjectively and objectively. There is no gold standard, but the easiest and most practical is the Epworth Sleepiness Scale (ESS). The major advantages of the ESS are that it is simple, quick, inexpensive, and has high test–retest reliability. Drawbacks include poor correlation with the severity of sleep apnea and the disadvantages that accompany any self-evaluated test such as misperception of sleep episodes. Input from the bed partner can be useful.

## POLYSOMNOGRAPHY

Attended full-channel PSG is considered the standard assessment for SDB. A full night-attended PSG is indicated for the diagnosis of SDB in the context of appropriate symptoms/comorbid factors.

- Electroencephalography (EEG), electro-oculography (EOG), electromyography (EMG) of muscle tone

(these first three variables required to allow stage of sleep to be determined), respiratory airflow, respiratory effort, arterial oxygen saturation, snoring intensity, electrocardiogram, and EMG of the anterior tibialis muscles are continuously monitored.

- The respiratory parameters provide useful information not only in the setting of uncomplicated SDB, but also track sleep-related problems in patients with underlying lung disease such as obstructive airway diseases (asthma, chronic obstructive airway disease), restrictive airway disease, pulmonary vascular disease, and congestive heart failure. Such respiratory measurements include monitoring of airflow, snoring, respiratory muscle activity, oxygenation and, at times, carbon dioxide levels.

### Positive Pressure Therapy Titration

Polysomnography is also recommended for positive pressure titration [i.e., continuous positive airway pressure (CPAP), or bilevel positive airway pressure (BPAP)] in order to determine the optimal therapeutic pressure. Full-night PSG with titration is indicated in patients with documented diagnosis of SDB for which therapy is indicated.

- Polysomnography with titration is recommended for the following: (a) apnea index (AI) at least 20 per hour or AHI greater than 30 per hour irrespective of the patient's symptoms; (b) AHI of at least 5 per hour in a patient with excessive daytime somnolence.
- More recent guidelines have also suggested that comorbidity such as hypertension, diabetes mellitus, stroke, and cardiovascular disease should also warrant treatment with positive pressure therapy, and therefore titration study in the setting of diagnosed SDB.
- An optimal titration study is defined as the presence of sufficient sleep time to determine the optimal pressure, normalization of the AHI, adequate rapid eye movement (REM)–supine time during the optimal pressure setting, elimination of audible snoring, and normal oxygen saturation levels (greater than 90%). In the case of respiratory arousals suggesting UARS, reduction of respiratory arousals and crescendo snore arousals should be documented.

### Split-Night Polysomnography

A split-night study involves an initial diagnostic PSG followed by positive pressure titration during PSG during the same study. This is a viable alternative to one full night of PSG followed by a second full night of titration.

- A split-night study may be performed if the following four criteria are met: (a) AHI of at least 40 per hour is documented during a minimum of 2 h of diagnostic PSG; it may also be considered if the AHI is 20–40 per hour in the context of clinical judgment such as for long events or severe oxygen desaturation; (b) positive pressure therapy titration is carried out for more than 3 h; (c) PSG documents that positive pressure titration eliminates or nearly eliminates respiratory events during REM and non-REM sleep, including REM sleep in the supine position; and (d) a second full-night study with positive pressure therapy titration is performed if the titration during the split-night study is less than 3 h or if there was no resolution or near-resolution of events during REM and REM-supine sleep.

### Multiple Studies

Sleep position, acclimatization to a foreign sleep environment, concurrent respiratory tract infections, and variable alcohol and drug use are thought to be responsible for night-to-night variability in both respiratory and sleep parameters.

- In patients with moderate to severe SDB, the reproducibility of the respiratory parameters from night to night is good. For milder SDB a single negative study may not exclude SDB, and a second study should be considered.

### Polysomnography Prior to Upper Airway Surgery

A preoperative clinical evaluation including PSG is routinely indicated to evaluate for the presence of SDB prior to upper airway surgery. This also provides a preoperative baseline for the patient to allow comparison to postoperative PSG that is prompted by recurrence of symptoms.

### Follow-up Polysomnography

Follow-up PSG is recommended after good response to oral appliance treatment in patients with moderate to severe SDB to ensure therapeutic benefit, after surgical treatment in patients with moderate to severe SDB to ensure satisfactory response, after surgical treatment of patients with SDB whose symptoms return despite initial success of treatment, after substantial weight loss or gain, and when clinical response is insufficient.

- Follow-up PSG is not recommended or routinely indicated for patients treated with positive pressure therapy whose symptoms continue to be resolved with treatment.

### EVALUATION OF SLEEP-DISORDERED BREATHING

Polysomnography involves the recording of multiple physiologic parameters during sleep. The following PSG channels are used to assess respiratory variables.

### Airflow Monitoring

Most airflow sensors detect apneas reliably, but the detection and quantification of decreased flow needed to diagnose a hypopnea depends on the type of sensor used. Hypopneas make up the majority of obstructive respiratory events and measurements, therefore, need to be reliable.

### Pneumotachometer

This method of airflow monitoring provides a direct quantitative measurement of airflow or tidal volume. This requires connection to a sealed mask placed over the nose or mouth. It is considered the reference standard for obstructive apnea and hypopnea detection.

- Pneumotachometers measure the flow rates of gases during breathing. The breath is passed through a short tube in which there is a fine mesh, which presents a small resistance to the flow. Flow ($V'$) is derived from the pressure difference over a small, fixed resistance, offered by a fine metal mesh. The pressure drop across the resistance relates linearly to flow at relatively low flows, when the flow pattern is laminar. Higher flows give rise to a turbulent flow pattern, where the pressure drop across the resistance changes proportionally greater with flow. Accurate measurements are best performed when the flow pattern is laminar, with flow linearly related to the pressure drop.

### Intranasal Pressure Transducer

This provides an indirect measurement of airflow by detecting pressure changes; it has an excellent response-to-airflow profile, and is capable of detecting airflow limitation. Changing pressures require a transducer that can respond to rapid changes. Nasal pressure transducers provide a significantly more sensitive measure of airflow than temperature-based transducers; pressure transducers may provide a measure of upper airway resistance as inspiration and expiration provide transducer signal fluctuations similar to airflow.

- The new transducers provide additional information for scoring hypopneas. If used for evaluation of sleep-related breathing disorders, the new level of sensitivity may lead to scoring of many more events than are typically scored with other methods of airflow detection (e.g., temperature-based devices). Nasal pressure sensors connected to the nose via nasal prongs are more accurate than thermo elements in detecting hypopneas.
- Nasal pressure monitoring is not recommended for patients who are predominantly mouth breathers or have nasal obstruction in which airflow may be underestimated. Mouth breathing can affect the measurement, but pure mouth breathing is uncommon. Nasal pressure is falsely increased in the presence of nasal obstruction, and there is a nonlinear relation between nasal pressure and nasal flow. Square root linearization of nasal pressure greatly increases the accuracy for quantifying hypopneas and detecting flow limitation.

- The American Academy of Sleep Medicine (AASM) recommends nasal pressure transducer (with or without square root transformation) as the airflow sensor for the detection of hypopnea.

### Nasal Thermocouple/Thermistor

This provides an indirect semiquantitative assessment of airflow that detects the relatively higher temperature of expired air compared to inspired ambient air. It is the recommended sensor to detecting apneas.

- Thermocouples consist of two different metal wires welded together at one end, which generate a thermoelectric voltage that changes according to the temperature difference between the two ends.
- Thermistors consist of a semiconductor material that exhibits a large change in resistance in proportion to a small change in temperature. Compared to thermocouples, thermistors have a more limited temperature range, but are highly sensitive within this range.
- Thermal sensors are nonlinearly related to airflow, generally overestimating ventilation compared to pneumotachography. Therefore, they cannot reliably detect hypopneas. Furthermore, their accuracy varies greatly depending on the position of the sensors, sleep position of the patient, presence of nasal obstruction, and type of thermoelement used.

### Respiratory Inductance Plethysmography

This provides an accepted semi-quantitative measure of ventilation that is assessed by changes in thoracic and abdominal pressures.

- Respiratory inductance plethysmography (RIP) is based upon the two-compartment model of thoracoabdominal movement during respiration. Transducers are placed at the level of the nipples and umbilicus to monitor their cross-sectional diameters reflected as variations in inductance, or resistance to change in flow of the transducers.
- Respiratory inductance plethysmography detects changes in the diameter of the chest and abdomen during inspiration and expiration and, when properly calibrated, the sum of the two signals can provide an estimate of tidal volume during sleep. An accurate initial calibration is needed to assure valid measurements. Measurement inaccuracies may occur due to displacement of transducer bands or to changes in sleep position. Calibration may be difficult to maintain throughout the night.

### Snore Monitoring

The snore microphone is used to detect snoring during PSG; it provides an output signal with easily identifiable waveforms. This tracing, in conjunction with sleep technician comments, may assist in the diagnosis of primary snoring. In addition, it is used during positive pressure titration to help determine the optimal pressure setting.

### Respiratory Muscle Monitoring

This provides an indirect measurement of respiratory effort via electrodes placed on the chest wall. However, it is not ideal for detecting respiratory event-related arousals (RERA) or central respiratory events; reliable recordings are difficult to obtain, it is prone to artifacts (e.g., electrocardiography and nonrespiratory muscle electromyography), and there are no data on its accuracy, reliability, or correlation with long-term outcomes.

### Esophageal Manometry

This is the reference standard for measuring respiratory efforts during PSG. Respiratory efforts are associated with changes in pleural pressure that can be accurately measured using esophageal manometry. This method is useful in distinguishing central versus obstructive apneas, and for detecting RERAs (i.e., increasingly more negative esophageal pressures immediately preceding an arousal, following which the esophageal pressure rapidly returns to normal levels).

### Piezoelectric Sensors, Strain Gauges, and Magnetometers

Other methods that can be used to assess airflow include piezoelectric sensors, strain gauges and magnetometers. Piezoelectric sensors may measure qualitative changes in airflow but are not reliable in distinguishing central from obstructive respiratory events.

### Pulse Oximetry Monitoring

The fundamental physical property that allows the measurement of arterial oxygen saturation is that the color of blood changes with the degree of its saturation. Hemoglobin, in its reduced form or oxygenated state absorbs light at wavelengths below approximately 630 nm, whereas hemoglobin absorbs more light near infrared region (810–1000 nm) when it is desaturated.

- Pulse oximeters usually are designed with two light-emitting diodes: one designed to emit light in the red region (∼660 mn) and the other in the near-infrared region (∼925 or 940 nm). In order to measure absorption of arterial blood only, without interference from venous blood, skin, and bone, and to minimize scatter effect, a differential absorption is calculated by dividing the small change in intensity by the total intensity of the output light.
- Chromophores other than oxyhemoglobin and reduced hemoglobin, such as carboxyhemoglobin and methemoglobin, may cause falsely elevated readings. Oximeters may be prone to artifact during states of poor perfusion, excessive patient motion (particularly at the probe site), and electrical noise, and also may be affected by changes in heart rate and circulation time. Overall, pulse oximetry is easy

to use, inexpensive, readily available, noninvasive, and permits continuous monitoring of oxygen saturation. Pulse oximetry sensitivity is improved with shorter sampling intervals, and minimal filtering in order to achieve the most rapid response.

## Carbon Dioxide Monitoring

This works by drawing a stream of air from the nose or mouth into a chamber in which light is shone through the air. The degree of absorption at a specific frequency of infrared light is proportional to the concentration of carbon dioxide ($CO_2$).

- Values for $CO_2$ are near or at zero at the start of inspiration, rise abruptly until the end of expiration when there is a plateau in the $CO_2$ level. The end-expiratory value is correlated with arterial $PaCO_2$ provided that there is complete gas emptying to functional residual capacity, and minimal ventilation–perfusion mismatch.

- End-tidal $CO_2$ monitoring may help identify hypoventilation in obesity hypoventilation syndrome, as well as in chronic obstructive pulmonary disease, congestive heart failure, and neurologic diseases that produce neuromuscular weakness. In addition, end-tidal $CO_2$ values can be helpful in assessing disorders of chronic hyperventilation, distinguishing pathophysiologic from psychogenic causes by the persistence or resolution of hypocapnia, respectively, during sleep.

- In general, end-tidal $CO_2$ monitoring tends to underestimate $PaCO_2$ values. Studies have demonstrated that the difference between arterial $CO_2$ measurements and end-tidal $CO_2$ values were $<5$ mm Hg in 50% of the time and $<10$ mm Hg in 80% of the time.

- A limitation of end-tidal $CO_2$ monitoring is the inability to measure levels in the setting of CPAP or bilevel pressure therapy to assess response to treatment.

- Capnography (breath-by-breath $CO_2$ measurement) may detect the absence of expiratory airflow and signal an apnea. Although there are no established criteria, an apneic event is commonly considered to be present when there is a failure of end-expiratory $CO_2$ to fall after expiration with a subsequent decline in $CO_2$ over the subsequent 10 s to values at or near zero. The end of the apneic episodes is suggested by a rapid rise in $CO_2$ with expiration. The duration of an event is defined from the peak of the preceding $CO_2$ rise to the peak of the next $CO_2$ rise.

- A cardiac oscillation in the capnography signal may indicate a patent airway during a central apneic event, but there can be expiratory puffs after an obstructed inspiratory effort.

- Capnography can also be used to identify obstructive hypopneas (i.e., persistent efforts characterized by asynchronous movements of the ribcage and abdomen with a rising end-tidal $CO_2$).

## Transcutaneous $CO_2$ Monitoring

There are two methods that may be employed for transcutaneous $CO_2$ monitoring. The first uses a silver electrode that measures $CO_2$, which had diffused from the skin through a gas-permeable membrane into a solution (response time less than 1 min); the other uses an infrared capnometer that analyzes $CO_2$ in the gas phase (response time more than 2 min). Neither end-tidal nor transcutaneous monitoring of $CO_2$ is an accurate reflection of $CO_2$ levels and are not used routinely during PSG. Transcutaneous $CO_2$ values tend to overestimate arterial $CO_2$ values, particularly in the setting of hypercapnia.

## CLASSIFICATION OF RESPIRATORY EVENTS

*Obstructive apnea* is defined as a drop in peak thermal sensor excursion by $\geq 90\%$ of baseline values, lasting at least 10 s, with at least 90% of the event's duration meeting the amplitude reduction criteria for apnea, associated with continued or increased inspiratory effort throughout the entire period of absent airflow. Event duration is measured from the nadir preceding the first breath that approximates the breathing amplitude. When baseline breathing amplitude cannot be easily determined, the termination of an event is defined by a clear and sustained increase in breathing amplitude or, an event-associated resaturation of at least 2% is observed, if there is an accompanying desaturation. The identification of an obstructive apnea does not require a minimum desaturation criterion.

*Central apnea* is defined as a drop in peak thermal sensor excursion by $\geq 90\%$ of baseline values, lasting at least 10 s, with at least 90% of the event's duration meeting the amplitude reduction criteria for apnea, associated with no inspiratory efforts throughout the entire period of absent airflow. Event duration is measured from the nadir preceding the first breath that approximates the breathing amplitude. When baseline breathing amplitude cannot be easily determined, the termination of an event is defined by a clear and sustained increase in breathing amplitude or, an event-associated resaturation of at least 2% is observed, if there is an accompanying desaturation. The identification of a central apnea does not require a minimum desaturation criterion.

*Mixed apnea* is defined as a drop in peak thermal sensor excursion by $\geq 90\%$ of baseline values, lasting at least 10 s, with at least 90% of the event's duration meeting the amplitude reduction criteria for apnea, associated with absent inspiratory effort during the initial portion of the respiratory event followed by resumption of inspiratory effort during the latter part of the event. Event duration is measured from the nadir preceding the first breath that approximates the breathing amplitude. When baseline breathing amplitude cannot be easily determined, the termination of an event is defined by a clear and sustained increase in breathing amplitude or, an event-associated resaturation of at least 2% is observed, if there is an accompanying desaturation. The identification of a mixed apnea does not require a minimum desaturation criterion.

*Hypopnea* is a drop of $\geq 30\%$ of the nasal pressure signal compared to baseline values, lasting at least 10 s, accompanied by a $>4\%$ oxygen desaturation from pre-event baseline and at least 90% of the event's duration meeting the amplitude criteria for hypopnea. An alternative definition is a drop of $\geq 50\%$ of the nasal pressure signal compared to baseline values, lasting at least 10 s, accompanied by a $\geq 3\%$ oxygen desaturation from pre-event baseline (or associated with an arousal), and at least 90% of the event's duration meeting the amplitude criteria for hypopnea.

*Respiratory-effort related arousal* is scored when there is a sequence of breaths lasting for at least 10 s characterized by increasing respiratory effort or flattening of the nasal pressure waveform leading to an arousal from sleep. The sequence of breaths does not meet criteria for an apnea or hypopnea.

*Cheyne–Stokes respiration* consists of at least three consecutive cycles of cyclical crescendo and decrescendo change in breathing amplitude, and at least one of the following: five or more central apneas or hypopneas/hour of sleep; or cyclic crescendo–decrescendo change in breathing amplitude has a duration of at least 10 consecutive minutes.

*Sleep-related hypoventilation* is defined as $\geq 10$ mm Hg increase in $PaCO_2$ during sleep in comparison to waking supine values.

## THERAPY OF SLEEP-DISORDERED BREATHING

### Lifestyle Modification Strategies

Optimal weight management, with diet, exercise, and, in appropriate cases, bariatric surgery, is important for patients with excess weight. Patients in whom SDB occurs either exclusively or predominantly in a supine sleep position should be counseled regarding positional therapy. Avoidance of sleep in a supine position can be accomplished using a wedge or cushion, or sewing a pocket filled with tennis balls on the back of a pajama's shirt.

- Individuals with SDB should also be advised to avoid substances that may reduce upper airway muscle tone, such as alcohol, sedatives, narcotics, and muscle relaxants. Drowsy driving precautions should be reviewed and documented.

### Positive Airway Pressure Therapy

This is the standard treatment for SDB. It acts by splinting all aspects of the airway; in contrast, oral appliances or upper airway surgery only address a limited aspect of the upper airway anatomy. A titration study is performed to determine the optimal pressure setting that reduces the number of apneas/hypopneas during sleep; improves hypoxia and sleep architecture; and reduces arousals.

### Oral Appliance Therapy

Oral appliances are typically reserved for mild SDB or as an adjunct in the treatment of moderate to severe SDB.

### Upper Airway Surgery

Upper airway or craniofacial surgical interventions may be an option for SDB treatment; however, they require careful assessment and evaluation, including a nasopharyngoscopic examination, by an experienced otolaryngologist. Outcomes are often suboptimal; the reported efficacy of uvulopalatopharyngoplasty is about 40.7%. Procedures, such as the Somnoplasty®, radiofrequency ablation, laser assisted uvulopalatoplasty, and palatal implants, can improve snoring but there is either no or minimal data to support their use for SDB.

## KEY POINTS

1. Sleep-disordered breathing is estimated to occur in 1 of 20 adults and remains underrecognized and underdiagnosed. With the increasing prevalence of obesity in the general population, the public health impact of SDB is becoming increasingly evident.

2. Although symptoms of habitual snoring, excessive daytime somnolence, obesity [defined as body mass index (BMI) $\geq 35$ kg/m$^2$], and witnessed apneas, when considered individually, have a low sensitivity and specificity for SDB, the presence of more than one factor increases the likelihood of the disorder.

3. Recurrent episodes of intermittent hypoxia, episodic arousals accompanied by sympathetic nervous system activation, and altered baroreflex control are likely physiologic contributors to cardiovascular morbidity associated with SDB.

4. The oronasal thermal sensor is the recommended sensor for detecting apneas, whereas the nasal pressure transducer is the sensor of choice for the detection of hypopneas.

5. Therapy of SDB includes lifestyle modification through exercise, optimal weight management, and the avoidance of substances that can potentially reduce upper airway muscle tone and, thereby, worsen SDB. Nasal positive airway pressure remains the gold standard of SDB treatment. Other treatment options include the use of oral devices and upper airway surgery.

## BIBLIOGRAPHY

American Academy of Medicine Task Force. Sleep-related breathing disorders in adults: Recommendations for syndrome definition and measurement techniques in clinical research. The Report of an American Academy of Sleep Medicine Task Force. *Sleep* 1999; 22:667–689.

Ayappa I, et al. Relative occurrence of flow limitation and snoring during continuous positive airway pressure titration. *Chest* 1998; 114:685–690.

Ayappa I, et al. Non-invasive detection of respiratory effort-related arousals (REras) by a nasal cannula/pressure transducer system. *Sleep* 2000; 23:763–771.

Ballester E, et al. Nasal prongs in the detection of sleep-related disordered breathing in the sleep apnoea/hypopnoea syndrome. *Eur Respir J* 1998; 11:880–883.

Chesson AL, et al. The indications for polysomnography and related procedures. *Sleep* 1997; 20:423–487.

Duran J, et al. Obstructive sleep apnea-hypopnea and related clinical features in a population-based sample of subjects aged 30 to 70 yr. *Am J Respir Crit Care Med* 2001; 163:685–689.

Farre R, et al. Accuracy of thermistors and thermocouples as flow-measuring devices for detecting hypopnoeas. *Eur Respir J* 1998; 11:179–182.

Hoekema A, et al. Efficacy and co-morbidity of oral appliances in the treatment of obstructive sleep apnea-hypopnea: A systematic review. *Crit Rev Oral Biol Med* 2004; 15:137.

Hosselet JJ, et al. Detection of flow limitation with a nasal cannula/pressure transducer system. *Am J Respir Crit Care Med* 1998; 157:1461–1467.

Iber C, et al. *The AASM Manual for the Scoring of Sleep and Associated Events: Rules, Terminology and Technical Specifications*, 1st ed. American Academy of Sleep Medicine, Westchester, I, 2007.

Kapur V, et al. The medical cost of undiagnosed sleep apnea. *Sleep* 1999; 22:749–755.

Le Bon O, et al. Mild to moderate sleep respiratory events: One negative night may not be enough. *Chest* 2000; 118:353–359.

Littner M. Polysomnography in the diagnosis of the obstructive sleep apnea-hypopnea syndrome: Where do we draw the line? *Chest* 2000; 118:286–288.

Mehra R, et al. Prevalence and correlates of sleep-disordered breathing in older men: Osteoporotic fractures in men sleep study. *J Am Geriatr Soc* 2007; 55:1356–1364.

Montgomery-Downs HE, et al. Snoring and sleep-disordered breathing in young children: Subjective and objective correlates. *Sleep* 2004; 27(1):87–94.

Netzer NC, et al. Using the Berlin Questionnaire to identify patients at risk for the sleep apnea syndrome. *Ann Intern Med* 1999; 131:485–491.

Pazos G, et al. Complications of radiofrequency ablation in the treatment of sleep-disordered breathing. *Otolaryngol Head Neck Surg* 2001; 125:462.

Peppard PE, et al. Longitudinal study of moderate weight change and sleep-disordered breathing. *JAMA* 2000; 284:3015–3021.

Phillips BA, et al. Monitoring sleep and breathing: Methodology. Part I: Monitoring breathing. *Clin Chest Med* 1998;19:203–212.

Polysomnography Task Force, American Sleep Disorders Association Standards of Practice Committee. Practice parameters for the indications for polysomnography and related procedures. *Sleep* 1997; 20:406–422.

Powell NB, et al. Radiofrequency volumetric tissue reduction of the palate in subjects with sleep-disordered breathing. *Chest* 1998; 113:1163–1174.

Redline S, et al. Effects of varying approaches for identifying respiratory disturbances on sleep apnea assessment. *Am J Respir Crit Care Med* 2000; 161:369–374.

Redline S, et al. The scoring of respiratory events in sleep: Reliability and validity. *J Clin Sleep Med* 2007; 3:169–200.

Rodenstein DO. Sleep apnoea syndrome: The health economics point of view. *Monaldi Arch Chest Dis* 2000; 55:404–410.

Rosner V, et al. Validity of transcutaneous oxygen/carbon dioxide pressure measurement in the monitoring of mechanical ventilation in stable chronic respiratory failure. *Eur Respir J* 1999; 13:1044–1047.

Rowley JA, et al. The use of clinical prediction formulas in the evaluation of obstructive sleep apnea. *Sleep* 2000; 23:929–938.

Series F, et al. Nasal pressure recording in the diagnosis of sleep apnoea hypopnoea syndrome. *Thorax* 1999; 54:506–510.

Terris DJ, et al. Occult mucosal injuries with radiofrequency ablation of the palate. *Otolaryngol Head Neck Surg* 2001; 125:468.

Thurnheer R, et al. Accuracy of nasal cannula pressure recordings for assessment of ventilation during sleep. *Am J Respir Crit Care Med* 2001; 164:1914–1919.

Whyte KF, et al. Clinical features of the sleep apnoea/hypopnoea syndrome. *Q J Med* 1989; 72:659–666.

# 16

## CENTRAL SLEEP APNEA

Shahrokh Javaheri

University of Cincinnati, College of Medicine, Cincinnati, Ohio, and Sleepcare Diagnostics, Mason, Ohio

### INTRODUCTION

Central apnea is due to a temporary failure in breathing rhythm generation resulting in the loss of ventilatory effort, lasting at least 10 s. During a central apnea, there is no medullary inspiratory neural output to the diaphragm and other inspiratory thoracic pump muscles. Therefore, central apnea is characterized polysomnographically by the absence of oronasal airflow and thoracoabdominal excursions.

- Central apnea could be due to a number of physiologic conditions and pathologic disorders. In part because central apneas may occur in normal individuals (i.e., physiologic central apnea), the minimum number of events required during sleep to represent a distinct pathologic disorder is not clear. More importantly, this issue is further compounded by: (a) difficulty in accurately distinguishing central hypopneas from obstructive hypopneas; the former which should be added to the number of central apneas and reported as a central apnea–hypopnea index; and (b) co-occurrence of that central and obstructive hypopneas, which like central and obstructive apneas, commonly present together in the same subject.

- The minimum central apnea–hypopnea index required to define the presence of a "clinically significant" sleep-related breathing disorder is not clear. Some researchers have arbitrarily employed an apnea–hypopnea index of 15 per hour or greater, but this may not be the appropriate threshold.

- Despite the varied causes of central apnea, a unified concept that explains the pathogenesis of central apnea during sleep in most (but not all) conditions has been described; this relates to the profound effect of sleep on control of breathing, the concept of an apneic threshold, the proximity of the prevailing (eupneic) $PCO_2$ to the apneic threshold $PCO_2$, and the increased $CO_2$ sensitivity below eupnea.

### CONTROL OF BREATHING

Three distinct control systems influence breathing; these include automatic/metabolic control of breathing, behavioral control of breathing, and the wakefulness drive to breathe.

- The automatic/metabolic control system reflects both the underlying automaticity of the breathing rhythm and its coupling to the metabolic rate. The various components of this system include the pontomedullary respiratory centers (a central pacemaker, presumably located in the pre-Botzinger complex and dorsal and ventral respiratory groups), and a number of receptors [peripheral arterial chemoreceptors (i.e., the carotid bodies located between internal and external carotid arteries), and the medullary central chemoreceptors] whose activities are regulated by a variety of physiologic variables, specifically $PO_2$ and $PCO_2/H^+$. This complex system is responsible for the act of breathing at all times, and for maintaining arterial $PO_2$ and $[H^+]$ relatively constant by coupling alveolar ventilation to metabolic rate (metabolic control). Any disturbance in breathing that changes $PO_2$, $PCO_2$, or $[H^+]$ will alter the activity of the system in such a way that the initial disturbance is minimized (i.e., a negative feedback system). Under normal circumstances, $PCO_2$ is the most important variable controlling breathing, and any small change in $PCO_2$ invariably affects ventilation.

- The behavioral control of breathing is best exemplified by circumstances when the respiratory system is used for nonrespiratory functions, such as talking, swallowing, or laughing.

- Wakefulness also influences breathing (wakefulness drive), and this is mediated through the ascending reticular activating system, located in the brainstem, as part of the brain arousal system, which consists of multiple neural aggregtes. However, the wakefulness drive to breathe along with the behavioral control are absent during sleep and, therefore, breathing becomes under the metabolic control system. This switch is critical because metabolic control system is sensitive to small changes in $PCO_2$, and sleep unmasks a very $PCO_2$-sensitive apneic threshold.

## APNEIC THRESHOLD AND THE GENESIS OF CENTRAL APNEA DURING SLEEP

The mechanisms involved in the genesis of central apnea relate specifically to the state of sleep and removal of the wakefulness drive on breathing. This unmasks the apneic threshold $PCO_2$, a $PCO_2$ level below which rhythmic breathing ceases resulting in central apneas.

- Normally, with onset of sleep, ventilation decreases and $PCO_2$ rises by a few mm Hg. If the spontaneous prevailing $PCO_2$, referred to as the eupneic $PCO_2$, decreases below the apneic threshold $PCO_2$, breathing ceases and central apnea occurs. As a result of central apnea, $PCO_2$ rises; breathing resumes after $PCO_2$ once again exceeds the apneic threshold. Therefore, the difference between the two $PCO_2$ set points, the $PCO_2$ at the apneic threshold minus the prevailing $PCO_2$, is a critical factor for the development of central apnea—the less this difference, the greater the likelihood of the occurrence of central apnea because small increases in ventilation could lower the prevailing $PCO_2$ below the apneic threshold. Conversely, when the apneic threshold $PCO_2$ is further from the eupneic $PCO_2$, large ventilatory changes are necessary to lower the $PCO_2$ below the apneic threshold $PCO_2$, and the likelihood of developing central apnea decreases. It must be emphasized that what is important in the genesis of central apnea, is the difference between the two $PCO_2$ set points, rather than the actual value of the prevailing $PCO_2$.

- Central apnea is precipitated by sleep because of an unmasking of the apneic threshold. It is rare to observe central apnea during wakefulness, independent of $PCO_2$ level. When central apnea occurs during "wakefulness," it is usually at a time when the patient is very relaxed and almost dozing. If such patients were being monitored electroencephalographically, slowing of brain waves are commonly observed when central apnea occurs. Central apnea is then followed by hyperpnea resulting in a shift in the frequency of brain waves.

## CLASSIFICATION OF CENTRAL SLEEP APNEA

| | |
|---|---|
| Physiologic central sleep apnea | At sleep onset |
| | Postarousal or postsigh |
| | During phasic rapid eye movement (REM) sleep |
| Eupneic–hypopcapnic (nonhypercapnic) central sleep apnea | Systolic heart failure |
| | Idiopathic central sleep apnea |
| | Idiopathic pulmonary arterial hypertension |
| | High altitude |
| | Cerebrovascular disorders |
| Hypercapnic central sleep apnea | Alveolar hypoventilation with normal pulmonary function |
| | Neuromuscular disorders |
| | Opioids (awake $PCO_2$ could be normal) |
| Central sleep apnea associated with endocrine disorders | Acromegaly |
| | Hypothyroidism |
| Central sleep apnea associated with obstructive sleep apnea | Minor component of obstructive sleep apnea |
| | With positive airway pressure therapy of obstructive sleep apnea/ posttracheostomy |
| | Postuvulopalatopharyngoplasty |
| Central sleep apnea associated with upper airway disorders | |

## PHYSIOLOGIC CENTRAL APNEA

The conditions causing or associated with central sleep apnea in this category are considered normal sleep phenomena. Not surprisingly, the frequency of occurrence of such central apneas is normally minimal. Such central apneas can occur with onset of sleep, after an arousal or a sigh, and occasionally during phasic REM sleep.

### Sleep-Onset Central Apnea

With removal of the wakefulness drive and onset of sleep, the $CO_2$-sensitive apneic threshold is exposed, and a higher than awake $PCO_2$ level is necessary to maintain rhythmic breathing. This is because the apneic threshold $PCO_2$ is normally close to the level of awake $PCO_2$. Consequently, with sleep onset, few central apneas (sleep-onset central apneas) occur, and, along with a decrease in ventilation, $PCO_2$ rises. When $PCO_2$ is above the apneic threshold, rhythmic breathing, at a ventilation less than that during wakefulness, is maintained.

### Postarousal/Postsigh Central Apnea

During an arousal, the prevailing sleeping $PCO_2$ (which is higher than awake $PCO_2$) is considered hypercapnic for the wake brain; therefore, ventilation rises and $PCO_2$ decreases (negative feedback system). When the arousal is over and sleep resumes, the prevailing $PCO_2$ is considered hypocapnic for the sleeping brain. Therefore, central apneas occur, as they do with sleep onset. Similarly, after a sigh, even without an arousal, central apnea occurs if $PCO_2$ decreases below the apneic threshold.

### Phasic REM Sleep

One of the unique features of phasic REM sleep is the variability in breathing pattern. The source of the variability does not depend on variations in chemoreceptor activity. These variations are intermittent and in animal studies are associated with ponto–geniculo–occipital (PGO) waves influencing medullary respiratory centers.

- Irregular breathing and sometimes central and obstructive apneas are commonly observed in humans during phasic REM sleep. These events most probably have to do with ponto-medullary electrophysiologic activity that occurs during phasic REM sleep. Central apneas occur with total inhibition of rhythmic breathing. On the other hand, obstructive apneas occur when there is a predominant inhibition of inspiratory drive to the muscles of the upper airway with relative preservation of diaphragmatic inspiratory activity. An arousal, characterized by appearance of $\alpha$ waves and an increase in chin electromyogram (EMG) commonly occur following these events, but is soon followed by sleep.

## EUPNEIC–HYPOCAPNIC (NONHYPERCAPNIC) CENTRAL SLEEP APNEA

These disorders are generally characterized by both an awake steady-state $PaCO_2$ that is either within or less than normal value ($<36$ mm Hg) and an increased ventilatory response to changes in $PCO_2$ and perhaps also to $PO_2$.

- During sleep, the prevailing $PCO_2$ may fall below the apneic threshold (resulting in a central apnea), either because of an inability to increase $PCO_2$ or because the apneic threshold $PCO_2$ rises (e.g., due to hypoxemia), or a combination of the two factors.
- Ventilatory response to $PCO_2$ below eupnea, if increased, it increases the likelihood of developing central apnea during sleep. This is an important mechanism mediating central sleep apnea in patients with systolic heart failure.
- The hypercapnic ventilatory response (above eupnea) if increased, it will increase the likelihood of developing central apneas. This is because anytime an arousal occurs, the immediate prearousal $PCO_2$ becomes hypercapnic for the aroused brain, and therefore, intense hyperventilation occurs that could drive the prevailing $PCO_2$ below apneic threshold, and subsequently causing a central apnea as sleep is resumed. Following a central apnea, $PCO_2$ increases until an arousal recurs. In this way, the cycle of apnea–hyperpnea is perpetuated. The disorders in this category are discussed below.

### Systolic Heart Failure

Heart failure is a highly prevalent disorder and is estimated to affect about 5 million Americans (about 2% of the population) with an approximate annual incidence of half a million people. It is projected that the prevalence of heart failure will continue to rise into the twenty-first century. Because heart failure is highly prevalent and central sleep apnea is common in the setting of the failing heart, heart failure is the most common cause of central sleep apnea in the general population.

- Hunter–Cheyne–Stokes breathing (HCSB) is a form of periodic breathing commonly with an intervening central apnea (or hypopnea) situated between the waxing and waning phases of breathing. The pattern of periodic breathing in this disorder is unique in that it has long crescendo–decrescendo phases in thoracoabdominal excursions and airflow due to a long arterial circulation time, a pathophysiologic feature of systolic heart failure. The prolonged waxing phase of HCSB distinguishes it from other forms of periodic breathing with central sleep apnea, such as the idiopathic form, and central apnea associated with use of opioids in which the recovery phase (out of apnea) is somewhat abrupt and short rather than smooth and prolonged.

### Mechanisms of Central Sleep Apnea and Periodic Breathing in Heart Failure

Normally, with onset of sleep, ventilation decreases and $PCO_2$ increases. This maintains the prevailing $PCO_2$ above the apneic threshold $PCO_2$, and rhythmic breathing occurs. However, in some patients with heart failure, the prevailing awake $PCO_2$ does not rise during sleep. Because of the proximity of the prevailing $PCO_2$ to the exposed apneic threshold, central sleep apnea occurs. Furthermore, some heart failure patients have enhanced $CO_2$ sensitivity below eupnea. This also increases the likelihood of developing central apnea. The reason for the lack of normally observed sleep-induced rise in $PCO_2$ in some patients with heart failure is not clear but could be due to the lack of normally observed sleep-induced decrease in ventilation. Presumably, in heart failure patients with severe left ventricular diastolic dysfunction (and a stiff left ventricle), which invariably accompanies systolic dysfunction, pulmonary capillary pressure could rise when venous return increases. This results in a small increase in respiratory rate and ventilation, preventing the normally observed rise in $PCO_2$.

- Several studies have shown that subjects with heart failure and low $PaCO_2$ have a high probability of developing central sleep apnea during sleep. The reason for this is not clear, but it may also have to do with the severity of the left ventricular diastolic dysfunction that invariably accompanies systolic dysfunction. Heart failure patients with hypocapnia have a more severe left ventricular diastolic dysfunction and a higher wedge pressure than eupneic heart failure patients. Diastolic dysfunction will be further unmasked during supine position as venous return rises. Consequently, such patients may not be able to normally decrease their ventilation with sleep onset and their $PCO_2$ remains close to apneic threshold.

- Although a low awake $PaCO_2$ is highly predictive of central sleep apnea, it is not a prerequisite. Many patients with heart failure and central sleep apnea have normal awake $PaCO_2$. Rather, it is the proximity of the apneic threshold to the $PaCO_2$ that is important.

- The gender difference in the prevalence of central apnea in congestive heart failure may also be related to the difference between apneic threshold and the prevailing $PCO_2$. Combining the results of several studies, 40% of the male subjects have central sleep apnea, which is significantly higher than the 18% prevalence of central sleep apnea in female subjects. However, in women with congestive heart failure and systolic dysfunction, the risk of central sleep apnea is six times higher in those 60 years or older when compared to those less than 60 years of age. Premenopausal women have a lower apneic threshold than men, and this may be in part the reason for a lower prevalence of central apnea in premenopausal females than in males with heart failure. The balance of female and male hormones could mediate the lower apneic threshold in women than in man.

- In systolic heart failure, central apnea occurs in the background of periodic breathing. Long crescendo–decrescendo ventilation arms characterize this unique pattern of periodic breathing. The mechanisms underlying this unique pattern of periodic breathing are to some extent distinct from those mediating development of central apnea, though some mechanisms overlap. Mathematical and experimental models of the negative feedback system controlling breathing homeostasis predict that increased arterial circulation time (which delays the transfer of information regarding changes in $PO_2$ and $PCO_2$ from pulmonary capillary blood to the chemoreceptors, increased mixing gain), enhanced gain of the chemoreceptors (enhanced $CO_2/O_2$ chemosensitivity), and enhanced plant gain (a large change in $PaCO_2$ for a small change in ventilation) collectively increase the likelihood of periodic breathing. All these three factors may be present in systolic heart failure. It is therefore not surprising that heart failure is so conducive to the development of period breathing.

- In systolic heart failure, effective arterial circulation time could be increased for a variety of reasons, such as pulmonary congestion, left atrial and ventricular enlargement, and diminished stroke volume. Plant gain is increased because of a low functional residual capacity due to the presence of pleural effusion, cardiomegaly, pulmonary congestion, or edema. Finally, in some patients with heart failure, hypercapnic ventilatory response is increased; this is one of the distinguishing features between those heart failure patients with or without significant periodic breathing and central apnea during sleep. In individuals with increased sensitivity to carbon dioxide, the chemoreceptors elicit a large ventilatory response whenever the partial pressure of carbon dioxide rises. The consequent intense hyperventilation, by driving the $PCO_2$ below the apneic threshold, results in central apnea. $PCO_2$ then rises due to the central apnea. Therefore, the cycles of hyperventilation and hypoventilation are maintained.

- These alterations in the negative feedback system controlling breathing are not necessarily state (sleep or wake)–specific, and periodic breathing may occur both during wakefulness and sleep, although more frequently during sleep. Sleep promotes periodic breathing because of both the assumption of supine position and also its own specific effects. In a supine position and during sleep, cardiac output decreases (further prolonging arterial circulation time), and both functional residual capacity and metabolic rate decrease, thereby, enhancing plant gain. All these alterations increase the likelihood of developing periodic breathing during sleep.

- Treatment of central sleep apnea in heart failure may be achieved in several ways. Since heart failure is the fundamental reason for development of periodic breathing and central sleep apnea, therapy of heart failure must be maximized first. If periodic breathing persists, several therapeutic options are available.

## THERAPY OF CENTRAL SLEEP APNEA IN SYSTOLIC HEART FAILURE

The following modalities have been used in the treatment of central sleep apnea in systolic heart failure. However, controlled long-term studies are necessary to determine if therapy affects the natural history (morbidity and mortality) of systolic heart failure.

Optimization of cardiopulmonary function including cardiac resynchronization therapy

Heart transplantation

Nocturnal administration of nasal supplemental oxygen

Theophylline

Acetazolamide

Positive airway pressure devices such as continuous positive airway pressure (CPAP) and pressure support servoventilation

Atrioventricular pacing devices

### Idiopathic Central Sleep Apnea

This is a rare disorder. Polysomnographically, it is characterized by repetitive episodes of central apnea. Patients are commonly older males and may present with complaints of restless sleep, insomnia, and/or daytime symptoms, such as sleepiness and fatigue related to sleep fragmentation caused by the arousals.

- By definition, idiopathic central apnea is a diagnosis of exclusion and other causes of central apnea need to be ruled out. Silent congestive heart failure and central nervous system disorders such as stroke and multiple small infarctions should be excluded, particularly in older patients.

- Patients with idiopathic central apnea commonly have a low arterial $PCO_2$, and increased hypercapnic ventilatory response during wakefulness. A heightened ventilatory response to $CO_2$ facilitates development of central apnea during arousals from sleep.

- Studies have reported that acetazolamide was effective in decreasing central apneas. Acetazolamide causes metabolic acidosis and decreases $PaCO_2$. In spite of a lower (than normal) $PaCO_2$, central apneas decrease because ventilatory response to $CO_2$ below eupnea remains unaffected and consequently the apneic threshold $PCO_2$ more than that of $PaCO_2$. This results in widening of the two $PCO_2$ set points, which will decrease the likelihood of developing central apnea. CPAP devices, supplemental nasal oxygen, and theophylline are other alternatives, but no systematic studies are available. In a case report, the use of bilevel positive airway pressure device resulted in worsening of central apnea, presumably by lowering the prevailing $PCO_2$ below apneic threshold.

### Idiopathic Pulmonary Arterial Hypertension

This is characterized by pulmonary arterial hypertension with normal pulmonary capillary pressure. It is a disorder of unknown etiology, although certain genetic factors have been found to be associated with the familial form of idiopathic pulmonary hypertension.

- In more advanced hemodynamic states of this disorder, there is severe pulmonary arterial hypertension, right ventricular failure, and diminished cardiac output. In one study, 30% of patients with idiopathic pulmonary artery hypertension had moderately severe sleep apnea with an apnea–hypopnea index of 37 per hour, resulting in oxygen desaturation; patients with periodic breathing had significantly more hemodynamic abnormalities than those without periodic breathing. Presumably, diminished stroke volume and increased arterial circulation time were the underlying mechanisms in mediating periodic breathing in this disorder.

- Nocturnal supplemental nasal oxygen has been recommended for the treatment of central sleep apnea in idiopathic pulmonary arterial hypertension. Interestingly, in one patient with idiopathic pulmonary hypertension, hypocapnia and low cardiac output, central sleep apnea was eliminated after lung transplantation. Use of positive airway pressure devices should be avoided; in a case report,

use of bilevel positive airway pressure therapy was associated with death; although cause and effect cannot be proven, possibilities include reduction in cardiac output with the use of bilevel device and worsening of central sleep apnea.

### High Altitude

The pattern of periodic breathing at high altitude resembles Hunter–Cheyne–Stokes breathing in heart failure, with one exception—the cycle of periodic breathing is short. As noted earlier, periodic breathing in heart failure has long crescendo–decrescendo phases because of an increased circulation time, a pathologic feature of systolic heart failure.

- The mechanism involves hypoxemia that occurs at high altitude. Hypoxemia narrows the difference between spontaneous $PCO_2$ minus apneic threshold $PCO_2$, and increases hypocapnic chemosensitivity below the eupnea. Furthermore, the frequency of periodic breathing during sleep at high altitude tends to be more in individuals with enhanced ventilatory response to both hypercapnia and hypoxia. The hypercapnic ventilatory response resembles that reported in patients with heart failure with central sleep apnea.

- During sleep at high altitude when the apneic threshold is unmasked, central apnea occurs as spontaneous $PCO_2$ falls below apneic threshold. $PCO_2$ rises with the apnea, and breathing resumes. The subsequent reduction in $PCO_2$ as breathing increases perpetuates the cycle.

- Inhalation of supplemental oxygen and small amount of $CO_2$ decreases periodic breathing. Furthermore, it has also been shown that administration of acetazolamide improves oxygen desaturation and ameliorates the symptoms of acute mountain sickness in humans at high altitude. Acetazolamide widens the difference between the two $PCO_2$ set points (in contrast to hypoxemia) resulting in improvement of periodic breathing at high altitude.

### Cerebrovascular Disorders

A number of studies have shown that patients with stroke (acute, chronic, ischemic, and nonischemic) have obstructive and central sleep apnea. In regard to obstructive sleep apnea, this disorder could either precede (cause or contribute to development of) or be caused by, stroke. In either case, obstructive sleep apnea may influence the outcome of patients with stroke.

- In contrast to obstructive sleep apnea, central apneas are most probably caused by the stroke and may decrease over time.

- A pattern of breathing similar to Hunter–Cheyne–Stokes breathing has also been reported in patients with stroke. This pattern of breathing appears to have no relation to the site of pathology. The mechanisms of central sleep apnea and periodic breathing in stroke are not well understood, although unrecognized systolic heart failure could also be a factor. Both supplemental nasal oxygen and theophylline are effective therapeutic modalities.

## HYPERCAPNIC CENTRAL SLEEP APNEA

These heterogeneous disorders are characterized by daytime steady-state hypercapnia, although in some $PaCO_2$ may be within upper normal range. According to the alveolar ventilation equation, $PaCO_2$ is directly proportional to $CO_2$ production and inversely related to alveolar ventilation. In the disorders in this category, the rise in $PaCO_2$ is due to decreased global ventilation.

- Effects of sleep on these disorders are multiple. The full impact of these disorders as manifested by pronounced hypercapnia becomes unmasked during sleep when wakefulness drive to breathe is absent and ventilation decreases.

- Normally, with sleep onset and the removal of the wakefulness drive, ventilation decreases and $PCO_2$ rises by 2–4 mm Hg. However, such a small physiological decrease in ventilation results in a large increase in $PCO_2$ when steady-state awake hypercapnia is already present. This is dictated by the alveolar ventilation equation and is related to the hyperbolic relation of $PCO_2$ with alveolar ventilation. Similarly, in the presence of hypercapnia, if an arousal occurs because of return of wakefulness drive to breathe, ventilation increases somewhat but $PCO_2$ decreases considerably (increased plant gain). This increases the probability of developing central apnea, if apneic threshold $PCO_2$ is also elevated. An increase in the apneic threshold and its proximity to a chronically elevated $PCO_2$ is critical and not yet proven. However, it is a likely assumption because it has been shown that steady-state acute hypercapnia results in an elevated apneic threshold $PCO_2$.

- The second effect of sleep on breathing in disorders in this category relates to the nature of the pathophysiologic process. In some of the disorders in which the lesion involves the brainstem medullary respiratory centers responsible for automatic breathing, central apneas may also occur during sleep, when the wakefulness drive to breath is absent.

- The third effect of sleep on these disorders involves the neurophysiologic changes associated with REM sleep. During REM sleep, there is costal muscle atonia. Therefore, in neuromuscular disorders involving the diaphragm, which normally is the only inspiratory thoracic pump muscle active during REM sleep, airflow ceases, and thoracoabdominal tracings can look like central apneas.

- Finally, severe oxygen desaturation could occur during sleep. This is related to the chronic steady-state hypercapnia, the hyperbolic nature of $PaCO_2$ in relation to alveolar ventilation, and that with sleep onset, ventilation decreases. Therefore, $PaCO_2$ rises considerably, and this, in turn, results in severe hypoxemia due to the reciprocal relation between alveolar $PCO_2$ and $PO_2$.

## Alveolar Hypoventilation Syndromes with Normal Pulmonary Function

These central nervous system disorders are characterized by daytime hypercapnia, diminished or absence $CO_2$ chemosensitivity, and normal pulmonary function.

- These disorders could be either genetic (congenital central hypoventilation syndrome and perhaps primary hypoventilation syndrome) or acquired (a variety of brainstem and spinal cord disorders). The unique feature of all of these disorders is the failure of automatic/metabolic control of breathing that becomes manifest during sleep when wakefulness drive to breathe is absent (Ondine's curse). Since the automatic/metabolic pathway controls breathing during sleep, a defect in this pathway will decrease ventilation dramatically and central apneas can develop.

- Congenital central hypoventilation syndrome (CCHS) is a rare genetic disorder commonly associated with other neurocristopathies, such as Hirschsprung disease. The disorder manifests itself after birth, although recently few adult cases have been reported. Investigators have reported a high prevalence of heterozygous de novo mutations in the homebox gene PHOX 2B in most (but not all) patients with CCHS. Most of the mutations consist of an expansion of a polyalanine stretch (5–9 alanine expansions within a 20-residue polyalanine tract), with the remaining being frame-shift or nonsense mutations after the PHOX 2B homedomain.

- Treatment of CCHS have included diaphragmatic pacing, or mechanical ventilation by mask, via tracheostomy, or by negative pressure ventilation. If diaphragmatic pacing or negative pressure ventilation unmask or result in an upper airway occlusion during sleep, positive airway pressure therapy should be considered; a tracheostomy may be necessary. Respiratory stimulants are generally ineffective. A recently developed positive airway pressure device, referred to as pressure support servoventilator with backup rate (Bipap Auto SV, Respironics, and VPAP Adapt SV, Res Med) could be the therapy of choice, though no studies have been reported. With these devices, during overnight titration, the expiratory pressure is progressively increased to eliminate obstructive apneas. The device provides variable inspiratory support, inversely proportional to the patient's breathing. Support increases with hypopneas and decreases when breathing is normal. The backup rate aborts any impending central apneas.

- Primary (idiopathic) alveolar hypoventilation syndrome is usually a disorder of adult males presenting in the third and fourth decades of life. This disorder is characterized by chronic hypercapnia in an adult without any demonstrable neuromuscular, thoracic, pulmonary, or central nervous system pathology. The mechanisms leading to chronic hypercapnia are not understood but could have a genetic basis.

- Treatment of idiopathic alveolar hypoventilation syndrome should be individualized. Treatment options include nocturnal supplemental oxygen, negative pressure ventilation, noninvasive nocturnal mechanical ventilation, or diaphragmatic pacing. If upper airway occlusion occurs with negative pressure ventilation or diaphragmatic pacing, positive airway pressure devices should be used; tracheostomy with mechanical ventilation may be required. Among the positive airway pressure devices, pressure support servoventilation is perhaps the treatment of choice. However, no studies using theses devices have been reported.

- Brainstem disorders can produce severe hypoventilation and central apneas during sleep since the central chemoreceptors and respiratory centers are located in this region. Furthermore, afferent inputs from peripheral chemoreceptors are also processed in this location. Various pathologic processes, such as compression, ischemia, infarct, tumor, and encephalitis (viral, bacterial, and Leigh's disease) involving the brainstem have been associated with central sleep apnea. Respiratory centers are bilateral and widespread, and infarcts causing apnea are usually bilateral. Unilateral infarcts rarely cause central apneas unless they are extensive and involve the medullary nerves above and below the medullary neuronal decussation. Treatment should be individualized along the lines described for CCHS and primary alveolar hypoventilation.

- Cervical cordotomy and anterior cervical spinal artery syndrome can result in failure of automatic breathing during sleep (Ondine's curse). In these two conditions, the process involves the descending pathways serving the automatic control of breathing. Spinothalamic cervical cordotomy has been performed for intractable pain in the past, and individuals would subsequently develop Ondine's curse. Anterior spinal artery syndrome gives rise to motor palsy and dissociated sensory loss below the level of the lesion, along with bladder dysfunction. Ondine's curse occurs when the anterior cervical spine is involved bilaterally, such as seen with thrombosis of the anterior spinal artery.

- Therapy should be individualized, as outlined above for CCHS and primary alveolar hypoventilation.

## Neuromuscular Disorders

This category includes a large number of neuromuscular disorders that may affect the respiratory muscles (muscular dystrophies such as myotonic dystrophy, and idiopathic diaphragmatic paralysis), neuromuscular junction (myasthenia gravis), phrenic and intercostal nerves (amyotrophic lateral sclerosis), or brainstem.

- A specific pathophysiologic breathing disorder could occur during sleep depending on the site of pathology. REM sleep hypoventilation or central apneas may occur with diaphragmatic involvement. In contrast, obstructive apneas and hypopneas may predominate during sleep with involvement of the pharyngeal muscles.

- As respiratory muscle weakness progresses and daytime hypercapnia develops, sleep-related breathing disorders manifest with more severe hypercapnia, oxygen desaturation, and central apneas.

- Treatment of sleep-related breathing disorders in neuromuscular diseases should be individualized. Two important factors determining the modality of therapy are the impairment in rhythmogenesis due to pathologic processes involving the respiratory centers and the presence of upper airway obstruction during sleep. The use of bilevel ventilation could be helpful for patients with hypercapnia if the brainstem is not involved. If rhythmogenesis is impaired and upper airway obstruction is present during sleep, bilevel ventilation with a backup rate, or tracheostomy with assisted ventilation may be necessary. As noted above, therapy with a proportional assist servoventilator could be the treatment of choice.

## Opioids

Ventilatory depression during wakefulness is a well-known effect of opioid drugs. This ventilatory depression is characterized by decreased tidal volume and minute ventilation, increased $PaCO_2$, and diminished hypercapnic and hypoxic ventilatory responses. However, normally with chronic use of opioids, respiratory tolerance develops such that daytime respiratory depression, that is, chronic hypercapnia, is either absent, or mild in nature. Unfortunately, however, respiratory depression in the form of central and obstructive apneas and hypopneas occur during sleep. In this regard, a few recent studies have demonstrated a high prevalence of sleep apnea (30–90%) in patients using opioids chronically for pain management. The prevalence of central sleep apnea is dose dependent and is increased particularly in these individuals taking more than 200 mg/day equivalent dose morphine.

- The mechanisms responsible for opioid-induced central (and obstructive) apneas have not been studied. The disordered breathing events could be due to both central and peripheral mechanisms. With removal of the wakefulness drive to breathing during sleep, rhythmic breathing is metabolically controlled, and respiratory depression manifested by more severe hypercapnia and cessation of breathing with central apneas could occur. Diminished central drive to muscles of the upper airway could result in obstructive apneas and hypopneas. It is also conceivable that opioids may suppress arousal reflexes that could prolong episodes of apneas and hypopneas as well as periods of hypoventilation. The presence of hypercapnia could also promote central apneas because of an increased plant gain.

- Treatment of sleep apnea associated with use of opioids has not been studied. Because there are mixed patterns of sleep apnea, that is, co-occurrence of both obstructive and central apneas and hypopneas, use of pressure support servoventilation, discussed above, could be an appropriate therapeutic modality.

## CENTRAL SLEEP APNEA IN ENDOCRINE DISORDERS

Central sleep apnea has been observed in patients with acromegaly or hypothyroidism. In both disorders, however, obstructive sleep apnea is the predominant form of sleep-disordered breathing.

### Acromegaly

Several studies have reported a relatively high prevalence of sleep apnea in patients with acromegaly. Both obstructive and central sleep apneas occur.

- Patients with acromegaly may suffer from central sleep apnea; this correlated with levels of human growth hormone, IGF-1, and hypercapnic ventilatory response. An enhanced ventilatory response could increase the likelihood of developing central sleep apnea.
- Treatment of acromegaly with octreotide, a somatostatin analog, could result in tissue regression and improvement in sleep apnea. However, this may take several months, and sleep apnea may persist despite therapy of acromegaly; therefore a trial of CPAP remains the therapy of choice.

### Hypothyroidism

Patients with hypothyroidism, particularly those with myxedema, may develop obstructive sleep apnea due to excess pharyngeal soft tissue, similar to patients with acromegaly. Central apneas may also be observed although it is much less frequent than obstructive apneas. The mechanism responsible for central apneas remains unclear.

## CENTRAL SLEEP APNEA WITH OBSTRUCTIVE SLEEP APNEA

Few central apneas can be observed in patients with obstructive sleep apnea, and also after treatment of obstructive sleep apnea with CPAP, tracheostomy, or uvulopalatopharyngoplasty. Most of central apneas that emerge with CPAP therapy are transitory, although in a small number of patients central apneas persist. Such patients may suffer from sever sleep apnea, atrial fibrillation, systolic heart failure, or be on opioids. A number of these patients have central apneas on initial polysomnograms.

## CENTRAL SLEEP APNEA WITH UPPER AIRWAY DISORDERS

There are many receptors in the nose, larynx, and pharynx, and animal studies have demonstrated that stimulation of upper airway receptors may cause central apneas. Apnea may be produced by water, chemical, or mechanical stimulation of the receptors. Central apnea has been also produced by stimulation of the superior laryngeal nerve.

- Human studies show that preterm infants develop central apneas in response to oropharyngeal stimulation by water or saline. Systematic studies in adults, however, are not available. Researchers have demonstrated that in normal adults, induced-nasal obstruction resulted in central apneas, although the predominant effect was obstructive sleep apnea. Another study showed a significant increase in the number of central apneas in normal individual during nasal obstruction.
- Further evidence of upper airway receptors mediating central apnea in humans stems from the effects of high-frequency (30 Hz) low-pressure ventilation in aborting central apneas. Similarly, application of CPAP could improve central apneas in disorders that are either idiopathic or due to systolic heart failure. It has been postulated that oropharyngeal closure may induce central apneas via upper airway receptor stimulation.

## KEY POINTS

1. Central apnea is due to a temporary failure in breathing rhythm generation resulting in the loss of ventilatory effort, lasting at least 10 s. A central apnea is characterized polysomnographically by the absence of oronasal airflow and thoracoabdominal excursions.
2. Central apneas occur in many pathophysiologic conditions. Depending on the cause or mechanism, central apneas may not be clinically significant. In contrast, in some disorders central apneas result in pathophysiologic consequences. Under such circumstances, diagnosis and treatment of central sleep apnea may improve quality of life, morbidity, and perhaps mortality.

## BIBLIOGRAPHY

Amiel J, et al. Polyalanine expansion and frameshift mutations of the paired-like homeobox gene PHOX2B in congenital central hypoventilation syndrome. *Nat Genet* 2003; 33:459–461.

Arzt M, et al. Suppression of central sleep apnea by continuous positive airway pressure and transplant-free survival in heart failure. *Circulation* 2007; 115:3173–3180.

Blanchi B, et al. Mutations of brainstem transcription factors and central respiratory disorders. *Trends Mol Med* 2005; 11:23–30.

Boden AG, et al. Apneic threshold for $CO_2$ in the anesthetized rat: Fundamental properties under steady-state conditions. *J Appl Physiol* 1998; 85:898–907.

Colas A, et al. Systemic complications of acromegaly: Epidemiology, pathogenesis, and management. *End Rev* 2004: 25:102–152.

Dauger S, et al. PHOX2B controls the development of peripheral chemoreceptors and afferent visceral pathways. *Development* 2003; 130:6635–6642.

Farber HW, et al. Pulmonary arterial hypertension. *N Engl J Med* 2004; 351:1655–1665.

Fareny RJ, et al. Sleep-disordered breathing associated with long-term opioid therapy. *Chest* 2003; 123:632–639.

Fries R, et al. Clinical significance of sleep-related breathing disorders in patients with implantable cardioverter defibrillators. *Pace* 1999; 22:223–227.

Garrigue S, et al. Benefit of atrial pacing in sleep apnea syndrome. *N Engl J Med* 2002; 346:404–412.

Herrmann BL, et al. Effects of octreotide on sleep apnea and tongue volume (magnetic resonance imaging) in patients with acromegaly. *Eur J Endocrinol* 2004; 151:309–315.

Hermann DM, et al. Sleep-disordered breathing and stroke. *Curr Opin Neurol* 2003; 16:87–90.

Hommura F, et al. Continuous versus bilevel positive airway pressure in patient with idiopathic central sleep apnea. *Am J Respir Crit Care Med* 1997; 155:1482–1485.

Javaheri S. A mechanism of central sleep apnea in patients with heart failure. *N Engl. J Med* 1999; 341: 949–954.

Javaheri S. Treatment of central sleep apnea in heart failure. *Sleep* 2000a; 23:S224–S227.

Javaheri S. Effects of continuous positive airway pressure on sleep apnea and ventricular irritability in patients with heart failure. *Circulation* 2000b; 101:392–397.

Javaheri S. Pembrey's Dream: The time has come for a long-term trial of nocturnal supplemental nasal oxygen to treat central sleep apnea in congestive heart failure. *Chest* 2003a; 123:322–325.

Javaheri S. Heart failure and sleep apnea: Emphasis on practical therapeutic options. *Clin Chest Med* 2003b; 24:207–222.

Javaheri S, et al. Association of low $PaCO_2$ with central sleep apnea and ventricular arrhythmias in ambulatory patients with stable heart failure. *Ann Intern Med* 1998a; 128:204–207.

Javaheri S, et al. Sleep apnea in 81 ambulatory male patients with stable heart failure: Types and their prevalences, consequences, and presentations. *Circulation* 1998b; 97:2154–2159.

Javaheri S, et al. Prevalence of obstructive sleep apnea and periodic limb movement in 45 subjects with heart transplantation. *Eur Heart J* 2004; 25:260–266.

Javaheri S, et al. Central sleep apnea, right ventricular dysfunction, and low diastolic blood pressure are predictors of mortality in systolic heart failure. *J Am Coll Cardiol* 2007; 49:2028–2034.

Kraus J, et al. Ondine's curse in association with diabetes insipidus following transient vertebrobasilar ischemia. *Clin Neurol Neurosurg* 1999; 101:196–198.

Manconi M, et al. Anterior spinal artery syndrome complicated by the Ondine Curse. *Arch Neurol* 2003; 60:1787–1790.

Manning HL, et al. Respiratory control and respiratory sensation in a patient with a ganglioglioma within the dorsocaudal brain stem. *Am J Respir Crit Care Med* 2000; 161:2100–2106.

Nakayama H, et al. Effect of ventilatory drive on $CO_2$ sensitivity below eupnea during sleep. *AM J Crit Care Med* 2002; 165:1251–1258.

Newson-Davis IC, et al. The effect of non-invasive positive pressure ventilation (NIPPV) on cognitive function in amyotrophic lateral sclerosis: A prospective study. *J Neurol Psychiatry* 2001; 71:482–487.

Parra O, et al. Time course of sleep-related breathing disorders in first-ever stroke or transient ischemic attack. *Am J Respir Crit Care Med* 2000; 161:375–380.

Rosenow F, et al. Sleep apnea in endocrine diseases. *J Sleep Res* 1998; 7:3–11.

Sasaki A, et al. Molecular analysis of congenital central hypoventilation syndrome. *Hum Gen* 2003; 114:22–26.

Schulz R, et al. Nocturnal periodic breathing in primary pulmonary hypertension. *Eur Respir J* 2002; 19:658–663.

Schulz R, et al. Central sleep apnoea and unilateral diaphragmatic paralysis associated with vertebral artery compression of the medulla oblongata. *J Neurol* 2003; 250:503–505.

Schulz R, et al. Reversal of nocturnal periodic breathing in primary pulmonary hypertension after lung transplantation. *Chest* 2004; 125:344–347.

Shahar E, et al. Sleep-disordered breathing and cardiovascular disease: Cross-sectional results of the Sleep Heart Health Study. *Am J Respir Crit Car Med* 2001; 163:19–25.

Shiomi T, et al. Primary pulmonary hypertension with central sleep apnea—Sudden death after bilevel positive airway pressure therapy. *Jpn Circ J* 2000; 64:723–726.

Sin DD, et al. Risk factors for central and obstructive sleep apnea in 450 men and women with congestive heart failure. *Am J Respir Crit Care Med* 1999; 160:1101–1106.

Solin P, et al. Influence of pulmonary capillary wedge pressure on central apnea in heart failure. *Circulation* 1999; 99:1574–1579.

Staniforth AD, et al. Nocturnal desaturation in patients with stable heart failure. *Heart* 1998; 79:394–399.

Teichtahl H, et al. Sleep-disordered breathing in stable methadone programme patients: A pilot study. *Addiction* 2001; 96:395–403.

Teschler H, et al. Adaptive pressure support servo-ventilation. *Am J Respir Crit Care Med* 2001; 164:614–619.

Trang H, et al. The French congenital central hypoventilation syndrome regise general date, phenotype, and genotype. *Chest* 2005; 127:72–79.

Tremel F, et al. High prevalence and persistence of sleep apnea in patients referred for acute left ventricular failure and medically treated over 2 months. *Eur Heart J* 1999; 20:1201–1209.

Vanderlaan M, et al. Epidemiologic survey of 196 patients with congenital central hypoventilation syndrome. *Pediatr Pulmonol* 2004; 37:217–229.

Walker M, et al. Chronic opioid use a risk factor for the development of central sleep apnea and ataxic breathing. *J Clin Sleep Med* 2007; 3:455–461.

Weese-Mayer DE, et al. Idiopathic congenital central hypoventilation syndrome: Analysis of genes pertinent to early autonomic nervous system embryologic development and identification of mutations in PHOX2B. *Am J Med Genet* 2003; 123:267–278.

Widdicombe J. Airway receptors. *Respir Physiol* 2001; 125:3–15.

Xie A, et al. Apnea-hypopnea threshold for $CO_2$ in patients with congestive heart failure. *Am J Respir Crit Care Med* 2002; 165:1245–1250.

Yaggi H, et al. Sleep-disordered breathing and stroke. *Clin Chest Med* 2003; 24:223–237.

Yaggi H, et al. Obstructive sleep apnoea and stroke. *Lancet Neurol* 2004; 3:333–342.

Zhou XS, et al. Effect of gender on the development of hypocapnic apnea/hypopnea during NREM sleep. *J Appl Physiol* 2000; 89:192–199.

Zhou XS, et al. Effect of testosterone on the apnea threshold in women during NREM sleep. *J Appl Physiol* 2003; 94:101–107.

# 17

## OBESITY HYPOVENTILATION SYNDROME

JOHN G. PARK

Center for Sleep Medicine, Division of Pulmonary and Critical Care Medicine,
Mayo Clinic College of Medicine, Rochester, Minnesota

### INTRODUCTION

- Obesity hypoventilation syndrome (OHS), also commonly referred to as Pickwickian syndrome, is broadly defined as hypercapnia during wakefulness in obese persons.

- The clinical features of OHS include marked obesity, hypersomnolence, periodic respiration, polycythemia, cyanosis, and right ventricular hypertrophy and failure.

- The prevalence of OHS is about 5–31% of obese adults, and it is uncommon, but possible, in obese children.

### PATHOPHYSIOLOGY

At least four different factors may influence the development of OHS.

- The first factor is morbid *obesity*, defined as a body mass index (BMI) $\geq 35 \text{ kg/m}^2$. The incidence of OHS increases with further weight gain. However, weight alone does not correlate with OHS, which is uncommon even among obese persons. Obesity increases metabolic demand due to the increased muscle work required to move the excess weight; this increased metabolic demand results in increased oxygen consumption and carbon dioxide production. Thus, minute ventilation needs to increase to maintain normocapnia.

- The required increase in minute ventilation may be hampered by *mechanical limitation*, the second factor contributing to overall hypoventilation. To adapt to the increased work of breathing due to increased elastic and nonelastic resistance, respiratory rate increases and tidal volume decreases. This adaptive mechanism is limited in obese persons because of their decreased expiratory reserve volume; it is further exacerbated in the supine position. The decrease in lung volume is partly a result of an elevated diaphragm due to truncal obesity. Because of increased resistive load and limited lung volume, the total work of breathing in patients with OHS can reach three times that of normal-weight subjects and 1.3 times that of subjects with simple obesity (obesity without OHS). It is postulated that rather than continuing to increase energy expenditure in breathing, patients with OHS tend to breathe at a much lower tidal volume, which, in turn, leads to increase in dead-space ventilation (airflow in regions of the airway not involved in gas exchange) and worsening of ventilation-perfusion mismatch. Arterial carbon dioxide is dependent on its production as well as its elimination by effective ventilation. Thus, obese persons are at risk for hypercapnia as a result of both increased carbon dioxide production and decreased ventilation. These adaptive measures ultimately result in poor ventilation and further increase in $PaCO_2$.

- The third factor contributing to OHS is *blunted central chemoreceptor response* to hypercapnia and hypoxemia. Mechanical limitation is not the sole cause of hypercapnia since patients with OHS can voluntarily hyperventilate to normalize their $PaCO_2$, and administration of progesterone, a respiratory stimulant, can normalize or, at least, decrease $PaCO_2$. Persons with OHS have decreased ventilatory drive in response to hypoxia and hypercapnia (one-sixth and one-third of that of normal persons, respectively).

- The fourth factor contributing to OHS may be the *coexistence of obstructive sleep apnea* (OSA). Some have suggested that OHS is a severe form of OSA and that, due to repeated hypoventilation during apneic phases,

OSA is a causative factor in the development of OHS. Other studies, however, have failed to show that OHS is related to the frequency, number, duration, or type of episodes of apnea or hypopnea. Furthermore, up to 25% of patients with OHS do not have OSA. Finally, hypercapnia does not respond to continuous positive airway pressure (CPAP) therapy or tracheostomy in all patients, so OSA, while not the sole cause, most likely contributes to the development of OHS.

- The true pathophysiologic mechanism(s) of OHS may vary from person to person. Depending on the person's susceptibility, one or all of the above-mentioned factors may contribute to chronic hypoventilation in the setting of obesity. Effective therapy, therefore, may depend on correction of multiple contributing factors.

## EVALUATION

In evaluating a patient with hypercapnia, multiple causes must be considered, including disorders of ventilatory control, anatomical defects, and electrolyte abnormalities.

- A complete medical history, physical examination, and an arterial blood gas determination are necessary. Guided by the initial evaluation, pulmonary function testing may help assess the functional capacity of the lungs, radiologic assessment may identify structural abnormalities, blood chemistries may identify electrolyte abnormalities, polysomnography will identify sleep-disordered breathing, and ventilatory response to hypercapnia and hypoxemia will help assess the integrity of the respiratory control system. Further neurologic or rheumatologic evaluation may be necessary, depending on the clinical suspicion.

## CAUSES OF CHRONIC HYPERCAPNIA

*Mechanical limitations*
  Kyphoscoliosis
  Chronic obstructive lung disease
  Advanced interstitial lung disease
  Postpneumonectomy
  Postthoracoplasty
  Myopathies: muscular dystrophies, myotonic dystrophies, acid-maltase deficiency
  Obesity hypoventilation syndrome
*Neuropathic limitations*
  Myasthenia gravis
  Eaton–Lambert syndrome
  Bilateral diaphragm paralysis
  Spinal cord injury
  Motor neuron disease (e.g., amyotrophic lateral sclerosis)
  Peripheral neuropathies (e.g., Guillain–Barré syndrome)

*Central control limitations*
  Primary alveolar hypoventilation
  Cerebrovascular accident
  Central nervous system neoplasm
  Arnold–Chiari malformation
  Bulbar poliomyelitis
  Neurosarcoidosis
  Carotid body dysfunction or trauma
  Prolonged hypoxia
  Obesity hypoventilation syndrome
  Drugs (e.g., narcotics, sedatives)
*Metabolic causes*
  Hypothyroidism/myxedema
  Electrolyte abnormalities (e.g., hypokalemia, hypophosphatemia)
  Chronic metabolic alkalosis

## THERAPY

Several different therapies have been used to control OHS.

- Progesterone has been tried with some short-term success in the past, but, because of lack of proven long-term efficacy and potential adverse effects, no pharmacologic agents are currently recommended for the treatment of OHS.

- Although CPAP is effective in decreasing daytime $PCO_2$ in some patients with OHS, other noninvasive positive-pressure ventilators are the preferred mode of respiratory support. Noninvasive ventilators, such as bilevel positive airway pressure (BPAP), are more effective than CPAP in improving hypercapnia, edema, hypersomnolence, and dyspnea. Some patients, however, may not respond completely to noninvasive ventilation.

- The most consistent benefit appears to result from significant weight loss, such as with bariatric surgery. According to the National Institutes of Health 1991 consensus statement regarding morbid obesity, patients with a BMI $\geq 35\,kg/m^2$ and an obesity-related comorbid condition, or those with a BMI $\geq 40\,kg/m^2$ should be considered for surgical treatment for obesity. Gastric surgery for weight loss has been shown to normalize lung volumes, normalize $PCO_2$ and $PaO_2$, significantly improve OSA, improve pulmonary hypertension, and improve polycythemia. Its benefits, however, must be considered in relation to the increased morbidity associated with surgery in obese persons.

## KEY POINTS

1. Obesity hypoventilation syndrome is defined by the presence of waking hypercapnia in obese persons.

2. At least four different factors may influence the development of OHS, including morbid obesity, mechanical limitation to breathing, blunted central chemoreceptor response to hypercapnia and hypoxemia, and coexistence of obstructive sleep apnea (OSA). Effective therapy, therefore, may depend on correction of multiple contributing factors.

3. Noninvasive positive airway pressure ventilation and optimal weight management, including bariatric surgery if necessary, have been shown to be effective in controlling OHS.

## BIBLIOGRAPHY

Alpert MA. Obesity cardiomyopathy: pathophysiology and evolution of the clinical syndrome. *Am J Med Sci* 2001; 321:225–236.

American Academy of Sleep Medicine Task Force. Sleep-related breathing disorders in adults: Recommendations for syndrome definition and measurement techniques in clinical research. The Report of an American Academy of Sleep Medicine Task Force. *Sleep* 1999; 22:667–689.

Berg G, et al. The use of health-care resources in obesity-hypoventilation syndrome. *Chest* 2001; 120:377–383.

Fitzpatrick M. Leptin and the obesity hypoventilation syndrome: A leap of faith? *Thorax* 2002; 57:1–2.

Kessler R, et al. The obesity-hypoventilation syndrome revisited: A prospective study of 34 consecutive cases. *Chest* 2001; 120:369–376.

Masa JF, et al. The obesity hypoventilation syndrome can be treated with noninvasive mechanical ventilation. *Chest* 2001; 119:1102–1107.

Nowbar S, et al. Obesity-associated hypoventilation in hospitalized patients: Prevalence, effects, and outcome. *Am J Med* 2004; 116:1–7.

# 18

## CARDIOVASCULAR COMPLICATIONS OF OBSTRUCTIVE SLEEP APNEA

PETER Y. HAHN, LYLE J. OLSON, AND VIREND K. SOMERS
Mayo Clinic College of Medicine, Rochester, Minnesota

### INTRODUCTION

Cardiovascular disease is highly prevalent in the United States, affecting 23% of the population. It is a significant source of decreased productivity, health care expenditure, and impaired quality of life. Most importantly, it results in considerable morbidity and mortality with approximately 38.5% of all deaths in the United States attributable to cardiovascular disease.

- There is growing awareness that obstructive sleep apnea (OSA) may be an important and treatable risk factor for cardiovascular disease. Large cross-sectional epidemiologic studies have shown that patients with OSA have increased rates of hypertension, ischemic heart disease, heart failure (HF), and stroke. Recent studies suggest that OSA may act through multiple mechanisms, including sympathetic activation, inflammation, endothelial dysfunction, disordered coagulation, metabolic dysregulation, and oxidative stress, to elicit cardiovascular dysfunction and disease.

### PHYSIOLOGIC EFFECTS OF OBSTRUCTIVE SLEEP APNEA

In general, sleep is characterized by a state of cardiovascular "relaxation." A decline in blood pressure (BP), heart rate (HR), systemic vascular resistance (SVR), and cardiac output (CO) is commonly observed with sleep onset. With deeper levels of nonrapid eye movement (NREM) sleep, these measures decline further and likely reflect a further decrease in sympathetic activity. During rapid eye movement (REM) sleep, however, sympathetic activity may increase, resulting in lability of HR and BP, both of which can approach relaxed waking levels.

- In OSA, the sleep-related state of cardiovascular relaxation is disrupted. Hypoxemia, hypercapnia, increased sympathetic activity, and dramatic swings in intrathoracic pressure during apneic events can lead to acute and chronic adverse cardiovascular effects.

- During recurrent apneas, hypoxemia and retained carbon dioxide ($CO_2$) can stimulate chemoreceptors leading to an increase in sympathetic nervous activity (SNA). Studies have shown that SNA progressively rises during obstructive apneas and peaks with arousal. This progressive rise in SNA increases SVR by peripheral vasoconstriction. Systemic BP subsequently also increases gradually during the apnea. Although CO and HR generally decrease during the apnea, both increase dramatically with arousal and apnea termination. The resumption of breathing at arousal results in further acute increases in BP, likely reflecting the increase in CO in the face of severe peripheral vasoconstriction. Oxyhemoglobin saturation also decreases during apnea and recovers only slowly after apnea termination. The sudden increase in CO with arousal means that myocardial oxygen demand increases at a time when oxyhemoglobin saturation is still low.

- In addition to increased sympathetic activity and its effects on HR, BP, SVR, and CO, the large swings in intrathoracic pressure during apneas also have acute cardiovascular effects. Inspiratory effort against a collapsed upper airway can result in impressive swings in intrathoracic pressure. Intrathoracic pressure during an apnea can be as low as $-80$ cm $H_2O$. Such dramatic negative intrathoracic pressure changes can result in distortion of intrathoracic structures and can impair cardiac filling and cardiac function. The negative intrathoracic pressure directly results in an increased left ventricular (LV) transmural pressure gradient, which effectively acts to increase LV afterload. LV relaxation is also affected, further impeding LV filling and preload. Increased afterload and reduced preload together lead to a reduction in stroke volume (SV) and CO during the apnea. With arousal and resumption of breathing, venous return increases, potentially distending the right ventricle and causing the interventricular septum to shift to the left, resulting in impairment of both LV compliance and LV diastolic filling.

## MECHANISMS LINKING OBSTRUCTIVE SLEEP APNEA AND CARDIOVASCULAR DISEASE

### Sympathetic Activation

Patients with OSA have been shown to have faster HR, decreased HR variability, and increased BP variability compared to matched controls. Decreased HR variability and increased BP variability have been shown to elevate cardiovascular risk. Normotensive individuals with decreased HR variability have a higher risk for future hypertension. Increased BP variability is associated with target organ damage.

- The decreased HR variability as well as increased BP variability seen in OSA is likely due to a heightened sympathetic drive. Interestingly, the heightened sympathetic drive is present even during awake normoxic conditions.

- This high level of tonic sympathetic excitation may, in part, be due to increased chemoreflex activation. Deactivating chemoreflex drive by having OSA patients breathe 100% $O_2$ results in a significant decrease in sympathetic activity, HR, and BP.

### Oxidative Stress, Inflammation, and Endothelial Dysfunction

Reactive oxygen species (ROS) and oxidative stress have been implicated in the development and progression of cardiovascular disease. ROS are highly reactive molecules that react with proteins, nucleic acids, and lipids, resulting in cell injury.

- Obstructive sleep apnea is characterized by repetitive episodes of hypoxia followed by reoxygenation. The repetitive hypoxia/reoxygenation in OSA may be analogous to tissue reperfusion injury, which is associated with the formation of reactive oxygen species and endothelial damage. The role of reactive oxygen species and oxidative stress, however, in the development of cardiovascular disease in patients with OSA remains controversial. Some studies have found increased levels of ROS breakdown products in patients with OSA, whereas others have not. Reactive nitrogen species (RNS) and nitrosative stress have also been implicated as possible mechanisms for the development of cardiovascular disease. However, it has recently been shown that OSA may not be accompanied by increased free nitrotyrosine, a marker for nitrosative stress.

- There is increasing evidence that inflammation plays an important role in the development of ather-

osclerosis and cardiovascular disease. C-reactive protein (CRP) and serum amyloid-A (SAA), both nonspecific markers of systemic inflammation, may be risk factors for cardiovascular disease. Patients with OSA have increased levels of both CRP and SAA. It has been suggested that CRP may decrease after continuous positive airway pressure (CPAP) therapy. The increased levels of these inflammatory markers suggest that OSA represents a state of heightened systemic inflammation. Further evidence of this is the observation that various cytokines, including TNFα, IL-8, and IL-6, have been found to be increased in OSA when compared to controls. IL-6 induces production of CRP from the liver. The primary stimulus for this state of heightened inflammation is unclear. ROS species may play a role by directly stimulating endothelial cells to produce proinflammatory cytokines and upregulate adhesion molecules. Low oxygen tension itself has also been shown to directly stimulate circulating leukocytes. Adherence of leukocytes to the endothelium is considered to be an important event in the development of endothelial dysfunction.

- Endothelial dysfunction is considered to be a nascent form of atherosclerosis and is thought to play a vital role in the development of a wide array of cardiovascular diseases. Endothelial dysfunction can be seen in patients with hypertension, hyperlipidemia, diabetes, and smoking. Patients with OSA who are free of any other overt cardiac or vascular disease have impaired endothelial function. This suggests that OSA itself may be an independent risk factor for the development of impaired endothelial function. Adhesion of leukocytes to vascular endothelium is thought to interfere with the ability of endothelial cell-derived nitric oxide (NO) to relax vascular smooth muscle. This results in impairment of endothelium-dependent vasodilation. Animals pretreated with blocking antibodies directed against adhesion molecules have shown attenuation of this impairment. Several studies have demonstrated that adhesion receptor expression e.g., intercellular adhesion molecule (ICAM), vascular cell adhesion molecule (VCAM), E-selectin is significantly increased in patients with OSA compared to obese controls. Although some studies have measured circulating adhesion receptors, this increase suggests that the endothelium is activated and "primed" for binding with leukocytes. It has also been shown that monocytes isolated from OSA patients have increased expression of adhesion molecules (CD15, CD11c) and demonstrate increased adherence to human endothelial cells in culture. Levels of adhesion receptors, proinflammatory cytokines, and monocyte adherence have been shown to decrease after therapeutic CPAP. Interestingly, leukocytes isolated from OSA patients show higher levels of ROS production, which may play a role in directly inactivating NO. Studies by several groups have also shown that NO breakdown products are reduced in OSA, suggesting an impairment of NO synthesis.

- Other abnormalities of the vascular endothelium associated with OSA have been described. Endothelin-1 is a potent long-acting vasoconstrictor important for regulating vascular tone and is elevated in OSA, which may contribute to sustained vasoconstriction. Furthermore, endothelin-1 concentration decreases with CPAP therapy. CRP may also contribute to vascular disease by its direct effects on the endothelium.

- Elevated homocysteine levels are also associated with endothelial dysfunction and the development of cardiovascular disease. It was recently demonstrated, however, that homocysteine levels are not elevated in OSA patients compared with controls.

- Vascular endothelial growth factor (VEGF) is a glycoprotein that plays an important role in angiogenesis by stimulating normal and abnormal vessel growth. A recent study found that in patients with OSA, VEGF levels are increased and are related to the severity of OSA. VEGF levels have been shown to decrease with CPAP therapy. A protective role for VEGF against cardiovascular disease has been postulated.

## Disordered Coagulation

Recent evidence suggests that OSA results in abnormalities of coagulation that may be important in the development of cardiovascular disease. Interpretation of many of these studies, however, presents difficulties due to the inclusion of patients with concomitant disease processes such as hypertension, hypercholesterolemia, and smoking that may also have effects on coagulation.

- Several studies have shown that platelet activation and aggregation are increased in patients with OSA. In one recent study, increased platelet activation appeared to be related to increased arousal index. This relationship may reflect sympathetic activation and increased nocturnal levels of catecholamines associated with arousals.

- Total serum fibrinogen and whole blood viscosity levels are also elevated in OSA, which, together with platelet activation, may contribute to a predisposition to clot formation.

- Several coagulation factors including factors XIIa and VIIa are higher in OSA patients. Patients with OSA have also been shown to have increased levels of thrombin breakdown products, D-dimer and thrombin-antithrombin complex (TAT), again implicating an underlying state of hypercoagulability.

- Fibrinolytic activity may also be reduced in OSA.

- Many of these abnormalities in coagulation including platelet activation appear to be alleviated after CPAP therapy. However, a recent study showed that elevated levels of factor XIIa and VIIa, TAT, and soluble P-selectin did not fall with one month of therapeutic CPAP.

## Metabolic Dysregulation

Diabetes and obesity are important risk factors for cardiovascular disease. Recent studies have investigated the possible association between OSA and glucose intolerance and found that OSA patients had higher levels of fasting blood glucose, insulin, and glycosylated hemoglobin compared with matched controls. These changes appeared to be independent of body weight, suggesting that OSA impairs glucose tolerance.

- The severity of OSA appears to correlate with the degree of insulin resistance, and severe OSA has been shown to greatly increase the risk of overt diabetes mellitus. The mechanism by which OSA is linked to impaired glucose tolerance is not fully understood but may be related to sympathetic activation and sleep deprivation. Leptin resistance may also play a role. Leptin, an adipocyte-derived hormone, suppresses appetite and promotes satiety. Obesity is associated with elevated leptin levels, suggesting resistance to the metabolic effects of leptin. Interestingly, men with OSA have higher leptin levels than matched obese individuals without OSA, suggesting an even greater resistance to leptin. Resistance to leptin in OSA patients may predispose to weight gain. Leptin may also predispose to platelet aggregation and has been implicated as an independent marker of increased cardiovascular risk. Recent evidence has shown an independent association between leptin and CRP, supporting a possible inflammatory role for leptin.

## POTENTIAL MECHANISMS LINKING OSA AND CARDIOVASCULAR DISEASE

    Increased sympathetic activation

    Oxidative stress

    Inflammation

    Endothelial dysfunction

    Disordered coagulation

    Metabolic dysregulation

## CARDIOVASCULAR DISEASES ASSOCIATED WITH OSA

### Hypertension

Several studies have demonstrated compelling evidence that implicates OSA in the development of hypertension. Experimentally induced OSA in dogs using intermittent and repetitive airway occlusion during sleep resulted in a 15% increase in both nocturnal and daytime BP within 5 weeks.

- In humans, four large cross-sectional population-based studies and one prospective population-based study have found associations between the apnea–hypopnea index (AHI) and daytime hypertension.

- The Sleep Heart Health Study examined the association between OSA and BP in over 6000 subjects. Results suggested that OSA was independently associated with hypertension. The odds ratio for the most severe group was 1.37, showing an overall small to moderate effect. More specifically, the prevalence of hypertension was found to progressively increase with severity of OSA (i.e., increasing AHI). The Sleep Heart Health Study and other cross-sectional studies have also found stronger associations between OSA and hypertension in less obese and younger subjects.

- Evidence that implicates OSA in the development of hypertension has come from the prospective findings of the Wisconsin Sleep Cohort. In this study, an AHI of 15 or greater was associated with a three fold increased risk of developing new hypertension when subjects were evaluated 4 years after the initial sleep study. Even subjects with minimally elevated baseline AHI (AHI >0 but <5) had a 42% increased odds of developing hypertension over the 4-year follow-up.

- The recent set of guidelines from the Joint National Committee on the Detection, Prevention, Evaluation and Treatment of High Blood Pressure (JNC VII) lists OSA as the first of the identifiable causes of hypertension.

- The mechanisms linking OSA with hypertension are complex and not fully elucidated. As discussed above, however, increased sympathetic activity, inflammation-mediated endothelial dysfunction, and predisposition to weight gain due to leptin resistance likely play important roles in the pathogenesis of hypertension in OSA.

- Although there is general consensus that CPAP treatment reduces nocturnal BP in patients with OSA, the effect on daytime BP is less clear. The effectiveness of CPAP in reducing daytime BP in hypertensive patients has been recently evaluated in several studies. Two randomized placebo-controlled trials using subtherapeutic or "sham" CPAP as a control demonstrated that several months of CPAP resulted in a reduction in daytime BP of between 1.3 and 5.3 mm Hg. The effect seemed to be greatest in patients with more severe OSA compared with those with mild OSA. A consistent decrease in diastolic BP after 24 h of CPAP has also been observed.

### Ischemic Heart Disease

There is a high prevalence of OSA in patients with coronary artery disease (CAD). This association is supported by several case-controlled and cross-sectional epidemiologic studies.

- In the Sleep Heart Health Study cohort, OSA was found to be an independent risk factor for CAD. The presence of OSA in patients with CAD may also be a prognostic indicator.

- There is also evidence supporting an association between OSA and myocardial infarction (MI). OSA has been shown to be very common in patients with prior MI. In these patients, OSA appears to be as strong a risk factor as obesity, smoking, and hypertension.

- Obstructive sleep apnea is associated with intermittent hypoxemia, $CO_2$ retention, sympathetic activation, surges in BP, and increases in LV afterload. Not surprisingly, all of these may predispose to the development of nocturnal myocardial ischemia. Studies have noted nocturnal ST-segment changes consistent with myocardial ischemia in patients with OSA who do not have clinically significant CAD. Patients with severe OSA demonstrate more frequent ST-segment depression, and CPAP has been shown to reduce the total duration of ST-segment depression in these patients. The ST-segment changes may be related to increased myocardial oxygen demand during the postapneic surge in BP and HR at a time when oxyhemoglobin saturation remains low. Although some patients with OSA may experience nocturnal ischemia, a recent study found that cardiac troponin T was not elevated in patients with severe OSA and coexistent CAD, suggesting that myocardial injury is not taking place.

### Heart Failure

Sleep-disordered breathing in patients with HF can be primarily obstructive, primarily central [e.g., Cheyne–Stokes respirations (CSR) or central sleep apnea (CSA)], or a combination of both. Epidemiologic studies suggest an association between OSA and HF.

- The Sleep Heart Health Study demonstrated that patients with OSA (defined as an AHI $\geq$ 11) were more than twice as likely to have heart failure. In this group of subjects, the odds ratio of having heart failure was higher than that for all other cardiovascular diseases.

- In other case-control studies, 11–37% of HF patients undergoing polysomnography (PSG) were found to have OSA. Although OSA has been associated with both systolic and diastolic dysfunction, patients with diastolic dysfunction may have an especially high likelihood of OSA. Diastolic dysfunction may be related to long-standing hypertension and the effects of increased afterload and transmural wall stress associated with the direct effects of recurrent apneas over a lengthy period. Acute exacerbations in HF can also occur due to the acute effects of OSA on LV function.

- Obstructive sleep apnea may contribute directly to the development of HF by its effects on sympathetic drive, endothelial function, hypertension, and ischemic heart disease, all of which are known to be important risk factors for HF. Activation of inflammation in OSA may also be an important factor as systolic dysfunction can be induced directly by inflammatory cytokines via their effects on myocardial contractility.

- Heart failure may, itself, predispose to the development of OSA. During sleep, the supine position may lead to redistribution of edema from the lower extremities to the upper airway. Upper airway soft tissue edema can result in increased upper airway resistance, increased inspiratory force, and potential collapse.

- Pulmonary congestion and stretch of pulmonary vagal receptors may lead to hyperventilation and daytime hypocapnia predisposing to periodic breathing during sleep. During periodic breathing, central respiratory drive and drive to the pharyngeal dilator muscles decline, which may result in collapse of the vulnerable upper airway. Interestingly, during PSG many of these patients will demonstrate predominantly periodic breathing in the first half of the night followed by predominantly obstructive apneas during the latter half. Therefore the coexistence of OSA and HF may result in a vicious cycle.

- Preliminary data suggest that treatment of OSA in patients with HF may have important beneficial effects. The physiologic effects of CPAP in OSA include reducing LV afterload, increasing SV, reducing myocardial oxygen demand, and reducing cardiac and peripheral sympathetic tone. In some respects, the effects of CPAP are analogous to the effects of β-blockers.

- Several small short-term studies of patients with HF and OSA have shown a modest improvement of both ejection fraction and functional class after treatment with CPAP for as little as one month.

- Larger randomized trials need to be done to determine whether specific treatment of OSA in HF patients will result in a reduction of long-term morbidity and mortality.

### Cardiac Arrhythmias

Obstructive sleep apnea patients undergoing PSG are frequently noted to have disturbances of cardiac rhythm.

- Sinus bradycardia, sinus pauses, and sinoatrial block are the most frequently observed nocturnal disturbances in rhythm. These bradyarrhythmias are associated with the apneic event and likely represent a form of the "diving response" whereby apnea and hypoxemia trigger a reflex increase in vagal tone. Effective treatment of OSA with CPAP results in resolution of these bradyarrhythmias.

- Supraventricular tachycardias have also been shown in patients with OSA. These appear to resolve after CPAP therapy as well.

- Evidence implicating OSA in the development of other serious arrhythmias including ventricular tachycardia remains unclear. Several studies have shown conflicting results regarding the association between OSA and ventricular tachycardia. Although it is generally thought to be more prevalent with

desaturations of < 65%, methodologic limitations, small sample sizes, comorbid conditions, and lack of control groups have allowed only limited conclusions.

- An association between OSA and atrial fibrillation (AF) has been noted. OSA appears to play a role in the recurrence of AF after cardioversion. One study showed that untreated OSA in patients cardioverted for AF doubled the likelihood of recurrence of AF within 12 months compared to patients receiving effective CPAP treatment. Another study found that close to half of patients with AF are likely to have OSA. This study also showed that the association of OSA with AF was even greater than the association of OSA with hypertension, body mass index, or neck circumference. Adrenergic activation, acute BP changes, and cardiac distortion induced by obstructive apneas may play a role in the association between OSA and AF.

### CARDIOVASCULAR DISEASES POTENTIALLY ASSOCIATED WITH OSA

Hypertension
Ischemic heart disease
Heart failure
    LV systolic dysfunction
    LV diastolic dysfunction
    Congestive heart failure
Bradyarrhythmias
    Sinus bradycardia
    Sinus pause
    Sinoatrial arrest
Atrial fibrillation
Stroke
Pulmonary hypertension

### KEY POINTS

1. Cardiovascular disease is a major cause of morbidity and mortality. Large epidemiologic studies show that patients with OSA have an increased risk of hypertension, ischemic heart disease, stroke, and heart failure.

2. Obstructive sleep apnea causes acute changes in cardiovascular regulation during sleep, disrupting the normal state of cardiovascular relaxation. Recent studies intimate an important role for sympathetic activation, inflammation and endothelial dysfunction, disordered coagulation, metabolic dysregulation, and, possibly, oxidative stress in the development of cardiovascular disease. However, whether treatment of OSA attenuates cardiovascular risk remains to be determined.

## BIBLIOGRAPHY

Becker HF, et al. Effect of nasal continuous positive airway pressure treatment on blood pressure in patients with obstructive sleep apnea. *Circulation* 2003; 107:68–73.

Bradley TD, et al. Sleep apnea and heart failure: Part I: Obstructive sleep apnea. *Circulation* 2003; 107:1671–1678.

Brooks D, et al. Obstructive sleep apnea as a cause of systemic hypertension. Evidence from a canine model. *J Clin Invest* 1997; 99:106–109.

Gami AS, et al. Cardiac troponin T in obstructive sleep apnea. *Chest* 2004a; 125:2097–2100.

Gami AS, et al. Association of atrial fibrillation and obstructive sleep apnea. *Circulation* 2004b; 110:364–367.

Hui DS, et al. The effects of nasal continuous positive airway pressure on platelet activation in obstructive sleep apnea syndrome. *Chest* 2004; 125:1768–1775.

Ip MS, et al. Obstructive sleep apnea is independently associated with insulin resistance. *Am J Respir Crit Care Med* 2002; 165:670–676.

Kanagala R, et al. Obstructive sleep apnea and the recurrence of atrial fibrillation. *Circulation* 2003; 107:2589–2594.

Kaneko Y, et al. Cardiovascular effects of continuous positive airway pressure in patients with heart failure and obstructive sleep apnea. *N Engl J Med* 2003; 348:1233–1241.

Kato M, et al. Impairment of endothelium-dependent vasodilation of resistance vessels in patients with obstructive sleep apnea. *Circulation* 2000; 102:2607–2610.

Lavie L, et al. Plasma vascular endothelial growth factor in sleep apnea syndrome: Effects of nasal continuous positive air pressure treatment. *Am J Respir Crit Care Med* 2002; 165:1624–1628.

Milleron O, et al. Benefits of obstructive sleep apnoea treatment in coronary artery disease: A long-term follow-up study. *Eur Heart J* 2004; 25:728–734.

Narkiewicz K, et al. Selective potentiation of peripheral chemoreflex sensitivity in obstructive sleep apnea. *Circulation* 1999; 99:1183–1189.

Nieto FJ, et al. Association of sleep-disordered breathing, sleep apnea, and hypertension in a large community-based study. Sleep Heart Health Study. *JAMA* 2000; 283:1829–1836.

Ohga E, et al. Increased levels of circulating ICAM-1, VCAM-1, and L-selectin in obstructive sleep apnea syndrome. *J Appl Physiol* 1999; 87:10–14.

Ohga E, et al. Effects of obstructive sleep apnea on circulating ICAM-1, IL-8, and MCP-1. *J Appl Physiol* 2003; 94:179–184.

Peled N, et al. Nocturnal ischemic events in patients with obstructive sleep apnea syndrome and ischemic heart disease: Effects of continuous positive air pressure treatment. *J Am Coll Cardiol* 1999; 34:1744–1749.

Peppard PE, et al. Prospective study of the association between sleep-disordered breathing and hypertension. *N Engl J Med* 2000; 342:1378–1384.

Pepperell JC, et al. Ambulatory blood pressure after therapeutic and subtherapeutic nasal continuous positive airway pressure for obstructive sleep apnoea: A randomised parallel trial. *Lancet* 2002; 359:204–210.

Phillips BG, et al. Increases in leptin levels, sympathetic drive, and weight gain in obstructive sleep apnea. *Am J Physiol Heart Circ Physiol* 2000; 279:H234–H237.

Punjabi NM, et al. Sleep-disordered breathing and insulin resistance in middle-aged and overweight men. *Am J Respir Crit Care Med* 2002; 165:677–682.

Robinson GV, et al. Circulating cardiovascular risk factors in obstructive sleep apnoea: Data from randomised controlled trials. *Thorax* 2004; 59:777–782.

Schulz R, et al. Enhanced release of superoxide from polymorphonuclear neutrophils in obstructive sleep apnea. Impact of continuous positive airway pressure therapy. *Am J Respir Crit Care Med* 2000; 162:566–570.

Shamsuzzaman AS, et al. Obstructive sleep apnea: Implications for cardiac and vascular disease. *JAMA* 2003; 290:1906–1914.

Sin DD, et al. Effects of continuous positive airway pressure on cardiovascular outcomes in heart failure patients with and without Cheyne-Stokes respiration. *Circulation* 2000; 102:61–66.

Wallace AM, et al. Plasma leptin and the risk of cardiovascular disease in the west of Scotland coronary prevention study (WOSCOPS). *Circulation* 2001; 104:3052–3056.

# 19

## NEUROCOGNITIVE AND FUNCTIONAL IMPAIRMENT IN OBSTRUCTIVE SLEEP APNEA

W. David Brown
Sleep Diagnostics of Texas, The Woodlands, Texas

### INTRODUCTION

The primary events of obstructive sleep apnea (OSA) include repetitive episodes of hypoxemia, hypercapnia, and arousals, the latter giving rise to sleep fragmentation. Apnea can also be associated with daytime sleepiness, transient blood pressure elevations, changes in serum chemistry, and, possibly, changes in brain morphology.

- Both the primary events and secondary consequences of obstructed breathing during sleep could theoretically lead to cognitive, emotional, and behavioral changes.

### NEUROCOGNITIVE FUNCTIONING

Among the major symptoms of OSA are intellectual deterioration and difficulty focusing and concentrating.

- Although cognitive impairment is often found in studies of patients with OSA, there is a great deal of discrepancy between studies, and the clinical significance of the changes noted is uncertain. This may reflect the difficulty in measuring a broad range of "cognitive" abilities, limitations of cognitive tests and study designs, differing severity of study groups, the presence of comorbid medical conditions, and the possible age-related effects on cognition. Attempts to attribute measured changes in cognition to a specific primary cause, such as sleep fragmentation or hypoxemia, have also proven difficult because of the interrelations of these factors.
- General intellectual functioning is the broadest measure that attempts to describe cognitive changes and is typically assessed with all or part of the Wechsler Adult Intelligence Scale (WAIS-R). Most studies that have used this inclusive measure find that OSA has a negative impact on intellectual functioning, and hypoxemia is the proposed mechanism

causing the impairment. However, a recent meta-analysis found that general intelligence and verbal intelligence are unaffected by OSA, and that patients with OSA perform better than both norm-referenced and control-referenced data. Visual intelligence produces a much greater effect size but has considerable variability.

- Frequent arousals from sleep, sleep stage deprivation, and transient hypoxemia have all been associated with memory impairment. As such, there is a great deal of interest in the role of apnea on memory. Memory is, however, a complex process, that is divided into different components such as short- and long-term, as well as, verbal and visual memory. Short-term memory can be further divided into working memory, and this memory can have further subdivisions.
- Most studies have found decrements in long-term memory in OSA patients. The majority of studies attribute the memory changes to hypersomnolence, but other studies have attributed the changes to hypoxemia. There is a small, but significant, association between polysomnographic (PSG) measures of sleep-disordered breathing (SDB) and a range of neuropsychological functions, including working memory, declarative memory, and signal discrimination; however, in one study, vigilance was negatively associated with sleepiness and was not explained by PSG variables.
- Even patients with mild apnea (apnea-hypopnea index (AHI) of 10–30 episodes/h without significant hypoxemia) may demonstrate vigilance and working memory deficits.
- Most studies are consistent in showing that OSA has pronounced effects on attention and vigilance. OSA markedly impairs sustained attention. The cause of the impairment remains controversial but may be due to chronic hypoxemia and/or excessive sleepiness. Attention returns to normal following treatment.

- Motor skills have also been found to be impaired in OSA patients. The major effects are seen in fine motor skills compared to gross motor speed. In some studies, manual dexterity did not return to normal following treatment, suggesting irreversible anoxic central nervous system (CNS) damage.

- Executive functions include skills such as problem solving, goal-oriented behavior, and mental flexibility. Most studies have found some impairment of executive functioning, but some studies have failed to find significant changes. Most authors consider the executive changes to be caused by hypoxemia, and functioning does not completely return following treatment; this suggests that impairment may be a permanent result of anoxic CNS damage.

## MOOD

Many studies have examined the psychological correlates of OSA. The tests typically used to assess emotional functioning are the Minnesota Multiphasic Personality Inventory (MMPI), Profile of Mood States (POMS), Beck Depression Inventory (BDI), and Symptom Checklist (SCL-90).

- Studies that used the MMPI typically find that patients with OSA have elevated scores on hypochondriasis (scale1), depression (scale 2), hysteria (scale 3), and social introversion (scale 0). This pattern suggests mild chronic dysphoria, tendency to focus on somatic problems, lowered activity level, difficulty expressing emotions, emotional apathy, and subjective helplessness. SCL-90 scores are often consistent with the MMPI, showing somatic concerns and dysphoric moods and suggesting that apnea patients have a "somatic-depressive" personality pattern.

- Researchers have demonstrated that BDI scores of depression correlated with the total number of obstructive apneas and with the AHI. Although OSA may not be a primary cause of psychiatric disorders, apneas can worsen mood. Other studies, however, have found no association with the existence or severity of OSA with either depression or anxiety. Sleep disruption is a common symptom of both depression and OSA, and some of the differences found may simply reflect the items on the instrument related to sleep quality and daytime sleepiness.

- Mood generally improves with treatment of OSA with continuous positive airway pressure (CPAP); however, this is not always the case.

## QUALITY OF LIFE

Obstructive sleep apnea can have a negative effect on cognitive functioning and emotion. The immediate symptoms of loud snoring, disturbed sleep, and daytime sleepiness, as well the stress of living with a chronic illness, can all conspire to diminish quality of life (QOL).

- Among the most common concerns raised by patients with severe OSA are abnormal fatigue and somnolence, obesity, snoring, depression, use of alcohol and antidepressants, frequent nocturnal awakenings, problems with CPAP (nasal mask and noise), relationship and sexual problems, loss of memory, and fear of death.

## MARITAL PROBLEMS

Several common symptoms of OSA can lead to adverse consequences in the family. Loud snoring, the most common symptom of OSA, is often the primary reason for patients to seek help. It has a disruptive effect on spouses' sleep and frequently results in couples sleeping in separate bedrooms; this puts an added burden on a marriage. In contrast to divorced individuals, married patients with OSA are more depressed, exhausted, and socially isolated. In one study, improvement in a patient's apnea hypopnea index reduced the bed partner's arousal index and improved the latter's sleep efficiency.

- Obstructive sleep apnea and sleepiness are important predictors of divorce, and the rate of divorce is two to three times higher in patients with OSA and sleepiness compared to normal individuals. In men, divorce rate is affected if OSA is severe enough to cause daytime sleepiness.

- Obstructive sleep apnea has a more pronounced effect on divorce rate in women, in whom OSA and sleepiness are associated with a seven times higher likelihood of being divorced at least twice.

- Erectile dysfunction (ED) and other sexual problems are common in men with OSA. ED has been reported in 30–68% of OSA patients. ED may be caused by hypertension or the use of hypertensive medication or, perhaps, a low testosterone level. A recent study suggests that ED is related, at least in part, to nerve alterations related to the severity of OSA and the degree of hypoxia. Conversely, there is no indication that men with ED are more likely to present with risk factors for OSA than those without ED.

## WORK AND HEALTH

- Daytime sleepiness associated with OSA often impairs the patient's ability to work, to solve problems at work or at home, or even perform simple tasks. Many have either lost their jobs or are on the verge of losing it due to their inability to adequately perform at the workplace. OSA patients perceive themselves as having poorer health and, as a result, have more sick leave than other workers. These patients may also limit their social activities due to embarrassment about falling asleep at inappropriate times.

- Studies that have systematically looked at the QOL in social, emotional, and physical domains using the Sickness Impact Profile (SIP) and the Medical

Outcomes Study SF-36 (SF-36) have demonstrated severely impaired QOL in patients with OSA. Even mild apnea may lead to diminished QOL in a number of areas.

## KEY POINTS

1. Obstructive sleep apnea appears to cause measurable changes in neurocognitive functioning. The most robust negative effects are seen in attention, vigilance, and executive functioning. Fine motor skills and manual dexterity are more impaired than gross motor speed. OSA has less clear effects on general intelligence and verbal fluency.

2. Effects on memory are difficult to interpret. Even mild OSA appears to negatively effect memory. Short-term visual memory appears to be most sensitive to the disorder, but long-term memory may also be affected. Some functioning returns to normal following treatment of OSA with nasal CPAP but other impairments remain, suggesting that sleep disruption, daytime sleepiness, and hypoxemia have differential effects on cognitive functioning, and that OSA may result in permanent anoxic central nervous system damage.

3. Individuals with moderate to severe OSA describe themselves as excessively sleepy. They report difficulty with attention, concentration, and planning. They work shorter hours or are working less efficiently, and acknowledge declines in recreation time and hobbies, as well as increases in interpersonal difficulties. They experience greater difficulty in performing everyday activities such as bathing and grocery shopping. They have more bodily pain and reduced energy levels and perceive their overall health to be poorer than the general population.

4. In an obese population with OSA, subjects reported more impaired work performance and increased sick leave, the best predictor of which is frequent sleepiness. OSA patients with sleepiness average 5 weeks more sick leave than individuals without OSA. This finding was independent of other medical conditions such as hypertension or diabetes.

5. Obstructive sleep apnea is also associated with increased accidents. Compared to those without SDB, men who are habitual snorers or have an AHI > 5 are at least three times as likely to have had at least one accident. Men and women with an AHI > 15 are seven times as likely to have had multiple accidents during a 5-year period compared to normal individuals, independent of age, average miles driven annually, alcohol use, body mass index, and education.

6. Quality of life issues may ultimately be the most interesting consequence of OSA. Loud snoring, erectile dysfunction, and daytime fatigue can place a significant strain on a marriage, resulting in marital problems or divorce. Daytime fatigue can result in increased accidents and diminished work performance resulting in fewer promotions or even loss of work. The stress of living with a chronic illness can result in increased anxiety and diminished QOL. These factors may be the initial concerns that lead individuals to seek treatment, and improvement in QOL may ultimately determine compliance with treatment.

7. Quality of life measures improve with optimal treatment; the largest effects are in the areas of sleep quality, rest, recreation, pastimes, and social functioning. There are moderately large improvements in psychological functioning, completion of household tasks, and work performance.

## BIBLIOGRAPHY

Adams N, et al. Relation of measures of sleep-disordered breathing to neuropsychological functioning. *Am J Respir Crit Care Med* 2001; 163:1626–1631.

Aikens JE, et al. A matched comparison of MMPI responses in patients with primary snoring or obstructive sleep apnea. *Sleep* 1999a; 22:355–359.

Aikens JE, et al. MMPI correlates of sleep and respiratory disturbance in obstructive sleep apnea. *Sleep* 1999b; 22:362–369.

Akashiba T, et al. Relationship between quality of life and mood or depression in patients with severe sleep apnea syndrome. *Chest* 2002; 122:861–865.

Baldwin CN, et al. The association of sleep-disordered breathing and sleep symptoms with quality of life in the sleep heart health study. *Sleep* 2001; 24:96–105.

Beebe DW, et al. The neuropsychological effects of obstructive sleep apnea: A meta-analysis of norm-referenced and case controlled data. *Sleep* 2003; 26:298–307.

Beninati W, et al. The effect of snoring and obstructive sleep apnea on the sleep quality of bed partners. *Mayo Clin Proc* 1999; 74:955–958.

Boland LL, et al. Measures of cognitive function in persons with varying degrees of sleep-disordered breathing: The Sleep Heart Health Study. *J Sleep Res* 2002; 11:265–272.

D'Ambrosio C, et al. Quality of life in patient's with obstructive sleep apnea. Effect of nasal continuous positive airway pressure—A prospective study. *Chest* 1999; 115:123–129.

Decary A, et al. Cognitive deficits associated with sleep apnea syndrome: A proposed neuropsychological test battery. *Sleep* 2000; 23:369–381.

Fanfulla F, et al. Erectile dysfunction in men with obstructive sleep apnea: An early sign of nerve involvement. *Sleep* 2000; 23:775–781.

Ferini-Strambi L, et al. Cognitive dysfunction in patients with obstructive sleep apnea (OSA): Partial reversibility after continuous positive airway pressure (CPAP). *Brain Res Bull* 2003; 61:87–92.

Jenkinson C, et al. Comparison of three measures of quality of life outcome in the evaluation of continuous positive airway pressure for sleep apnoea. *J Sleep Res* 1997; 6:199–204.

Macey PM, et al. Brain morphology associated with obstructive sleep apnea. *Am J Respir Crit Care Med* 2002; 166:1382–1387.

Naegele B, et al. Cognitive dysfunction in patients with obstructive sleep apnea syndrome (OSAS) after CPAP treatment. *Sleep* 1998; 21:392–397.

Pillar G, et al. Psychiatric symptoms in sleep apnea syndrome: Effects of gender and respiratory disturbance index. *Chest* 1998; 114:697–703.

Redline S, et al. Neuropsychological function in mild sleep-disordered breathing. *Sleep* 1997; 20:160–167.

Roth T, et al. Sleep and cognitive (memory) function: Research and clinical perspectives. *Sleep Med* 2001; 2:379–387.

Sateia MJ. Neuropsychological impairment and quality of life in obstructive sleep apnea. *Clin Chest Med* 2003; 24:249–259.

Seftel AD, et al. Erectile dysfunction and symptoms of sleep disorders. *Sleep* 2002; 25:643–647.

Smith R, et al. What are obstructive sleep apnea patient's being treated for prior to this diagnosis? *Chest* 2002; 121:164–172.

Vandeputte M, et al. Sleep disorders and depressive feelings: A global survey with the Beck depression scale. *Sleep Med* 2003; 4:343–345.

Veale D, et al. Identification of quality of life concerns with obstructive sleep apnoea at the time of initiation of continuous positive airway pressure: A discourse analysis. *Qual Life Res* 2002; 11:389–399.

Weaver TE. Outcome measurement in sleep medicine practice and research. Part 1: Assessment of symptoms, subjective and objective daytime sleepiness, health-related quality of life and functional status. *Sleep Med Rev* 2001a; 5:103–128.

Weaver TE. Outcome measurement in sleep medicine practice and research. Part 2: Assessment of neurobehavioral performance and mood. *Sleep Med Rev* 2001b; 5:223–236.

Young T, et al. Sleep-disordered breathing and motor vehicle accidents in a population-based sample of employed adults. *Sleep* 1997; 20:608–613.

Yu BH, et al. Effect of CPAP treatment on mood states in patients with sleep apnea. *J Psychiatr Res* 1999; 33:427–432.

# 20

## POSITIVE AIRWAY PRESSURE THERAPY FOR OBSTRUCTIVE SLEEP APNEA

MAX HIRSHKOWITZ
Baylor College of Medicine and the Michael E. DeBakey VAMC, Houston, Texas

TEOFILO LEE-CHIONG AND DANIEL SMITH
National Jewish Health, Denver, Colorado

## INTRODUCTION

Positive airway pressure therapy is the treatment of choice for most patients with obstructive sleep apnea (OSA). It involves providing a fan or turbine generated air-flow through the nose (and sometimes the nose and mouth) in order to maintain airway patency. There are four general types of positive airway pressure devices.

- *Continuous positive airway pressure* (CPAP) maintains a constant set pressure throughout both inspiration and expiration and currently is the most common therapeutic modality.
- *Bilevel positive airway pressure* (BPAP) provides two pressure levels set differently for inspiration and expiration. The changes in pressure between inspiration and expiration can also be used to assist ventilation.
- *Autotitrating positive airway pressure* (APAP) utilizes variable, automatically self-adjusting air-way pressures that are determined by algorithms that respond to the patient's breathing patterns. APAP is associated with lower mean airway pressures compared to CPAP.
- *Adaptive servo ventilation* delivers varying amounts of ventilatory support as needed based on the presence of apneas or hypopneas (i.e., increasing ventilatory support during periods of central apneas and hypopneas and reducing support during periods of normal respiration or hyperventilation) based on a calculated target minute ventilation that may vary throughout the entire sleep period.

## METHODS OF DETERMINING OPTIMAL POSITIVE AIRWAY PRESSURE

With CPAP, the patient sleeps with a single constant pressure throughout the night. Several methods have been developed for pressure selection; these include the following:

- Attended full-night laboratory polysomnography during which a technologist adjusts the pressure until obstructive respiratory events are minimized.
- Attended split-night laboratory polysomnography during which the first two, or more, hours are used to diagnose obstructive sleep-disordered breathing, and the remainder of the night is used to adjust pressures until the obstructive respiratory events are maximally diminished. The goal is to obtain a fixed single pressure that eliminates apnea, hypopnea, snoring, and respiratory effort-related arousals (RERAs) in all body positions and sleep stages. In general, higher pressures are required to prevent airway occlusion during rapid eye movement (REM) sleep than during non-REM sleep, except in patients with congestive heart failure. Additionally, sleep-disordered breathing is usually worse when an individual sleeps supine. The optimal pressure determined during this titration procedure is thereafter administered therapeutically nightly at home.
- Formulas-derived pressures from clinical, polysomnographic, and/or anthropometric variables. The calculated pressure can also be used as a starting CPAP pressure for laboratory titration.
- Unattended, and sometimes without even minimal, cardiopulmonary monitoring in the home or in a sleep laboratory using autotitrating devices.

## POSITIVE AIRWAY PRESSURE MECHANISM OF ACTION

It is generally held that the positive pressure creates a pneumatic splint for the vulnerable portions of the

*Sleep Medicine Essentials*, edited by Teofilo L. Lee-Chiong

nasopharyngeal airway. One explanatory model posits that the upper airway functions as a Starling resistor with a collapsible segment in the oropharynx. Airway collapse occurs when the intraluminal pressure is less than the critical opening pressure ($P_{crit}$, or the pressure required to keep it open). As nasal pressure is raised above $P_{crit}$ by positive airway pressure, inspiratory airflow increases in proportion to the level of positive pressure applied until airway occlusions are abolished.

- Upper airway (UA) patency is presumably maintained by head and neck muscle activity. This includes cervical muscles that provide caudal traction on the UA.
- Inspiratory increases in UA patency cannot be attributed solely to activity of UA muscles. The thorax also applies caudal traction to the UA. Tonic thoracic traction on the trachea increases with inspiration and demonstratively improves upper airway patency. This force acts through the pull of mediastinal and pulmonary structures transmitted through the carina as well as intrathoracic pressure changes acting independently to either draw the trachea into or push the trachea out of the thorax.

## EFFICACY OF CPAP IN PATIENTS WITH OBSTRUCTIVE SLEEP APNEA

Overall, CPAP is extremely safe and effective in patients with moderate and severe OSA. Furthermore, the beneficial effects of CPAP are sustained over time with continued use.

- In patients with moderate to severe OSA, CPAP improves sleep quality (e.g., decrease in number of arousals), nocturnal oxygen saturation, daytime alertness (e.g., driving stimulator steering performance), health care utilization (reduction in physician claims and hospitalization), blood pressure control, and mortality.
- Continuous positive airway pressure improves quality of life in patients with moderate to severe sleep apnea.
- Although efficacy is well established in patients with moderate and severe disease, the benefit to patients with mild OSA is less certain. A pathophysiologically defined diagnostic threshold for CPAP providing beneficial outcomes is not well characterized.

## THERAPEUTIC ADHERENCE

Continuous positive airway pressure therapy is only as beneficial as its utilization, and nonadherence to therapeutic regimen is a significant problem in clinical practice. To a large extent, the level of use has as much to do with the individual as it does with the therapy.

- While a noticeably beneficial therapy may lead to somewhat greater adherence in willing patients, a noxious intervention can discourage use in even the most ardent and willing participant. Therefore,

correcting mask problems, discomfort, nasal allergies, and other barriers to utilization, especially during the first few weeks, is critical to achieve therapeutic adherence. By reducing discomfort and immediately attending to difficulties, the clinician can remove barriers to regular use. Improving fit and feel of the mask will help optimize use. In one study, the most common complaints reported by patients on CPAP therapy were nocturnal awakenings and nasal problems, such as dryness, congestion, and sneezing.

- Adherence during the first month of therapy predicts later use through the law of initial effects. Usage level at the start of therapy provides a baseline for how much an individual is likely to accept any therapy or be driven off by its associated difficulties.
- Several factors can improve CPAP adherence, including airway humidification, proper selection of the CPAP interface, and prompt and aggressive management of adverse effects related to CPAP use.
- Utilization of CPAP can also be improved by educational programs (e.g., outpatient group clinics designed to encourage CPAP use, home CPAP education, providing written information about OSA and the importance of regular CPAP use, verbal reinforcement with phone calls, motivational enhancement to reduce ambivalence regarding treatment, and desensitization).

### Nasal Masks, Nasal Pillows, and Full-Face Masks

There is a huge assortment of masks available for delivering positive airway pressure. CPAP is usually applied via a nasal mask. However, some patients have nasal congestion, physically compromised nasal airways, or open their mouths (producing mouth leaks). Mouth leaks often cause discomfort and dissatisfaction with CPAP. Chin straps can sometimes correct mouth leaks, but a full-face mask may be needed. Full-face masks may help patients who are obligate mouth breathers, have chronic nasal congestion, or who are intolerant of nasal masks. Finally, some patients have an aversion to sleeping with a mask that produces a fear response. Desensitization is sometimes helpful; however, the use of a smaller apparatus that provides the airflow directly in the nares sometimes remedies this problem. Such nasal pillows or prongs also provide comfort to patients whose masks seem to continually leak notwithstanding careful sizing and adjustment.

### Humidifiers

Humidification is an important adjunct to CPAP therapy. A large percentage of individuals using CPAP complain of nasal symptoms that in turn adversely affect utilization. Problems may include nasal dryness, rhinorrhea, nasal congestion, sneezing, and epistaxis. Humidification can ameliorate these problems by reducing CPAP-related drying of nasal passages. This result is best achieved with heated humidification. Factors predicting the need for heated humidification include age >60 years, use of drying medications, presence of mucosal disease, and previous uvulopalatopharyngoplasty.

## Nasal Lubrication

A variety of salves, nose drops, and oils are available that purportedly decrease upper airway dryness. However, in one study, heated humidification reduces airway dryness more than oily nose drops.

## Pressure Ramp

Many CPAP machines come equipped with a "pressure ramp." The pressure ramp sets an initial low pressure and then gradually increases pressure to therapeutic level. The amount of time and rate of increase is usually adjustable. Pressure ramps are proposed to improve patient comfort by allowing a patient sufficient time to fall asleep before higher pressures are reached. However, subjective patient responses have been variable. Having lower pressures at sleep onset may permit obstructive events during subtherapeutic CPAP levels and allow sleep-onset central apnea episodes to occur, and repeated activation of the ramp can decrease effective CPAP therapy.

## Using Sedative-Hypnotics

Sedative-hypnotic medications (i.e., benzodiazepine receptor agonist sleeping pills) are sometime prescribed for patients that have difficulty sleeping with CPAP. These sedating medications are sometimes used to assist patients during the acclimatization phase of initial CPAP use or to treat insomnia that might be unmasked by CPAP therapy's ability to resolve accumulated sleep debt. The clinician must exercise great caution whenever sedative-hypnotics are used in OSA because these medications can increase arousal threshold, prolonged apnea duration, decrease respiratory drive, and worsen oxygen desaturation.

## OTHER MODES OF POSITIVE AIRWAY PRESSURE

### Autotitrating PAP

Optimal CPAP pressure may vary significantly over the course of a single night depending on the different sleep stages and changes in body position. Night-to-night variability can also be provoked by a host of factors (e.g., drinking alcohol near bedtime or being acutely sleep deprived). Using a fixed single pressure based on supine REM sleep (when pressure requirement is often maximal) usually involves using more pressure than needed for most of the night. Using higher than needed pressure increases the propensity of mask leaks, mouth leaks, and pressure intolerance. APAP devices use a variety of algorithms to adjust flow; therefore, patients with conditions and comorbidities that potentially interfere with adjustment accuracy are contraindicated.

- Autotitrating PAP titration and treatment are not currently recommended for (a) patients with heart failure, (b) patients with significant lung disease (e.g., chronic obstructive pulmonary disease, daytime hypoxemia, and respiratory failure from any cause),

(c) patients taking medication that decreases respiratory drive, (d) patients who have undergone upper airway surgeries, (e) patients with neuromuscular disease, or (f) patients with prominent nocturnal arterial oxygen desaturation due to conditions other than OSA (e.g., obesity hypoventilation syndrome).
- Autotitrating PAP efficacy in autoadjusting mode (APAP treatment) matches conventional constant-pressure CPAP in reducing the apnea-hypopnea indices, improving sleep quality, and adherence to use.
- Another application of APAP technology involves using the device to identify a fixed single pressure for subsequent treatment with a conventional CPAP device (APAP titration), and several studies have found that APAP titration compares favorably to conventional CPAP titration.
- There is an uncertain equivalence in performance of APAP machines made by different manufacturers or even between different APAP models made by the same manufacturer. Research outcomes with one APAP brand and model do not necessarily generalize to other devices because each manufacturer has different computer algorithms controlling pressure adjustment.
- Patients who do not snore (either due to palate surgery or naturally) should not be titrated with an APAP device that relies on vibration or sound in the device's algorithm.

### Bilevel Positive Airway Pressure

Bilevel positive airway pressure (BPAP) devices provide two pressure levels, one during inhalation and a lower one during exhalation. Complaints of dyspnea or discomfort during CPAP use, especially during expiration (against the continuous pressure) may represent a barrier to CPAP adherence in some patients, and BPAP therapy may be considered for them. BPAP therapy may also benefit patients with hypoventilation that persists despite CPAP.

### Noninvasive Positive Pressure Ventilation

Nocturnal noninvasive positive pressure ventilation (NIPPV) can be tried in patients with sleep-related hypoventilation and $CO_2$ retention despite treatment with CPAP and supplemental oxygen. Short-term NIPPV can result in improvements in both nighttime ventilation and daytime blood gas parameters, and permit patients to eventually resume CPAP therapy.

## KEY POINTS

1. Positive airway pressure is the preferred treatment for moderate or severe OSA.
2. There are several varieties of positive pressure devices; however, continuous positive airway pressure (CPAP) is currently the most commonly prescribed.

3. Continuous positive airway pressure improves airway patency during sleep, sleep quality, sleep continuity, daytime alertness, and overall quality of life in symptomatic patients with moderate or severe OSA.

4. Further studies are needed to assess the benefits of CPAP in less severe OSA and to better specify positive cardiovascular outcomes.

5. Continuous positive airway pressure effectiveness is compromised by nonacceptance and nonadherence.

6. Adherence is improved by careful interface selection, optimal mask fit, patient education, heated humidification, and prompt correction of mask and machine-related adverse events.

7. Automatic self-adjusting positive pressure devices (APAP) show great promise; however, at present they are not recommended as a replacement for laboratory titration, particularly in patients with significant cardiovascular and respiratory comorbidities.

8. Adaptive servo ventilation may be considered for patients with complex sleep apnea, a distinct form of sleep-related breathing disorder characterized by the development of central apneas or Cheyne-Stokes pattern of respiration with acute application of CPAP therapy in patients with predominantly obstructive or mixed apneas during the initial diagnostic study.

## BIBLIOGRAPHY

Akashiba T, et al. Nasal continuous positive airway pressure changes blood pressure "non-dippers" to "dippers" in patients with obstructive sleep apnea. *Sleep* 1999; 22:849–853.

Bahammam A, et al. Health care utilization in males with obstructive sleep apnea syndrome two years after diagnosis and treatment. *Sleep* 1999; 22:740–747.

Ballester E, et al. Evidence of the effectiveness of continuous positive airway pressure in the treatment of sleep apnea/hypopnea syndrome. *Am J Respir Crit Care Med* 1999; 159:495–501.

Barnes M, et al. A randomized controlled trial of continuous positive airway pressure in mild obstructive sleep apnea. *Am J Respir Crit Care Med* 2002; 165:773–780.

Berry RB, et al. The use of auto-titrating continuous positive airway pressure for treatment of adult obstructive sleep apnea. An American Academy of Sleep Medicine review. *Sleep* 2002; 25:148–173.

Brown LK. Back to basics: If it's dry, wet it: The case for humidification of nasal continuous positive airway pressure air. *Chest* 2000; 117:617–619.

Chervin RD, et al. Compliance with nasal CPAP can be improved by simple interventions. *Sleep* 1997; 20:284–289.

Dimsdale JE, et al. Effect of continuous positive airway pressure on blood pressure: A placebo trial. *Hypertension* 2000; 35:144–147.

d'Ortho MP, et al. Constant vs. automatic continuous positive airway pressure therapy: Home evaluation. *Chest* 2000; 118:1010–1017.

Engleman HM, et al. Effect of CPAP therapy on daytime function in patients with mild sleep apnoea/hypopnoea syndrome. *Thorax* 1997; 52:114–119.

Engleman HM, et al. Randomized placebo-controlled crossover trial of continuous positive airway pressure for mild sleep apnea/hypopnea syndrome. *Am J Respir Crit Care Med* 1999; 159:461–467.

Faccenda JF, et al. Randomized placebo-controlled trial of continuous positive airway pressure on blood pressure in the sleep apnea-hypopnea syndrome. *Am J Respir Crit Care Med* 2001; 163:344–348.

Hack M, et al. Randomised prospective parallel trial of therapeutic versus subtherapeutic nasal continuous positive airway pressure on simulated steering performance in patients with obstructive sleep apnoea. *Thorax* 2000; 55:224–231.

Hirshkowitz M, et al. Positive airway pressure therapy of OSA. *Semin Respir Crit Care Med* 2005; 26: 68–79.

Hoy CJ, et al. Can intensive support improve continuous positive airway pressure use in patients with the sleep apnea/hypopnea syndrome? *Am J Respir Crit Care Med* 1999; 159:1096–1100.

Hui DS, et al. Effects of augmented continuous positive airway pressure education and support on compliance and outcome in a Chinese population. *Chest* 2000; 117:1410–1416.

Jenkinson C, et al. Comparison of therapeutic and subtherapeutic nasal continuous positive airway pressure for obstructive sleep apnoea: A randomised prospective parallel trial. *Lancet* 1999; 353:2100–2105.

Jenkinson C, et al. Long-term benefits in self-reported health status of nasal continuous positive airway pressure therapy for obstructive sleep apnoea. *QJM* 2001; 94:95–99.

Kingshott RN, et al. Predictors of improvements in daytime function outcomes with CPAP therapy. *Am J Respir Crit Care Med* 2000; 161:866–871.

Lavie P, et al. Obstructive sleep apnoea syndrome as a risk factor for hypertension: Population study. *BMJ* 2000; 320:479–482.

Likar LL, et al. Group education sessions and compliance with nasal CPAP therapy. *Chest* 1997; 111:1273–1277.

Loredo JS, et al. Effect of continuous positive airway pressure vs placebo continuous positive airway pressure on sleep quality in obstructive sleep apnea. *Chest* 1999; 116:1545–1549.

Martins De Araujo MT, et al. Heated humidification or face mask to prevent upper airway dryness during continuous positive airway pressure therapy. *Chest* 2000; 117:142–147.

Massie CA, et al. Effects of humidification on nasal symptoms and compliance in sleep apnea patients using continuous positive airway pressure. *Chest* 1999; 116:403–408.

McArdle N, et al. Long-term use of CPAP therapy for sleep apnea/hypopnea syndrome. *Am J Respir Crit Care Med* 1999; 159:1108–1114.

Mortimore IL, et al. Comparison of nose and face mask CPAP therapy for sleep apnoea. *Thorax* 1998; 53:290–292.

Naughton MT, et al. Sleep apnea in congestive heart failure. *Clin Chest Med* 1998; 19:99–113.

Pepin JL, et al. Effective compliance during the first 3 months of continuous positive airway pressure. A European prospective study of 121 patients. *Am J Respir Crit Care Med* 1999; 160:1124–1129.

Rakotonanahary D, et al. Predictive factors for the need for additional humidification during nasal continuous positive airway pressure therapy. *Chest* 2001; 119:460–465.

Redline S, et al. Improvement of mild sleep-disordered breathing with CPAP compared with conservative therapy. *Am J Respir Crit Care Med* 1998; 157:858–865.

Rosenthal L, et al. CPAP therapy in patients with mild OSA: Implementation and treatment outcome. *Sleep Med* 2000; 1:215–220.

Schafer H, et al. Failure of CPAP therapy in obstructive sleep apnoea syndrome: Predictive factors and treatment with bilevel-positive airway pressure. *Respir Med* 1998; 92: 208–215.

Standards of Practice Committee of the American Academy of Sleep Medicine. Practice parameters for the use of auto-titrating continuous positive airway pressure devices for titrating pressures and treating adult patients with obstructive sleep apnea syndrome. An American Academy of Sleep Medicine Report. *Sleep* 2002; 25:143–147.

Stradling JR, et al. Automatic nasal continuous positive airway pressure titration in the laboratory: Patient outcomes. *Thorax* 1997; 52:72–75.

Weaver TE, et al. Night-to-night variability in CPAP use over the first three months of treatment. *Sleep* 1997; 20:278–283.

Wiest GH, et al. A heated humidifier reduces upper airway dryness during continuous positive airway pressure therapy. *Respir Med* 1999; 93:21–26.

Wright J, et al. Health effects of obstructive sleep apnoea and the effectiveness of continuous positive airways pressure: A systematic review of the research evidence. *BMJ* 1997; 314:851–860.

# 21

## ORAL DEVICES FOR OBSTRUCTIVE SLEEP APNEA

DENNIS R. BAILEY
Englewood, Colorado

### INTRODUCTION

An oral device (OD) is a reasonable means by which sleep-related breathing disorders (SRBD) may be managed. ODs are indicated for snorers and patients with mild to moderate obstructive sleep apnea (OSA) who prefer these devices, are intolerant of positive airway pressure (PAP) therapy, or have failed upper airway surgery for OSA. These devices improve upper airway space by repositioning the mandible both downward (open) and forward.

### TYPES OF ORAL DEVICES

Mandibular repositioners, which fit both the upper and lower teeth for the purpose of repositioning the mandible, can either be a one-piece design (monobloc) for both the upper and lower teeth that stabilized the mandible in a predetermined position (e.g., nocturnal airway patency appliance, or NAPA) or composed of two separate pieces, one for the upper and one for the lower teeth, that are attached in some fashion and allow for movement of the mandible during sleep to varying degrees. An advantage of a two-piece OD is that it allows for a greater ability to adjust and modify the appliance with the intent of achieving the most optimum effectiveness and patient comfort. The two-piece OD can also be used to address comorbid sleep bruxism, if present.

- Certain design characteristics of OD are recommended to maximize its efficacy, reduce adverse effects, and allow alterations of jaw position, when necessary.

*Adjustability* allows for modification of the OD whenever needed in specific situations such as:

- If dental work is done, the OD no longer fits over the teeth and must be adjusted (modified) or realigned

to adapt to the changes that were done (e.g., a crown or large restoration filling).

- The OD becomes loose and needs to be relined to improve its retention.
- If a tooth is lost, the area needs to be sealed or made more secure.

*Titratability* relates to the potential future need to alter the vertical opening of the OD, or if the degree of advancement needs to be changed. Unlike PAP, it is not practical to titrate for effectiveness of the OD during a polysomnography. Sequential adjustments need to be done over time as the patient becomes accustomed to using the appliance, and when changes are indicated to improve results. There are two forms of changes:

- To affect the degree of advancement, including altering an elastic type force or adjusting a screw
- To affect the vertical opening, most commonly by adjusting the contact in the posterior supporting areas of the device

*Full–tooth coverage* is important. The OD should cover all existing teeth since this aids in the prevention of undesirable tooth movement when using the OD.

*Posterior support* is customarily achieved by using flat pads in the posterior aspect of both the upper and lower components that are in contact when the OD is in place. This support is intended to stabilize and support the temporomandibular joints, and to allow the OD to function as a bite splint for the management of comorbid sleep bruxism, if present.

*Jaw mobility* allows for mandibular movement during sleep. Patients, even if they do not have sleep bruxism, experience some degree of jaw movement during sleep and may coexist with swallowing or lip licking.

*Patent nasal passage* is important. Patients should be able to breathe through their nose and have minimal nasal resistance when the OD is in place. This improves oxygen

*Sleep Medicine Essentials*, edited by Teofilo L. Lee-Chiong
Copyright © 2009 John Wiley & Sons, Inc.

levels during sleep, reduces mouth breathing, and may, itself, contribute to the reduction in the respiratory disturbance index.

## INDICATIONS FOR ORAL DEVICES

The generally accepted indications for OD based on the Standards of Practice for oral appliances from the American Academy of Sleep Medicine (AASM) are:

- Snoring when OSA is not present or has been ruled out with a sleep study
- Mild to moderate OSA when weight loss and/or positional therapy is not an option
- Severe OSA when patients are intolerant of, or refuse, PAP therapy
- Obstructive sleep apnea when patients are not candidates for, refuse, or have failed upper airway surgery

## CONTRAINDICATIONS FOR ORAL DEVICES

Oral devices are not indicated for use in the following situations:

- Central sleep apnea
- In patients who are compromised dentally (e.g., loose teeth that have inadequate support, teeth that are diseased or are otherwise compromised, broken teeth, or where there is an inadequate number of teeth to support the OD) for mandibular repositioners
- In patients who have severe temporomandibular joint (TMJ) dysfunction or other types of orofacial pain complaints; however, in many cases, OD may be helpful in comanaging TMJ dysfunction. In cases of severe or chronic TMJ dysfunction management and resolution of the TMJ complaints initially may allow patients to then proceed into OD treatment.

## AVAILABLE ORAL DEVICES FOR SLEEP APNEA

Currently, it is estimated that there are over 40 different ODs available on the market. The most popular and frequently utilized ODs are those that have received clearance from the Federal Drug Administration (FDA) for the management of snoring and OSA. ODs have a class II rating and are viewed as regulated medical devices.

- The FDA recognizes OD in three distinct categories: tongue retaining devices (TRD), mandibular repositioning devices (MRD), and palatal lifting devices. The MRD are the most commonly utilized devices. The TRD may be indicated in select situations such as in patients with compromised dentition or who are edentulous. Palatal lifting devices are infrequently used at this time.

## ORAL DEVICES FOR SPECIAL CIRCUMSTANCES

Two distinct patient types require custom design and fabrication of ODs, namely children or adolescents who have OSA and edentulous patients. On occasion, TRDs may be an effective alternative but many patients do not tolerate this device long term.

- For adolescents, the design of OD is similar to the monobloc appliance used to address malocclusion and to promote jaw growth. These devices will need to be remade over time as the individual grows to address the changes in dentition and occlusion. The use of more conventional FDA-cleared devices becomes possible as the adolescent patient acquires a full adult dentition and where growth and development is completed.
- In the edentulous patient, a form of denture without teeth and with posterior support may be utilized. The posterior support has flat surfaces that are in contact in order to support the mandible vertically and improve the retrolingual space. An alternative design positions the posterior surfaces of the dentures in such a way that it supports the mandible vertically and also is able to advance it when the posterior surfaces come in contact.
- Some patients with OSA may experience improvement in their upper airway space by simply wearing their dentures during sleep. Removing dentures during sleep may lead to airway compromise and worsen existing OSA. Studies have shown that both apnea frequency and oxygen saturation improve when dentures are worn during sleep.

## FUNCTION OF ORAL DEVICES

The primary function of the OD is to open and improve the upper airway during sleep by repositioning the mandible and the tongue to prevent these structures from collapsing into the airway during sleep.

- For an OD to be effective, the lateral dimension of the airway is the critical area where improvement needs to occur.
- The airway of patients with OSA is narrower during sleep compared to controls. The retropalatal and retroglossal airspaces are decreased the most; dimensions of the lateral walls are diminished as well. Studies have demonstrated that with mandibular repositioners, the improvement in the lateral aspect of the retropalatal and retroglossal spaces is greater than the anterior-posterior dimension of the airway.

## EFFECTIVENESS OF ORAL DEVICES

In one study involving patients with a respiratory disturbance index (RDI) < 10, a satisfactory outcome was seen in 57% of patients. At 5 years, RDI decreased from $22 \pm 17$ to

$4.9 \pm 5.1$, demonstrating that there was continued compliance with consistent use and ongoing adjustment or replacement, as needed.

- Patients with OSA appear to tolerate ODs better than PAP therapy.
- Oral devices have improved outcomes over surgery. Because they are less invasive and are reversible, they may be considered over surgery and are reasonable alternatives in the management of OSA when surgery has failed.

## DETERMINING POTENTIAL EFFECTIVENESS OF ORAL DEVICES

It is important to be able to determine the potential effectiveness of an OD prior to its use. In some instances, patients can simply open their mouth and advance the mandible to determine if it is easier to breathe, as well as more difficult to make a snoring sound.

- Another option is the use of sound waves to acoustically image the airway (pharyngometry). Generated sound waves are projected via a soft elastic mouthpiece that, once in contact with the structures in the airway, are reflected back; a computer then interprets the data to determine the anatomical location of collapse. With the mandible repositioned, the test is repeated to determine if there is improvement in the airway dimensions, particularly at the site of narrowing. This technology can be helpful in determining the optimum starting mandibular position when utilizing OD.

## ADVERSE EFFECTS AND THEIR MANAGEMENT

Side effects of OD most often occur early during treatment.

- *Excess salivation* is often present at the initiation of the treatment and usually resolves within the first week once the patient becomes accustomed to the OD. An adequate lip seal with the OD in place can help prevent excess salivation.
- *Dry mouth* is usually related to ongoing mouth breathing. Having a lip seal with the OD in place and being able to breath nasally generally resolve this complication.
- *Tooth movement* is generally minor in nature and not a long-term problem. This is often associated with advanced mandibular repositioning and is less likely with repositioning in the vertical plane. Also, patients may feel as if there is tooth movement when, in fact, they are experiencing minor bite changes.
- *Bite changes* are usually most common in the first half hour following removal of the OD in the morning. These changes are usually subtle and resolve

spontaneously. If they persist, exercises and the use of mild muscle relaxants may be helpful. However, medications, if required, are usually only necessary for a brief period of time until the patient becomes accustomed to the OD.

- *Jaw and/or temporomandibular joint pain* may occur in the early stages of OD use. Often, this is due to strain on the head and neck muscles, and pain from the muscles is felt in the area of the TMJ due to referred pain patterns. Actual joint problems are rare. This pain usually resolves over time. Exercises, muscle relaxant medications, and, at times, physical therapy may be indicated to manage the pain. Specially compounded transdermal medications, such as analgesics or muscle relaxers, applied in the area of the pain may also be helpful.

## KEY POINTS

1. Oral devices are indicated for snorers and patients with mild to moderate obstructive sleep apnea (OSA) who prefer these devices, are intolerant of positive airway pressure (PAP) therapy, or have failed upper airway surgery for OSA.
2. These devices improve upper airway space by repositioning the mandible both downward (open) and forward and prevent the collapse of the tongue and oropharyngeal tissues during sleep.
3. Mandibular repositioners, which fit both the upper and lower teeth for the purpose of repositioning the mandible, can either be a one-piece design (monobloc) for both the upper and lower teeth that stabilizes the mandible in a predetermined position or composed of two separate pieces, that fit over the upper and lower teeth and are connected together in a specific fashion.
4. Oral devices are contraindicated for the management of patients with predominantly central sleep apnea, a compromised dentition (periodontal disease, loose teeth or an insufficient number of teeth), and severe or chronic TMJ dysfunction and some types of orofacial pain complaints.

## BIBLIOGRAPHY

Bucca C, et al. Edentulism and worsening of obstructive sleep apnea. *Lancet* 1999; 353:121.

Center for Devices and Radiological Health, U.S. Food and Drug Administration. Class II special controls guidance document: Intra-oral devices for snoring and/or obstructive sleep apnea: Guidance for industry and FDA. Bulletin, Novemebr 12, 2002.

Endeshaw YW, et al. Association of denture use with sleep-disordered breathing among older adults. *J Public Health Dent* 2004; 64:181–183.

Fransoon A, et al. Influence of mandibular protruding device on airway passages and dentofacial characteristics in obstructive sleep apnea and snoring. *Ann J Orthod Dentofacial Orthop* 2002; 122:371–379.

Frantz D. The difference between success and failure. *Sleep Rev* 2001; 2:20–23

Hibi H, et al. Body posture during sleep and disc displacement in the temporomandibular joint: A pilot study. *J Oral Rehabil* 2005; 32(2):85–89.

Kushida CA, et al. Practice parameters for the treatment of snoring and obstructive sleep apnea with oral appliances: An update for 2005. *Sleep* 2006; 29(2):240–243.

Kyung SH, et al. Obstructive sleep apnea patients with the oral appliance experience pharyngeal size and shape changes in three dimensions. *Angle Orthod* 2005; 75(1):15–22.

Li HY, et al. Nasal resistance in patients with obstructive sleep apnea. *Otorhinolaryngol Relat Spec* 2005; 67:70–74.

Marklund M, et al. Mandibular advancement device in patients with obstructive sleep apnea. *Chest* 2001; 120:162–169.

Marklund M, et al. Mandibular advancement devices in 630 men and women with obstructive sleep apnea and snoring. *Chest* 2004; 125:1270–1278.

McLean HA, et al. Effect of treating severe nasal obstruction on the severity of obstructive sleep apnea. *Eur Respir J* 2005; 25:521–527.

Mehata M, et al. An oral elastic mandibular advancement device for obstructive sleep apnea. *Am J Respir Crit Care Med* 2000; 161:420–425.

Mehata M, et al. A randomized, controlled study of a mandibular advancement splint for obstructive sleep apnea. *Am J Respir Crit Care Med* 2001; 163:1457–1461.

Millaman R, et al. The efficacy of oral appliances in the treatment of persistent sleep apnea after uvulopalatopharyngoplasty. *Chest* 1998; 113:992–996.

Ohayaon M, et al. Risk factors for sleep bruxism in the general population. *Chest* 2001; 119:53–61.

Ribeiro De Alameida F, et al. Effects of mandibular posture on obstructive sleep apnea severity and the temporomandibular joint in patients fitted with an oral appliance. *Sleep* 2002; 25:507–513.

Rose E, et al. Occlusal and skeletal effects of an oral appliance in the treatment of obstructive sleep apnea. *Chest* 2002; 122:871–877.

Schmidt-Nowara W. Recent developments in oral appliance therapy of sleep disordered breathing. *Sleep Breath* 1999; 3:103–106.

Schwab R. Imaging for the snoring and sleep apnea patient. *Dent Clin N Am* 2001; 45: 759–796.

Tan Y, et al. Mandibular advancement splints and continuous positive airway pressure in patients with obstructive sleep apnea: A randomized cross-over trial. *Eur J Orthod* 2002; 24:239–249.

Uzun L, et al. Effectiveness of the jaw-thrust maneuver in opening the airway: A flexible fiberoptic endoscopic study. *J Otorhinolaryngol Relat Spec* 2005; 67:39–44.

Wilhelmsson B, et al. A prospective randomized study of a dental appliance compared with uvulopalatopharyngoplasty in the treatment of obstructive sleep apnea. *Acta Otolaryngol* 1999; 119:503–509.

# 22

# CIRCADIAN RHYTHM SLEEP DISORDERS

YARON DAGAN
Institute for Sleep Medicine, Assuta Medical Center, Tel Aviv, Israel, and Department of Medical Education,
Sackler Faculty of Medicine, Tel Aviv University, Tel Aviv, Israel

KATY BORODKIN
Department of Psychology, Bar Ilan University, Ramat Gan, Israel

LIAT AYALON
Department of Psychiatry, University of California San Diego and Veterans Affairs San Diego Healthcare System,
San Diego, California

## INTRODUCTION

In humans, sleep and wake episodes occur at regular times that match the 24-h day–night cycle. This temporal organization is known as circadian rhythmicity (from the Latin *circa-* "about", *dies-* "day"), which is present in many behavioral and physiological functions, such as fluctuations of body temperature and melatonin secretion. Circadian timing system is thought to play a central role in the generation, maintenance, and synchronization of circadian rhythms to each other and to the environmental 24-h period. The core component of this system is the suprachiasmatic nuclei (SCN) of the hypothalamus, which generate the endogenous circadian rhythms of the organism. The SCN is entrained by environmental factors, the most prominent of which is light.

- The delicate interplay of endogenous and exogenous factors, required to maintain normal sleep–wake rhythm, can become recurrently or chronically impaired in some individuals, leading to a group of disorders called circadian rhythm sleep disorders (CRSDs). CRSDs are characterized by an alteration of the circadian timing system or a misalignment between the timing of the individual's sleep–wake rhythm and the 24-h social and physical environment. In patients with CRSD, sleep episodes occur at inappropriate times, often causing wake periods to occur at undesired times. Consequently, the patient complains of insomnia or excessive daytime sleepiness and impairment in various areas of functioning.
- Circadian rhythm sleep disorders can be classified based on etiology either as behaviorally induced or physiologic disorders. CRSD of physiologic origin can occur as a primary condition or as a result of a medical disorder or drug use. These disorders are considered to be a malfunction of the biological clock per se and presumably can be distinguished from behaviorally induced CRSDs by inflexibility of the sleep–wake cycle. Behaviorally induced CRSDs are a consequence of maladaptive behaviors, such as individual's voluntary choice to create a temporal mismatch between internal and external factors, or environmental conditions, as it occurs in shift work and jet lag.

## DELAYED SLEEP PHASE DISORDER

Delayed sleep phase disorder (DSPD), also known as delayed sleep phase syndrome, is characterized by habitual sleep–wake times that are delayed, usually more than 2 h, relative to conventional or socially acceptable times.

- Sleep onset is typically delayed until 2:00–6:00 AM, and wake time occurs in the late morning or afternoon (Figure 22.1). Although delayed, the sleep–wake cycle is stable, with little day-to-day variability in sleep-onset times. Attempts to advance the sleep–wake phase to earlier hours by enforcing conventional sleep and wake times yield little permanent success. Sleep architecture is usually reported to be normal for age. The disturbance of sleep–wake cycle is strongly associated with severe impairments of social, occupational, and domestic functioning.

*Sleep Medicine Essentials*, edited by Teofilo L. Lee-Chiong
Copyright © 2009 John Wiley & Sons, Inc.

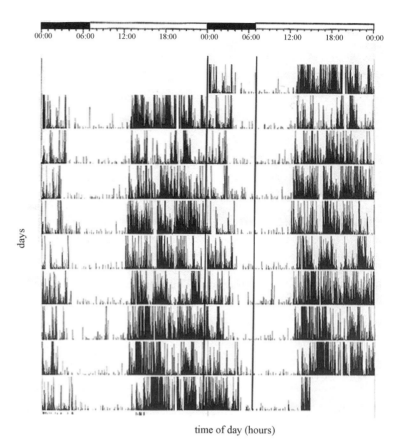

time of day (hours)

**Figure 22.1** Actogram of Delayed sleep phase type. Sleep episodes are represented by white areas, black areas stand for wake episodes. The 24-h period is double-plotted in a raster format. Note that in DSPT, the timing of sleep onset and offset is delayed relative to the circadian night (indicated by two continuous vertical lines along the actogram).

- Delayed sleep phase disorder is more common in adolescents and young adults, with an estimated prevalence of 7–16% in these age groups. It is the most frequent diagnosis (83.5%) among patients with CRSD presenting to sleep clinics for help.
- Pathophysiology of DSPD is largely unknown. Several studies suggest that DSPD is associated with phase changes of the circadian timing system. Familial DSPD has been described in which an autosomal dominant mode of inheritance is evident. Structural polymorphisms in the human period3 gene (hper3) are implicated in the pathogenesis of DSPD.

### ADVANCED SLEEP PHASE DISORDER

Advanced sleep phase disorder (ASPD), also known as advanced sleep phase syndrome, is a stable advance of the major sleep period, characterized by habitual sleep onset and wake-up times that are several hours earlier than desired or socially accepted.

- Typical sleep-onset times are between 6:00 and 9:00 PM, and wake times are between 2:00 and 5:00 AM (Figure 22.2). Patients with ASPD complain of early morning insomnia and excessive evening sleepiness. No abnormalities in sleep architecture are reported if the individual is allowed to maintain an advanced schedule.

- Thought to be less common than DSPD, ASPD is very rare in adolescents and young adults. A prevalence of 1% has been reported in middle-aged adults, and 1.2% in patients with CRSD who presented to sleep clinics. However, the prevalence of this disorder might be underestimated since ASPD is better tolerated than DSPD.
- It is assumed that the pathophysiology of ASPD involves altered phase relationships of endogenous circadian rhythms. Several pedigrees of familial ASPD with advanced melatonin and temperature rhythms has been reported in which the ASPD phenotype segregated as an autosomal dominant mode of inheritance. Although a mutation of human period2 (hper2) gene has been described in a large family with ASPD, other findings indicate genetic heterogeneity in this disorder.

### FREE-RUNNING (NONENTRAINED) TYPE

Free-running type, also known as non-entrained-type or non-24-h sleep–wake syndrome, is marked by sleep–wake cycles that are usually longer than 24 h. Due to this, sleep and wake episodes are delayed each day to later hours, thus alternating between synchrony and complete asynchrony with the environmental schedule (Figure 22.3). Attempts to adopt regular sleep–wake times are associated with difficulties initiating sleep at

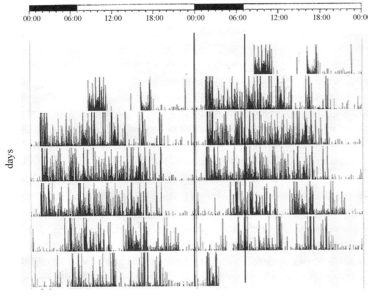

time of day (hours)

**Figure 22.2** Actogram of Advanced sleep phase type. Sleep episodes are represented by white areas, black areas stand for wake episodes. The 24-h period is double-plotted in a raster format. Note that in ASPT, the timing of sleep onset and offset is advanced relative to the circadian night (indicated by two continuous vertical lines along the actogram).

night coupled with daytime sleepiness. The inability to adhere to a scheduled lifestyle often leads to severe impairment of educational, occupational, social, and domestic functioning. This condition is associated with personality disorders.

- The incidence of the disorder in the general population is unknown. The nonentrained type is thought to occur in over half of totally blind individuals. Among patients with CSRD who present to sleep clinics, 12.1% receive a diagnosis of non-entrained-

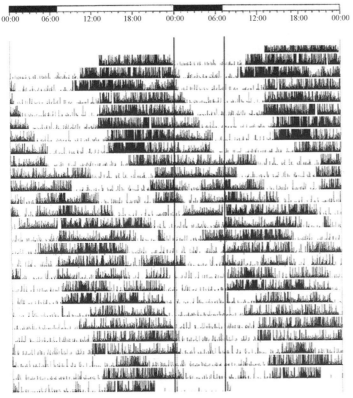

time of day (hours)

**Figure 22.3** Actogram of Non-entrained type. Sleep episodes are represented by white areas, black areas stand for wake episodes. The 24-h period is double-plotted in a raster format. Note that in Non-entrained type, sleep onset and offset are delayed each day by approximately one hour. As a result of this pattern, sleep episodes and night hours (indicated by two continuous vertical lines along the actogram) sometimes coincide and sometimes are completely out of phase.

type circadian rhythm sleep disorder. Onset may occur at any age in blind people.

- In blind people, a lack of photic input to the circadian pacemaker may readily account for the free-running rhythms. In sighted individuals, both a reduced sensitivity to the entraining influences of light and an endogenous circadian period longer than 24 h have been suggested. Altered phase relationships of endogenous circadian rhythms are also present. Thus far, genetic screening analyses have not yield any persistent association with the disorder.

## IRREGULAR SLEEP–WAKE TYPE

Irregular sleep–wake type, also known as irregular or disorganized sleep–wake pattern, is characterized by lack of a clearly defined sleep–wake circadian rhythm. The timing and the length of sleep and wake episodes are variable and unpredictable throughout the 24-h period (Figure 22.4). These patients are likely to manifest inability to initiate and maintain sleep at night, frequent daytime napping, and excessive daytime sleepiness. Other circadian rhythms, such as endocrine and body temperature, may also show a loss of diurnal variability.

- Irregular sleep–wake type is a rare condition, which can begin at any age. It is associated with neurologic disorders such as dementia and mental retardation. Anatomical or functional abnormalities of the endogenous pacemaker or weakened environmental entraining factors may be involved in the pathology of this disorder.

## SECONDARY CIRCADIAN RHYTHM SLEEP DISORDERS

Disruption of the circadian sleep–wake cycle may arise from an underlying primary medical or neurologic condition. Patients may display a variety of symptoms, including insomnia and excessive sleepiness. The disruption of sleep–wake cycle may range from an altered phase to irregular sleep–wake patterns. Impairment in major areas of functioning and quality of life is evident. Demographics are largely unknown. Causes include dementia, movement disorders, hepatic encephalopathy, traumatic head injury, and brain tumors.

- Secondary CRSD can also occur as a result of psychoactive substance abuse or dependency, or as a side effect of a drug (e.g., haloperidol or fluvoxamine). It has been suggested that these drugs alter the circadian sleep–wake cycle through their effects on serotonin and melatonin levels.

## EVALUATION

Diagnosis of CRSD is based largely on recognizing the characteristics and patterns of sleep disturbances. A clinical interview should refer to the patient's sleep–wake habits and difficulties in various areas of functioning (e.g., social, educational, occupational, and domestic). Patients should be asked about their hours of alertness and mealtimes; family history; ability to adjust sleep-wake cycles to changes in environmental demands; history of head injury or brain tumors; and use of psychoactive and neuroleptic medications.

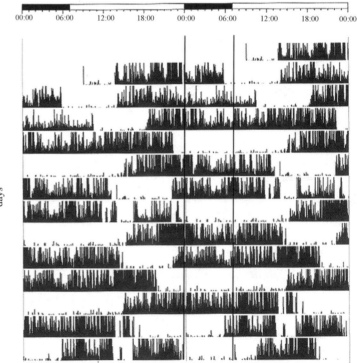

**Figure 22.4** Actogram of Irregular sleep-wake type. Sleep episodes are represented by white areas, black areas stand for wake episodes. The 24-h period is double-plotted in a raster format. Note the variability in the timing and length of sleep and wake episodes characteristic of this disorder.

time of day (hours)

- Diagnosis is aided by collection of 7–14 days of sleep logs and/or actigraphic monitoring. The actigraph is a watch-sized device worn on the wrist that monitors hand motion and provides data on sleep and wake periods. Actigraphic monitoring must be conducted during routine conditions since sleep–wake schedules obtained under forced conditions can mask the inherent pattern and lead to an erroneous diagnosis. In most cases, polysomnography is not required.

## KEY POINTS

1. Circadian rhythm sleep disorders are characterized by an alteration of the circadian timing system or a misalignment between the timing of the individual's sleep–wake rhythm and the 24-h social and physical environment. Sleep episodes occur at inappropriate times, often causing wake periods to occur at undesired times.

2. Delayed sleep phase disorder is characterized by habitual sleep-wake times that are delayed, usually more than 2 h, relative to conventional or socially acceptable times. On the other hand, advanced sleep phase disorder is a stable advance of the major sleep period, characterized by habitual sleep onset and wake-up times that are several hours earlier than desired or socially accepted.

3. Free-running type, also known as non-entrained-type or non-24-h sleep–wake syndrome, is marked by sleep–wake cycles that are usually longer than 24 h. Due to this, sleep and wake episodes are delayed each day to later hours.

4. Irregular sleep–wake type, also known as irregular or disorganized sleep–wake pattern, is characterized by lack of a clearly defined sleep–wake circadian rhythm. The timing and the length of sleep and wake episodes are variable and unpredictable throughout the 24-h period.

## BIBLIOGRAPHY

Ancoli-Israel S, et al. A pedigree of one family with delayed sleep phase syndrome. *Chronobiol Int* 2001; 18:831–840.

Ancoli-Israel S, et al. The role of actigraphy in the study of sleep and circadian rhythms. *Sleep* 2003; 26:342–392.

Ayalon L, et al. Case study of circadian rhythm sleep disorder following haloperidol treatment: Reversal by risperidone and melatonin. *Chronobiol Int* 2002; 19:947–959.

Ayalon L, et al. Circadian rhythm sleep disorders following mild traumatic brain injury. *Neurology* 2007; 68:1136–1140.

Cajochen C, et al. Role of melatonin in the regulation of human circadian rhythms and sleep. *J Neuroendocrinol* 2003; 15: 432–437.

Cermakian N, et al. A molecular perspective of human circadian rhythm disorders. *Brain Res Rev* 2003; 42:204–220.

Chesson AL, et al. Practice parameters for the nonpharmacologic treatment of chronic insomnia. An American Academy of Sleep Medicine report. Standards of Practice Committee of the American Academy of Sleep Medicine. *Sleep* 1997; 22:1128–1133.

Dagan Y, et al. Evaluating the role of melatonin in the long-term treatment of delayed sleep phase syndrome (DSPS). *Chronobiol Int* 1998; 15:181–190.

Dagan Y, et al. Circadian rhythm sleep disorders: Toward a more precise definition and diagnosis. *Chronobiol Int* 1999; 16:213–222.

Dagan Y, et al. Sleep-wake schedule disorder disability: A lifelong untreatable pathology of the circadian time structure. *Chronobiol Int* 2001; 18:1019–1027.

Ebisawa T, et al. Association of structural polymorphisms in the human period3 gene with delayed sleep phase syndrome. *EMBO Rep* 2001; 2:342–346.

Hermesh H, et al. Circadian rhythm sleep disorders as a possible side effect of fluvoxamine. *CNS Spectrums* 2001; 6:511–513.

Jones CR, et al. Familial advanced sleep-phase syndrome: A short-period circadian rhythm variant in humans. *Nat Med* 1999; 5:1062–1065.

Nagtegaal JE, et al. Delayed sleep phase syndrome: A placebo-controlled cross-over study on the effects of melatonin administered five hours before the individual dim light melatonin onset. *J Sleep Res* 1998; 7:135–143.

Reiter RJ. Melatonin: Clinical relevance. *Best Practice Res Clin Endocrinol Metab* 2003; 17:273–285.

Sack RL, et al. Entrainment of free-running circadian rhythms by melatonin in blind people. *N Engl J Med* 2000; 343:1070–1077.

Satoh K, et al. Two pedigrees of familial advanced sleep phase syndrome in Japan. *Sleep* 2003; 26:416–417.

Seabra ML, et al. Randomized, double-blind clinical trial, controlled with placebo, of the toxicology of chronic melatonin treatment. *J Pineal Res* 2000; 29:193–200.

Uchiyama M, et al. Altered phase relation between sleep timing and core body temperature rhythm in delayed sleep phase syndrome and non-24-hour sleep-wake syndrome in humans. *Neurosci Lett* 2000; 294:101–104.

Van Gelder RN. Recent insights into mammalian circadian rhythms. *Sleep* 2004; 27: 166–171.

Wirz-Justice A, et al. Disturbed circadian rest-activity cycles in schizophrenia patients: An effect of drugs? *Schizophr Bull* 2001; 27:497–502.

# 23

## JET LAG

Timothy H. Monk
Human Chronobiology Research Program, Western Psychiatric Institute and Clinic,
University of Pittsburgh Medical Center, Pittsburgh, Pennsylvania

## INTRODUCTION

The human biological clock, or "circadian system," is located in the suprachiasmatic nuclei (SCN) of the hypothalamus. One function of the biological clock is to prepare the individual for restful sleep at night and active wakefulness during the day. This is done through daily or "circadian" rhythms, which are generated by the SCN and which can be observed in many different physiological measures (e.g., body temperature, plasma cortisol level, and plasma melatonin level) as well as psychological measures (e.g., mood, alertness, and performance). There are two properties of the biological clock that are important when considering the effects of travel across several time zones, or jet lag.

- First, the clock is endogenous and self-sustaining, with a momentum of its own. This means that the SCN will continue to generate circadian rhythms, even if the individual is continuously awake and is unaware of the time of day. Thus, circadian rhythms are not simply the result of changes in waking state, ambient light, posture, or activity, although these factors do have some influence on the observed rhythms. For some rhythms (e.g., core body temperature) the influence of external factors can be equivalent to the influence of the SCN; for other rhythms (e.g., cortisol) they are minimal.

- Second, the SCN is resistant to changes in timing, taking several days to realign to a new routine (as is required when crossing time zones). While this process of realignment is taking place, the biological clock will not be functioning appropriately, leading to impairments in both nocturnal sleep and daytime wakefulness. There may also be malaise and irritability resulting from a loss in the temporal harmony of the different component rhythms.

## DEFINITION

The label "jet lag" refers to the lag between the time frame of the biological clock and that of the destination time zone. Because the biological clock is slow to adjust, there will be several days after arrival in the new time zone before the biological clock "catches up" with the new routine.

- During this adjustment process, sleep is impaired, with nocturnal awakenings related to hunger, need to void, or a simple lack of sleepiness. During the day, there may be a lack of alertness and performance ability, not only because of the partial sleep loss but also because the biological clock is (inappropriately) preparing the individual for sleep.

- There is also malaise and loss of concentration, which may result from a loss of the normal phase interrelationships between the various rhythmic processes. This has been likened to a symphony orchestra after the arrival of a second conductor, beating a different time. Until all of the instruments switch to the new conductor, there is a cacophony of noise. In biological terms, this is described as "internal desynchrony."

## IS EASTBOUND WORSE THAN WESTBOUND?

- Each postflight day allows 90 min of phase changes toward the new zone with flights in a westbound direction, but only 60 min with flights in an eastbound direction. For instance, a 6-hour phase delay (e.g., flight from Paris to New York) would require 4 days to recover completely, whereas a 6-h phase advance (e.g., flight form New York to Paris) would require 6 days for full recovery. Thus, the westward direction is associated with fewer jet lag symptoms than an eastward direction of travel.

- In contrast to the effects due to direction of travel (east- versus westbound), the effects due to traveling away from versus returning home are minimal.

## EFFECT OF AGING

There is little evidence from field studies of the effects of aging on jet lag. Laboratory simulations have shown that middle-aged men suffer more jet lag symptoms that younger men. Among older adults (over 70 years of age), sleep appears to be even more disrupted, even if the pacemaker can phase adjust at more or less the same rate. The same directional asymmetry (i.e., advancing phase being more difficult than delay in phase) observed in young and middle-aged subjects is also present in the elderly.

## CHRONIC JET LAG

A chronic jet lag syndrome is experienced by many business executives whose jobs require them to travel to many different time zones per month, as well as by airline personnel. It is likely that such individuals are in a semi-permanent state of circadian desynchrony.

- The health consequences of rotating shift work include gastrointestinal disorders, cardiovascular disorders, cancer, and depression. It is likely that patients suffering from chronic jet lag syndrome are equally at risk for these disorders.
- Recent studies have demonstrated the presence of cognitive deficits in these individuals, and have shown brain changes (e.g., temporal lobe atrophy) associated with such deficits.

## JET LAG COUNTERMEASURES

A number of different countermeasures for jet lag have been proposed, including behavioral techniques, use of bright light, and use of medications, such as hypnotic agents and melatonin.

### Behavioral Countermeasures

- The traveler should, if possible, anticipate the phase changes required by the trip by retiring to bed and getting up earlier for several days before an eastward trip or later before a westward trip. This should be done without truncating the sleep episode.
- Upon boarding the plane, the traveler should change his or her wristwatch to the destination time zone and attempt to follow a schedule indicated by that time (i.e., stay awake during the "daytime" and sleep during the "night").
- Caffeine and alcohol should be avoided, and liberal amounts of fluids should be taken.

- It is important for the traveler to recognize the potential fragility of his or her sleep after arrival and to adopt good sleep hygiene principles accordingly. These should include avoiding caffeine within 5 h of bedtime, eating and drinking in moderation, and avoiding heavy physical exercise close to bedtime. The traveler should have earplugs to counter the effects of noisy air conditioners, and a snack (but not chocolate) available if she or he gets hungry during the night. It may also be helpful to bring along a nightlight or dim flashlight to avoid switching on the bright room lights.
- The traveler should select a schedule that allows an early evening arrival. If this is not possible, or should remain awake until 10:00 PM local time. If sleep is irresistible, a short nap, not lasting more than 2 h, is permitted in the early afternoon. Light exercise in the daylight is encouraged and the traveler should avoid remaining indoors.
- A strategy that may be tried for short trips (<3 days) is remaining on the home time, and scheduling sleep periods, meals, and meetings to coincide with the "daytime" of the home time zone.

### Light Therapy and Light Restriction

Daylight illumination is a powerful synchronizer of the human biological clock.

- Being out and about in the daylight at one's destination is beneficial. Bright light exposure at the end of the biological day tends to delay circadian rhythms, whereas exposure at the beginning of the biological day tends to advance them. Thus, appropriately timed exposure to daylight (or very bright artificial lights) can be used to move the biological clock to the desired phase position. This can be used in conjunction with dark goggles to restrict daylight exposure at the other end of the day.

### Melatonin

Melatonin, a pineal hormone, is an important component of the circadian system. On a normal routine, production of the hormone is "switched on" at 8:00–11:00 PM, and "turned off" at 4:00–5:00 AM. Melatonin can cause drowsiness, and melatonin pills can be used to counter the effects of jet lag, particularly when administered at bedtime. Additionally, melatonin is a chronobiotic agent that directly affects the timing of the biological clock.

- Although not as powerful as daylight in phase shifting the sleep–wake rhythm, melatonin can, when administered at the correct circadian time, effect a phase change in the SCN.
- Melatonin pills have not always been successful as a countermeasure for jet lag, and some experts discourage their regular use.

## Hypnotic Agents

Sleeping pills (hypnotics) are best used short term to counter transient insomnia.

- Hypnotic agents may help consolidate sleep but do not appear to influence the rate at which the biological clock adjusts to the new time zone.
- Hypnotics with a duration of action of about 3–5 h are likely to be helpful in alleviating jet lag symptoms. Nonetheless, hypnotics should only be used sparingly and in conjunction with behavioral countermeasures.

## KEY POINTS

1. Jet lag involves sleep disruptions and impairments in mood and daytime functioning.
2. A number of possible treatment strategies are available for jet lag, including behavioral modification, optimal sleep hygiene, timed daylight exposure, and the judicious use of hypnotic agents and melatonin.

## ACKNOWLEDGMENTS

Sincere thanks are due to Melissa L. Clark for research assistance. Primary support for this work was provided by NASA Grants NAG9-1234 and NNJ04HF76G, National institute on Aging Grants AG-13396 and AG-020677, and by CTRC Grant RR-024153.

## BIBLIOGRAPHY

Arendt J. Jet lag/night shift, blindness and melatonin. *Trans Med Soc Lond* 1997; 114:7–9.

Barnes RG, et al. Adaptation of the 6-sulphatoxymelatonin rhythm in shiftworkers on offshore oil installations during a 2-week 12-h night shift. *Neurosci Lett* 1998; 241:9–12.

Cho K. Chronic "jet lag" produces temporal lobe atrophy and spatial cognitive deficits. *Nat Neurosci* 2001; 4:567–568.

Costa G. Shift work and occupational medicine: An overview. *Occup Med (Lond)* 2003; 53:83–88.

Edwards BJ, et al. Use of melatonin in recovery from jet-lag following an eastward flight across 10 time-zones. *Ergonomics* 2000; 43:1501–1513.

Lowden A, et al. Retaining home-base sleep hours to prevent jet lag in connection with a westward flight across nine time zones. *Chronobiol Int* 1998; 15:365–376.

Monk TH, et al. Inducing jetlag in older people: Directional asymmetry. *J Sleep Res* 2000; 9:101–116.

Moore RY. Circadian rhythms: Basic neurobiology and clinical applications. *Annu Rev Med* 1997; 48:253–266.

Sack RL, et al. Melatonin as a chronobiotic: Treatment of circadian desynchrony in night workers and the blind. *J Biol Rhythms* 1997; 12:595–603.

Shanahan TL, et al. Melatonin rhythm observed throughout a three-cycle bright-light stimulus designed to reset the human circadian pacemaker. *J Biol Rhythms* 1999; 14:237–253.

Sharkey KM, et al. Effects of melatonin administration on daytime sleep after simulated night shift work. *J Sleep Res* 2001; 10:181–192.

Spitzer RL, et al. Jet lag: Clinical features, validation of a new syndrome-specific scale, and lack of response to melatonin in a randomized, double-blind trial. *Am J Psychiatry* 1999; 156:1392–1396.

Stone BM, et al. Promoting sleep in shiftworkers and intercontinental travelers. *Chronobiol Int* 1997; 14:133–143.

Terzano MG, et al. New drugs for insomnia: Comparative tolerability of zopiclone, zolpidem and zaleplon. *Drug Safety* 2003; 26:261–282.

# 24

## SHIFT WORK SLEEP DISORDER

GARY S. RICHARDSON
Henry Ford Hospital, Detroit, Michigan

### INTRODUCTION

Shift work is generally defined as any schedule that requires work outside a broadly defined "day shift," usually 6:00–6:00 PM. Evening shifts, typically those between 2 PM and midnight, are generally well tolerated, allowing later times of arising and longer typical sleep durations than even typical day shifts. Night shifts, those between 9:00 PM and 8:00 AM are less well tolerated.

- As of 1997, 16.8% of full-time U.S. workers regularly worked shifts other than the day shift. Schedules that regularly include night shifts (straight night and rotating shift schedules) together comprise 6.4%, or 5.8 million full-time U.S. workers.

- The biological difficulties posed by night shift stem from the modulation of physiologic processes, including those governing sleep and wakefulness, by the endogenous circadian clock. When the circadian orientation of night workers is examined, it is out of phase with both day and night schedules and is much more variable than that of day workers. This is because light provides an intensity-dependent orienting, or phase-setting, signal for the internal clock, and even incidental exposure to bright sunlight, such as might occur during the drive home after the night shift, or in the fulfillment of family or household responsibilities throughout the day, will undermine efforts to entrain the circadian clock to a nocturnal orientation. Only extraordinary control of the light–dark environment both at home and at work allows stable and complete circadian adaptation to night shift.

### CONSEQUENCES OF SHIFT WORK

There is significant morbidity associated with shift work exposure given the impediments to physiologic adaptation to night work. Most prominently, shift work is associated with both increased difficulty sleeping and with increased sleepiness during waking hours.

- Sleepiness on the job, reflecting both the effects of sleep deficits accumulated during day sleep and the clock-mediated impairment of alertness during the night, results in a significantly greater risk of accidents.

- Shift workers are also at increased risk for a variety of adverse health outcomes including cardiovascular disease, ulcer disease, and breast cancer in women. Unlike the link between shift work and accidents where sleepiness clearly plays an important role, it is unclear how shift work may predispose to these other medical problems. Both chronic sleep deprivation, with attendant changes in immunological activity, and circadian misalignment with alterations in melatonin secretion have been proposed as possible pathologic mechanisms.

### DIAGOSIS OF SHIFT WORK SLEEP DISORDER

Although epidemiological studies suggest the difficulty with sleep and alertness at work is common among shift workers, a subset experience difficulty severe enough to warrant the clinical diagnosis of shift work sleep disorder (SWSD). Diagnostic criteria for SWSD established by the American Academy of Sleep Medicine requires the presence of either insomnia during day sleep or a complaint of excessive sleepiness during night work hours. The complaint(s) should not be adequately explained by another medical, psychiatric, or primary sleep disorder and must be temporally associated with shift exposure.

- Using this definition, work using a representative U.S. sample, aged 18–65 years, has established an overall prevalence of SWSD of 10% (14.1% among night workers, and 8.1% among workers on rotating shift schedule). Those with SWSD have significantly

*Sleep Medicine Essentials*, edited by Teofilo L. Lee-Chiong
Copyright © 2009 John Wiley & Sons, Inc.

higher rates of sleepiness-related accidents, ulcer disease, and depression than did workers on the same schedule but without SWSD.

## RISK FACTORS FOR SHIFT WORK SLEEP DISORDER

The epidemiology available for SWSD is limited. Studies suggest that SWSD is more common in night workers than in those on rotating shift schedules, though the difference is not statistically significant. Other potential risk factors for SWSD, such as age and gender, have not been examined extensively.

- Some studies that used "shift work intolerance" or dissatisfaction with the shift schedule, rather than SWSD, as the endpoint in risk factor assessments, have implicated a number of factors including female gender, increasing age, and duration of shift work exposure as possible risk factors.
- It is reasonable to assume that any factor that might limit the duration or quality of daytime sleep, and/or impair alertness during working hours, will increase the risk of SWSD. For example, female shift workers obtain significantly less sleep than their male counterparts, apparently because additional home and family responsibilities limit the time available for day sleep.
- The specific shift schedule may also be a risk factor for SWSD. It has generally been held that forward rotating shifts (day to evening to night) are more readily tolerated than backwards rotation (day to night to evening), and that slow rotation (changing every week) is less adverse than a rapidly changing schedule. However, recent data have challenged the significance of these features of the shift schedule. Instead, it appears that more specific features of the schedule (i.e., start times and the number of consecutive days off) are much more important in predicting worker satisfaction and sleep parameters than is the direction or speed of rotation.

## DIAGNOSIS OF SHIFT WORK SLEEP DISORDER

The diagnosis of SWSD is made on the basis of a clinical history of significant insomnia and/or significant sleepiness during work hours that occurs in the setting of shift work. The significance of the complaint is generally assessed in terms of interference with function on the job or family and social activities. Symptoms should be temporally associated with shift work, that is, sleep and alertness should improve during periods of day work or time off from work.

- Sleep diaries are particularly helpful in establishing the temporal pattern of the complaint.
- Polysomnography during day sleep and the Multiple Sleep Latency Test (MSLT) assessments at normal work times are included in the formal

definition of SWSD, but the absence of relevant normal values for either measure at these times substantially limits their diagnostic utility. In clinical practice, these measures are typically used only to evaluate the possible contribution of other sleep disorders.

- Actigraphy can be helpful if available and may also be useful in assessing the impact of interventions.

## MANAGEMENT OF SHIFT WORK SLEEP DISORDER

Management of SWSD should follow an ordered approach.

- The first step is to verify the diagnosis and identify contributory medical, psychiatric, or sleep disorders. While the existence of other primary sleep disorders would formally exclude the diagnosis of SWSD, in clinical practice this distinction is often difficult to make. Symptoms related to mild sleep apnea, for example, may be exacerbated by shift work, resulting in apparent temporal coincidence with the shift schedule. Similarly, it is often difficult to determine whether difficulty sleeping during the day reflects a contribution of underlying primary insomnia.

## APPROACH TO PATIENT WITH SHIFT WORK SLEEP DISORDER

I. Verify diagnosis and rule out other primary sleep disorders.
   A. If present, treat primary disorder and reevaluate.
II. If no primary sleep disorder, or if disorder adequately treated:
   A. Optimize day sleep.
      (1) Evaluate sleep conditions and general sleep hygiene.
      (2) Consider alternate sleep timing and/or addition of second sleep episode.
III. Consider pharmacological treatment.
   A. Improve duration and quality of day sleep (e.g., use short-acting BzRA such as zaleplon or zolpidem).
   B. Improve alertness during work at night (e.g., use modafinil before night shift).

- The second step in managing SWSD is optimizing the duration and quality of day sleep. This should begin with a "sleep audit" to establish the degree of sleep limitation imposed by the work schedule. A modified sleep diary, the sleep audit focuses on the timing and duration of attempted sleep over a representative sample of the work schedule. In rotating or variable schedules, the audit should be continued until at least one full rotation of the schedule is completed. The average number of hours per day for each shift serves as a rough measure of the severity of sleep limitation. The audit should be reviewed with the SWSD patient to develop specific sleep scheduling decisions.

- An alternate timing strategy can be devised to increase the time available for sleep. Most commonly, this involves the addition of a second sleep episode, or nap, in the evening before work, but it should be emphasized that there is no "correct" remedy to day sleep. Morning sleep, afternoon sleep, and split sleep schedules may all be used to help the shift worker obtain a reasonable amount of sleep in the setting of competing practical limitations. The goal is to maximize sleep duration, and empirical trials may be necessary to find the optimal solution for each patient. Repeat sleep audits are used to assess results.

- The quality of sleep obtained during the day is also a problem for shift workers. Attention to caffeine and nicotine use, as well as identification and elimination of counterproductive sleep treatments, is essential. For the day sleeper, phone ringers and cell phones should be switched off, and answering machine/voicemail messages explaining the schedule should be prepared. Family, neighbors, and friends need to be educated about the importance of adequate, uninterrupted day sleep.

- A persistent area of controversy in the practical management of SWSD is the extent to which light exposure should be regulated. While maintenance of a dark sleeping room has a clear benefit, if only for its direct impact on sleep quality, it is less clear whether shift workers should be counseled to limit light exposure for the rest of the day. While limitation of light exposure during the day and enhancement of light exposure at night can produce circadian phase shifts that are significantly more conducive to day sleep, shift workers are generally resistant to such restrictions, perceiving flexibility during their time off as one of the few advantages of night work. However, light exposure during days between night shifts should be as consistent as possible, fitting into a routine that includes the scheduled sleep hours.

- The third step in managing SWSD is the use of pharmacologic interventions. Reserved for patients in whom symptoms do not respond to reasonable efforts to optimize day sleep, pharmacologic options include both hypnotics to increase the quality and duration of day sleep and wake-enhancing medications to increase alertness during night work hours. In the former group, hypnotic BzRAs have been shown to improve day sleep in objective assessments, but the impact on alertness during the following night is limited. Newer selective agents, particularly those with shorter half-lives, such as zolpidem or zaleplon, are now the drugs of choice in this setting.

- Melatonin, a hormone with sedative and chronobiotic (direct circadian phase shifting) properties, offers theoretical advantages in the treatment of sleep disruption associated with SWSD. However, while there is substantial support for its use, many of the field and laboratory trials are difficult to interpret because they have also incorporated strict control of light exposure. When the contribution of the two interventions is separated, there appears to be little benefit in melatonin treatment. Consistent with this interpretation, placebo-controlled trials in real shift work settings without control of light–dark exposure have generally been negative.

- Wake-enhancing medications are the most common pharmacologic intervention if the category is expanded to include caffeine. Caffeine can clearly have a beneficial effect on alertness, but its use is limited by tolerance and side effects. Stimulants such as d-amphetamine, methylphenidate, and pemoline are also limited by side effects, as well as by significant risk of abuse. More recently, modafinil has been approved for use in the treatment of SWSD. Clinical experience with modafinil in SWSD remains limited, but the substantial advantages of this drug over older stimulants in the risk of abuse and side effects dictate that it is the treatment of choice for this indication.

## KEY POINTS

1. Shift work sleep disorder affects approximately 10% of full-time workers on night or rotating shifts.
2. Risk factors for SWSD include increasing age, female gender, and any predisposition to sleep disturbance or impaired alertness.
3. Shift work sleep disorder increases the risk of morbidity associated with shift work, such as ulcer disease and sleepiness-related accidents.
4. Treatment for SWSD should follow a stepwise approach in which the contribution of coexisting medical, psychiatric, or sleep disorders is first addressed; day sleep quality and quantity is optimized; and pharmacologic interventions to improve day sleep and enhance nocturnal alertness are then employed.

## BIBLIOGRAPHY

Akerstedt T. Shift work and disturbed sleep/wakefulness. *Sleep Med Rev* 1998; 2:117–128.

Akerstedt T, et al. Alertness-enhancing drugs as a countermeasure to fatigue in irregular work hours. *Chronobiol Int* 1997; 14:145–158.

Arendt J, et al. Efficacy of melatonin treatment in jet lag, shift work, and blindness. *J Biol Rhythms* 1997; 12:604–617.

Axelsson J, et al. Tolerance to shift work—How does it relate to sleep and wakefulness? *Int Arch Occup Environ Health* 2004; 77:121–129.

Beers TM. Flexible schedules and shift work: Replacing the 9-to-5 workday? *Monthly Labor Rev* 2000; 23:33–40.

Boivin DB, et al. Circadian adaptation to night-shift work by judicious light and darkness exposure. *J Biol Rhythms* 2002; 17:556–567.

Burgess HJ, et al. Bright light, dark and melatonin can promote circadian adaptation in night shift workers. *Sleep Med Rev* 2002; 6:407–420.

Cruz C, et al. Clockwise and counterclockwise rotating shifts: Effects on sleep duration, timing, and quality. *Aviat Space Environ Med* 2003; 74:597–605.

Folkard S, et al. Shift work, safety and productivity. *Occup Med (Lond)* 2003; 53:95–101.

Hansen J. Increased breast cancer risk among women who work predominantly at night. *Epidemiology* 2001a; 12:74–77.

Hansen J. Light at night, shiftwork, and breast cancer risk. *J Natl Cancer Inst* 2001b; 93:1513–1515.

Porcu S, et al. Performance, ability to stay awake, and tendency to fall asleep during the night after a diurnal sleep with temazepam or placebo. *Sleep* 1997; 20:535–541.

Richardson G, et al. Hormonal and pharmacological manipulation of the circadian clock: Recent developments and future strategies. *Sleep* 2000; 23:S77–85.

Sack RL, et al. Melatonin as a chronobiotic: Treatment of circadian desynchrony in night workers and the blind. *J Biol Rhythms* 1997; 12:595–603.

Smith PA, et al. Change from slowly rotating 8-hour shifts to rapidly rotating 8-hour and 12-hour shifts using participative shift roster design. *Scand J Work Environ Health* 1998; 24:55–61.

Tucker P, et al. Effects of direction of rotation in continuous and discontinuous 8 hour shift systems. *Occup Environ Med* 2000; 57:678–684.

Vgontzas AN, et al. Adverse effects of modest sleep restriction on sleepiness, performance, and inflammatory cytokines. *J Clin Endocrinol Metab* 2004; 89:2119–2126.

Wright SW, et al. Randomized clinical trial of melatonin after night-shift work: efficacy and neuropsychologic effects. *Ann Emerg Med* 1998; 32:334–340.

# 25

## THERAPY OF CIRCADIAN SLEEP DISORDERS

Robert L. Sack and Kyle Johnson
Department of Psychiatry Oregon Health and Sciences University, Portland, Oregon

### INTRODUCTION

Circadian rhythm sleep disorders (CRSDs) have a common underlying mechanism; namely, a misalignment between the timing of internal circadian rhythms and the normal, desired, or required time for sleep and wake.

- In some cases, the misalignment stems from abnormalities of endogenous circadian mechanisms [e.g., advanced sleep-phase disorder (ASPD) or non-24-h free-running rhythms]. In others, the circadian system is normal, but external circumstances exceed the limits of adaptation [e.g., shift work sleep disorder (SWSD)].

- There are two general treatment strategies: (1) resetting the clock or (2) overriding the clock. With clock resetting, the phase (timing) of the circadian pacemaker is shifted (reset) so that the output signals for sleep and wake are more congruous with a person's desired sleep–wake schedule. Clock resetting involves entrainment using light exposure and/or melatonin administered at the optimal circadian phase. In cases where circadian resetting is impractical or undesirable, overriding the circadian signal with a hypnotic or alerting medication may be the preferred strategy. Clock resetting and clock overriding can be used concurrently.

### CIRCADIAN SCIENCE

Mammalian circadian rhythms are generated by intracellular protein transcriptional feedback mechanisms in the neurons of the suprachiasmatic nucleus (SCN) of the hypothalamus. Output signals from the SCN not only modulate daily rhythms in alertness but also core body temperature and the secretion of certain hormones such as melatonin and cortisol (see Figure 25.1).

- In humans, the intrinsic rhythm of the clock is slightly longer than 24 h so that precise synchronization to a 24-h day (entrainment) depends on exposure to environmental circadian time signals (*Zeitgebers*), most importantly, the solar light–dark cycle. Nonphotic time cues (e.g., scheduled sleep and activity) may have some influence on the clock, but their potency, compared to light, appears to be relatively weak.

- Phase resetting is a normal, daily function of the circadian system. In the absence of timing signals or light (e.g., in totally blind people), circadian rhythms typically "free-run" on a non-24-h cycle (in the blind, the average is 24.5 h), expressing the intrinsic rhythm of the clock without the normal fine-tuning effects (phase resetting) of light exposure.

- The circadian visual system utilizes specialized (nonrod, noncone) receptors in the ganglion cells of the retina that are sensitive to environmental brightness. Photic information is conveyed to the SCN by a specific pathway (the retinohypothalamic tract) that is separate from the pathway mediating vision (see Figure 25.1). The SCN also has a dense population of melatonin receptors that presumably play a role in normal circadian regulation and mediate the phase-resetting effects of melatonin administration (see Figure 25.2)

### PHASE-RESETTING EFFECTS OF LIGHT

The phase-resetting effects of light are dependent on intensity, duration, timing, and wavelength.

#### Intensity

Compared to some other species (e.g., rodents), humans are relatively insensitive to light. Consequently, effective

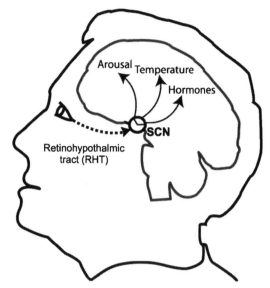

**Figure 25.1** Light and circadian system. The suprachiasmatic nucleus (SCN) of the hypothalamus contains the circadian clock. The intrinsic period of the clock is slightly longer than 24 h. Entrainment to an exact 24-h period involves photic input to the clock via a special pathway, the retinohypothalamic tract (RHT). Efferent pathways from the clock are widespread and regulate the circadian rhythms of sleep–wake (level of arousal), core body temperature, and the secretion of certain hormones such as melatonin and cortisol.

therapeutic phase shifting requires light exposure that approaches solar intensity. In addition to absolute intensity, the contrast between therapeutic light exposure and background ambient light may be important;

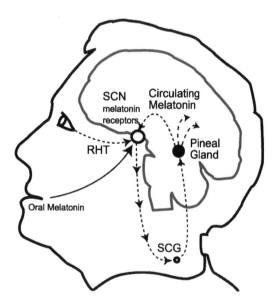

**Figure 25.2** Melatonin and the circadian system. The timing of melatonin secretion by the pineal gland is controlled by the circadian pacemaker, located in the suprachiasmatic nucleus (SCN) of the hypothalamus. Efferents pass from the SCN to the superior cervical ganglion (SCG) in the spinal cord, and postsynaptic sympathetic neurons enervate the pineal. Circulating melatonin from the pineal or from oral administration activates melatonin receptors on SCN neurons.

even relatively dim light can promote phase shifting if the exposure occurs in the context of almost complete darkness.

- If solar light is available, phase shifting can be promoted by simply going outside, even on cloudy days. If therapeutic light exposure is needed during the hours of darkness, an artificial light source can be used. Light sources vary in size from a large light box to a compact visor. A device that mimics the gradually increasing intensity of dawn sunlight (called a *dawn simulator*) has been shown to cause phase shifting.

- Appropriately timed avoidance of light can also promote phase resetting. Wearing goggles on the commute home from a night shift can promote an adaptive phase delay. Goggles presumably block the expected phase advance produced by morning sunlight, thereby permitting a greater phase delay.

### Duration

The initial exposure to a bright light stimulus may be the most potent component with diminishing returns as the duration of the stimulus is prolonged. Durations have varied from 15 min to 2 h in clinical studies. Intermittent light exposure can be about as effective as continuous light exposure.

- In clinical settings, it is important that the prescribed duration of treatment be realistic and consistent with the lifestyle of the patient. Bright light fixtures can be placed in settings where the patient can carry out other activities, such as putting on makeup, reading, or watching television.

### Timing

The phase-shifting effects of light and melatonin on the circadian clock are critically dependent on the time of day (i.e., the phase of the 24-h cycle).

- Light exposure around dusk (in normally entrained individuals) shifts the clock later, producing a phase delay. Light exposure around dawn shifts the clock earlier, producing a phase advance. Light exposure in the middle of the day has little phase-shifting effect. These time-dependent effects of light can be plotted as a phase response curve (PRC) (see Figure 25.3).

- If an individual's clock has been reset, the light PRC will be shifted as well. Consequently, light exposure can have unexpected effects; for instance, in a night worker who has made a significant circadian adaptation (i.e., resetting the clock to be congruent with his night-work/day-sleep schedule), light exposure at dawn may *hit* the phase delay, rather than a phase advance, portion of the light PRC. If the phase of the pacemaker is unknown, it may be necessary to measure some circadian marker (e.g.,

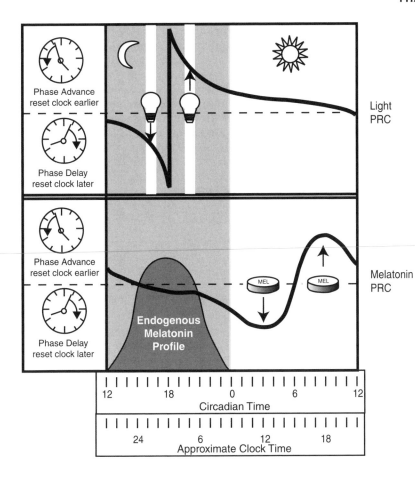

**Figure 25.3** Schematic phase response curves (PRCs) for light exposure and melatonin administration. The effects of light and melatonin on the circadian system are dependent on the time of administration. This relationship can be shown as a phase response curve. In summary, light exposure late in the day or melatonin administration in the morning will shift the circadian clock later (cause a phase delay), while light exposure in the morning or melatonin late in the day will cause the circadian clock to shift earlier (cause a phase advance). Both PRCs have an inflexion point, the time that advance responses become delay responses. According to convention, circadian time 0 is the beginning the light phase (daytime) of the 24-h cycle, and circadian time 12 is the beginning of the dark phase (night).

melatonin onset) in order to predict the effects of light.

- Persons ordinarily sleep in darkened rooms with their eyes closed, thereby limiting their exposure to light. Thus, sleep times can reset the clock indirectly, by gating a person's exposure to light.

### Wavelength

Retinal ganglion cells have an essential role in mediating the circadian effects of light, and two candidate photopigments, melanopsin and cryptochrome, may be involved in this process. The action spectrum indicates a peak sensitivity of about 500 nm (blue green light).

- There is no scientific basis for using *full spectrum* light sources; in fact, these sources emit significant amounts of ultraviolet (UV) light that may be toxic to the retina. Plexiglass diffusers, typically used in fixtures, filter out most of the UV spectrum.

### PHASE-RESETTING EFFECTS OF MELATONIN

Melatonin is a hormone normally produced by the pineal gland at night in the dark. Plasma levels rise sharply at about 9:00 PM ($\pm$2 h) and remain elevated for about 12 h. Measurement of the melatonin profile in either plasma or saliva (under dim light conditions) has become the preferred research method for assessing circadian phase.

- Daily administration of melatonin has been shown to entrain free-running rhythms in totally blind people. The melatonin PRC in sighted people is about 180° out of phase with the light PRC; thus, melatonin appears to be a darkness signal, causing a phase delay at the same times that light causes a phase advance (and visa versa) (see Figure 25.3)

- Initial human trials with melatonin employed doses (3–10 mg) that produced plasma levels many times higher than physiologic concentrations. Entrainment of blind free-runners was possible with much lower doses (less than 0.5 mg) that produced plasma levels in the physiologic range.

- Although melatonin appears to have significant phase shifting (*chronobiotic*) properties, it remains unclear whether it can overcome the effects of a competing bright light stimulus. In sighted people, melatonin administration probably works best in situations where the competing light signals are minimized.

- In the United States, melatonin is not classified as a drug; it is sold as a nutritional supplement. Although the Food and Drug Administration (FDA) does not license it as a treatment for any disorder, there have been no serious side effects or complications reported to date.

## PHASE RESETTING WITH SCHEDULED REST AND ACTIVITY

A few studies have suggested that vigorous exercise can shift circadian rhythms, and some field trials have showed that physical training improved sleep quality and performance on the job. However, a recent study showed no added benefit of exercise when combined with appropriately timed, bright light exposure.

## OVERRIDING CIRCADIAN SYSTEM

### Hypnotic Agents

In certain CRSDs (e.g., jet lag or short runs of night work), circadian desynchrony is self-limited, and hypnotics may be used short term to promote sleep when it is attempted at an unfavorable circadian phase. Rapidly metabolized hypnotics with a short half-life are preferred in order to minimize residual drowsiness during the subsequent wake period. In some instances, long-term use of hypnotics for CRSDs, ideally on an intermittent schedule, may be justified for patients who are unable to reset their clocks to fit their required sleep schedule.

### Alerting Agents

Although sleep promotion with hypnotics can be useful, awake-time sleepiness may remain a problem because of the persistence of a misaligned circadian system. The addition of alerting agents may be required to promote wakefulness.

- Caffeine is the most widely used alerting drug in the world and has been shown to improve alertness in simulated night work. Tolerance can develop. When caffeine intake is discontinued, rebound sleepiness can develop.
- Modafinil, a nonamphetamine alerting drug initially licensed for the treatment of narcolepsy, has recently been approved by the FDA for the treatment of SWSD.

## HOMEOSTAT–CIRCADIAN INTERACTION

In addition to the circadian clock, the sleep–wake cycle is driven by the buildup of sleep drive that is dependent on the duration of prior wakefulness (the homeostatic process of sleep regulation). The normal buildup of sleep drive sufficient to exceed the threshold for sleep takes about 16 h and is discharged during the sleep period. Normally, the homeostatic and circadian processes operate in tandem. The circadian alerting process drops away at bedtime at about the same time that a substantial drive for sleep has accumulated. However, in CRSDs, the circadian and homeostatic mechanisms are, by definition, uncoordinated, resulting in shortened, nonrefreshing sleep, resulting in an accumulation of homeostatic sleep drive.

## CLINICAL CONSIDERATIONS

### Counseling and Education

It is worthwhile to spend some time educating patients about the circadian system prior to initiating treatment. Most people are intuitively aware of the homeostatic regulation of sleep (i.e., not getting enough sleep will cause sleepiness), but the circadian regulation of sleep can be more difficult for patients to grasp (i.e., after staying awake for the entire night, it is not necessarily easy to sleep the following day because of the circadian alerting process).

### Shift Work Sleep Disorder

Therapy for SWSD often needs to be customized because work schedules vary so widely, ranging from an occasional or intermittent night duty to a steady five (or more) nights per week. In many occupations, night work can be unpredictable and erratic. Furthermore, night workers typically adopt day-active schedules on their days off so that even regular night workers alternate between diurnal and nocturnal orientation; as a result, circadian adaptation during a run of night work can quickly reverse during off days. Evening (swing) shift workers often adopt a delayed sleep phase, citing a need to "wind down" after getting home from work.

- Bright light exposure benefits phase shifting and promotes adaptation in SWSD. Avoidance of bright light in the morning is also useful.
- Melatonin administration is convenient although it may not be able to override a strong light stimulus. Melatonin may benefit daytime sleep in night workers by an additional direct sleep-promoting action.

### Delayed Sleep Phase Disorder

Delayed sleep phase disorder may be primary (perhaps related to a circadian period that is very long) or secondary (e.g., consistently staying up late and sleeping late in order to avoid school). In either case, the treatment challenge is to shift the sleep and circadian cycle to a time frame congruent with the patient's wishes and role in society. Treatment success will depend heavily on the patient's motivation so that time spent explaining the mechanism involved in DSPD, and the rationale for treatment, are well worthwhile.

- *Chronotherapy* is based on the formulation that patients with DSPD have an exceptionally long circadian period that makes it much easier for them to delay than to advance. Patients are prescribed a sleep schedule that regularly shifts later by about 3 h per day, around the clock, until the sleep is occurring at the desired time.
- Alternatively, treatment can involve bright light exposure in the morning and melatonin administration in the evening, aimed to promote phase advances to a desired sleep time. Because phase advances in DSPD are difficult, they must be gradual, and the use of an hypnotic drug may be indicated during the transition from a delayed to a desired phase. The rate of change is negotiated with the patient (from 15 min every 3 days to 30 min every other day). Patients can be given a spreadsheet that provides a schedule for medications and bed times. Timed light exposure and melatonin administration are used for clock resetting, while an hypnotic is used to ensure sleep at the desired time.

## PATIENT INSTRUCTIONS FOR DELAYED SLEEP PHASE DISORDER

1. Obtain a baseline assessment of sleep–wake schedule (keep a sleep diary, or wear an actigraph, if available).
2. Keep a consistent sleep schedule.
3. Reset the internal body clock. Get at least 30 min of bright light exposure promptly on awakening (e.g., going for a walk in the sunlight, or sitting by a bright light fixture). Take melatonin (0.5–3.0 mg) 2 h before bedtime. Shift the sleep schedule earlier using a predetermined plan (e.g., moving bedtime and wake time 15 min earlier every other day).
4. If still awake 30 min after lights out, take a sleeping medication (prescribed by a physician).
5. After regular sleep at the desired time is attained, keep the same schedule, even on weekends and vacation. Use the sleeping medication as little as possible.
6. If relapse occurs, start at step 2 again.

### Advanced Sleep Phase Disorder

This disorder is uncommon although a tendency for ASPD often occurs in older people. Because early morning awakening is not likely to interfere with employment or academic obligations, patients are less likely to seek attention.

- The recommended treatment is essentially the mirror image of the treatment for DSPD, involving bright light exposure in the evening and, if indicated, melatonin in the morning. The dose of morning melatonin should be very low (0.5 mg or lower) to minimize daytime sedation.

### Non-24-H Sleep–Wake Syndrome

In this disorder, circadian rhythms fail to entrain, and *free-run* on a non-24-h cycle, expressing the intrinsic period of the body clock. Some degree of relative coordination to a 24-h rhythm may occur. The pattern is readily demonstrated by serial assessments of the endogenous melatonin profile. The majority of patients are totally blind, and the failure to entrain is related to the lack of photic input to the circadian clock.

- Treatment, using low doses of melatonin at the same time of day, has been found to be very effective in the majority of these cases.
- There are some case reports of sighted individuals with this disorder. The etiology is unclear, but it has been suggested that these patients have an endogenous circadian period that is beyond the range of entrainment. In these patients, bright light exposure as well as melatonin administration timed to produce phase advances (see treatment of DSPS) have been helpful.

### Irregular Sleep–Wake Pattern

This diagnosis that can apply to patients who have very poor sleep hygiene but no discernable pathology of the circadian system. It can also apply to neurologically impaired patients (e.g., Alzheimer disease) who are presumed to have lesions affecting the SCN.

- Treatment involves good sleep hygiene combined with melatonin administration in the evening and bright light in the morning to reinforce their circadian rhythms.

### Jet Lag

This condition is self-limited; however, travel time is precious. In some people (e.g., airline crews), jet lag may be recurrent or even chronic. Although appropriately timed light exposure and melatonin treatment can accelerate circadian adaptation, there is an inevitable lag period until clock resetting is complete. Consequently, hypnotic medications, and possibly alerting agents, can help to control symptoms until circadian synchronization has been restored.

## PATIENT INSTRUCTIONS FOR JET LAG

### Before Trip

If possible, start the adaptation process 2–3 days before leaving on a long journey.

- If traveling eastward, start shifting lights out and wakeup time *earlier* by about 30 min per day. Obtain bright light exposure on awakening, either by going outside into the sunlight, or, if it is still dark outside, with a bright artificial light.

- If traveling westward, shift sleep time 30 min *later* each day and get as much light exposure in the evening as possible.
- If the trip is shorter (3 time zones or less), and the duration of the trip is short, it may be better to try to keep sleep synchronized to the home time zone while away.

### While in Flight

Because sleep deprivation is one of the causes of jet lag, consider using a sleeping medication to help with sleep during the flight. A short-acting agent, such as zaleplon, is preferred. Avoid drinking alcohol if using a sleeping medication. Leg compression from sitting (and sleeping) in an airplane seat for a long time can increase the risk of blood clot formation (deep vein thrombosis); occasionally walking about the cabin can reduce the risk.

### Upon Arrival at Destination

#### Eastward Flight

- *Light exposure*—In general,* morning light exposure will facilitate resetting the internal body clock to an earlier time. Go for a walk outside in the morning on awakening.
- *Melatonin*—Take melatonin (0.5–3.0 mg) about 2 h prior to the local bedtime to help reset the body clock to local time.
- *Hypnotic agent*—Consider taking a sleeping medication at bedtime until adaptation to the local time is attained.
- *Alerting medication*—Modafinil, an alerting medication, can be taken in morning. Do not take it later in the day as it might cause insomnia.

#### Westward Flight

- *Light exposure*—In general,* evening light exposure will facilitate resetting the internal body clock to a later time. If possible, stay outdoors until dusk and/or be in a brightly lit indoor space until bedtime.
- *Melatonin*—Take melatonin (0.5 mg) if early awakening is problematic (to be expected with westward travel). This will help reset the clock later. Do not take melatonin at bedtime; it can inhibit the adaptation process. Taking melatonin in the morning hours may cause some daytime sleepiness, but if the dose is very low (0.5 mg or less), the hypnotic effect is minimal.
- *Hypnotic agent*—If one wakes up early and cannot get back to sleep (and it is several hours before one is expected to be up), take a short-acting sleeping medication.
- *Alerting medication*—Modafinil can be taken in the morning to promote daytime alertness. Do

not take it later in the day as it might cause insomnia.

### After a Few Days at Destination

It takes about a day per time zone of travel to reset the body clock, so, depending on the distance and direction of travel, it may be a week (or more) before one is completely adapted to local time. Jet lag symptoms will recede as one becomes adapted to local time. However, sleeping in an unfamiliar environment may be difficult and justify the use of a sleeping medication for the duration of the trip. When a sleeping medication is discontinued, expect a few nights of lighter sleep before returning to baseline.

### KEY POINTS

1. Circadian rhythm sleep disorders (CRSDs) are caused by a misalignment between the timing of internal circadian rhythms and the normal, desired, or required time for sleep and wake.
2. There are two general treatment strategies for CRSDs, namely resetting the clock or overriding the clock. With clock resetting, the phase (timing) of the circadian pacemaker is shifted so that the output signals for sleep and wake are more congruous with a person's desired sleep–wake schedule. Clock resetting involves entrainment using light exposure and/or melatonin administered at the optimal circadian phase. When circadian resetting is impractical or undesirable, overriding the circadian signal with a hypnotic or alerting medication may be helpful. Clock resetting and clock overriding can be used concurrently.

### BIBLIOGRAPHY

Berson DM. Strange vision: Ganglion cells as circadian photoreceptors. *Trends Neurosci* 2003; 26:314–320.

Burgess HJ, et al. Preflight adjustment to eastward travel: 3 days of advancing sleep with and without morning bright light. *J Biol Rhythms* 2003; 18:318–328.

Danilenko KV, et al. The human circadian pacemaker can see by the dawn's early light. *J Biol Rhythms* 2000; 15:437–446.

Dijk DJ, et al. Integration of human sleep-wake regulation and circadian rhythmicity. *J Appl Physiol* 2002; 92:852–862.

Duffy JF, Wright KP Jr. Entrainment of the human circadian system by light. *J Biol Rhythms* 2005; 20:326–338.

Eastman CI, et al. How to use light and dark to produce circadian adaptation to night shift work. *Ann Med* 1999; 31:87–98.

Gronfier C, et al. Efficacy of a single sequence of intermittent bright light pulses for delaying circadian phase in humans. *Am J Physiol Endocrinol Metab* 2004; 287:E174–E181.

Lewy AJ, et al. The human phase response curve (PRC) to melatonin is about 12 hours out of phase with the PRC to light. *J Biol Rhythms* 1999; 14:227–236.

Lewy AJ, et al. Capturing the circadian rhythms of free-running blind people with 0.5 mg melatonin. *Brain Res* 2001; 918: 96–100.

---

*If travel involves crossing more than 8 time zones, this rule may not be valid for the first few days because light exposure will be on an unfavorable portion of the light PRC.

Lockley SW, et al. High sensitivity of the human circadian mel-atonin rhythm to resetting by short wavelength light. *J Clin Endocrinol Metab* 2003; 88:4502–4505.

Nagtegaal JE, et al. Delayed sleep phase syndrome: A placebo-controlled cross-over study on the effects of melatonin adminis-tered five hours before the individual dim light melatonin onset. *J Sleep Res* 1998; 7:135–143.

Sack RL, et al. Entrainment of free-running circadian rhythms by melatonin in blind people. *N Engl J Med* 2000; 343:1070–1077.

Sharkey KM, et al. Melatonin phase shifts human circadian rhythms in a placebo-controlled simulated night-work study. *Am J Physiol Regul Integr Compar Physiol* 2002; 282:R454–R463.

# 26

## DISORDERS OF AROUSAL AND SLEEP-RELATED MOVEMENT DISORDERS

KEITH CAVANAUGH AND NORMAN R. FRIEDMAN
Rocky Mountain Pediatric Sleep Disorders, The Children's Hospital, Aurora, Colorado

## INTRODUCTION

An arousal disorder is characterized by an incomplete awakening from sleep where the individual has voluntary movements but no awareness of their actions. There are three types of arousal disorders including confusional arousals, sleep terrors, and sleepwalking (somnambulism). Nocturnal leg cramps and rhythmic movement disorders are classified as sleep-related movement disorders and consist of relatively simple movements that disturb sleep.

## DISORDERS OF AROUSAL

### Confusional Arousals

Confusional arousals are characterized by episodes of mental confusion on arousal or awakening. They consist of confusion during, and following arousal from, sleep, usually from deep sleep in the first part of the night. They have also been labeled sleep drunkenness and excessive sleep inertia.

- Typically, individuals will display disorientation to time and space and disruption of speech. Memory impairment is present with both retrograde and anterograde types seen. Other clinical manifestations include perceptual impairment, inappropriate behavior, aggressive behavior, and errors of logic. These episodes are typically not associated with fear, walking behavior, or intense hallucinations.
- Although prevalence rates for other parasomnias such as night terrors and somnambulism have been estimated between 1 and 30% during childhood, the prevalence of confusional arousals is unknown. Less common in older children and rarely reported in adults, they are almost universally seen in young children before 5 years of age. Gender has not been shown to play a role.

- Overall, they are generally benign and tend to cease by adolescence. However, personal injury has been reported. Confused individuals may resist and become aggressive when restrained.
- Predisposing factors can be any factor that deepens sleep and impairs ease of awakening. This includes, but is not limited to, young age, recovery from sleep deprivation, circadian rhythm disorders, medications, and encephalopathic conditions. Abnormalities in areas impairing arousal (periventricular gray, the midbrain reticular area, and the posterior hypothalamus) have been identified in rare organic cases. Spontaneous confusional episodes can be induced by force arousal.
- Differential diagnosis would include sleep terrors, somnambulism, rapid eye movement (REM) sleep behavior disorder, and sleep-related epileptic seizures (e.g., complex partial associated with ictal discharges).
- Polysomnographic studies show confusional events occur during slow-wave sleep. They typically occur during the first third of the night but have been seen in awakening from lighter stages of sleep and very rarely during REM awakenings. Electroencephalographic (EEG) monitoring during the confusion period may show brief episodes of delta activity, stage 1 theta patterns, repeated microsleeps, or a diffuse and poorly reactive alpha rhythm.
- Treatment primarily involves reassurance, avoiding facilitating causes [e.g., sleep deprivation, central nervous system (CNS) depressants or stress], and medications. Mild stimulants are utilized to lighten deep sleepers.

### Sleep Terrors

A child who wakes up within the first few hours of the night with a piercing scream or cry is most likely experiencing a sleep terror. The child appears to be in fear of something.

Tachycardia, tachypnea, skin flushing, diaphoresis, dilated pupils, and increased muscle tone may be present. The child is unresponsive to his or her parents and is inconsolable. Inconsolability is a key feature.

- Except for some brief dream images, the child is amnesic to the episode. The memories include the need to act against "monsters" or other threats. He or she may have some incoherent vocalizations or call out to the parents, but they are not awake. The attacks may last 30 s to 5 min and usually occur within the first third of the night.

- The typical age of onset is 4–12 years with spontaneous resolution with onset of puberty. The prevalence is 3% for children and 1% for adults, and is more common in males. Ninety percent of patients have a family history of either sleepwalking or sleep talking.

- Sleep terrors are not associated with a higher incidence of psychopathology. Sleep-disordered breathing, restless legs syndrome, sleep deprivation, fever, distended bladder, or CNS depressant medications are potential precipitants.

- On polysomnography, one has an abrupt awakening during slow-wave sleep with sympathetic hyperactivity.

- The differential diagnosis includes nightmares, confusional arousals, and sleep-related epilepsy. The distinction between sleep terrors and nightmares is straightforward. A child who experiences a nightmare will remember the dream content, is consolable, and does not have a large sympathetic discharge. Nightmares tend to occur during REM sleep so they are more common during the last one third of the night. A confusional arousal does not have the associated terror.

- To manage sleep terrors one should treat the predisposing factors. Identify and treat sleep-disordered breathing. Avoid excessive tiredness. Prompted night awakenings have been effective. During an attack, instruct the parents to protect their child from injury but do not try to awaken the child. Make soothing comments and speak calmly and repetitively. Typically, a child does not want to be touched but others seem to feel better when being held. Another treatment option is scheduled nighttime awakenings.

## Sleepwalking

Sleepwalking or somnambulism consists of ambulation occurring during sleep associated with an altered state of consciousness. Other key features are diminished arousability, impaired judgment, inappropriate behavior, and partial or complete amnesia of the event.

- Sleepwalking can either be calm or agitated, but, in contrast to sleep terrors, autonomic activation is generally minimal. Attempts to communicate with the sleepwalker are generally unsuccessful.

Duration of each episode vary widely from several minutes to an hour.

- Sleepwalking typically occurs during slow-wave sleep in the first third or first half of the night but can arise throughout the entire sleep period in adults.

- Sleepwalking has been reported in up to 17–40% of children, with prevalence peaking between 11 and 12 years, and usually disappearing by adolescence. It is less common in adults, with a prevalence of about 0.5–4% in this age group.

- Predisposing factors for sleepwalking include sleep deprivation, febrile illness, stress, alcohol use, and obstructive sleep apnea. Certain medications, such as lithium or tricyclic antidepressants may also trigger episodes of sleepwalking.

- A positive family history of sleepwalking is common, and the prevalence increases progressively in relation to the number of affected parents: 22% if none of the parents had a history of sleepwalking, 45% if one parent sleepwalked, and 60% if both parents sleepwalked.

- Diagnosis is commonly made by history alone. Polysomnography may be indicated in patients with atypical clinical features, if sleepwalking has resulted in significant injuries, or there is poor response to therapy.

- No specific treatment is necessary in most cases. Therapy, if necessary, includes optimal sleep hygiene, environmental safety precautions, and scheduled awakenings.

## SLEEP-RELATED MOVEMENT DISORDERS

### Nocturnal Leg Cramps

Nocturnal leg cramps involve intensely painful sensations accompanied by muscle tightness or tension in the calf, with a majority being unilateral, and occasionally involving the foot, which occur during sleep. They are also referred to as "charley horses," nocturnal leg pain, and muscle hardness.

- Duration of symptoms vary from a few seconds to up to 30 min; symptoms then spontaneously remit. The sensation leads to an arousal or awakening from sleep. Frequency is usually from one to two episodes nightly, occurring several times a week. Some individuals experience them primarily in the daytime and do not report sleep disturbances.

- Symptoms of nocturnal leg cramps have been identified between 16 and 37% of healthy individuals, particularly following exercise. Although incidence is increased in the elderly, the exact prevalence of leg cramps is not known. Symptoms can wax and wane over many years. There appears to be a female predominance in prevalence, as they are often reported during pregnancy.

- Predisposing factors include pregnancy, diabetes mellitus, metabolic disorders, prior vigorous activity, fluid and electrolyte abnormalities, endocrine disorders, neuromuscular disorders, peripheral vascular disease, and disorders of decreased mobility (i.e., Parkinson's disease and arthritis). Medications that have been reported to cause leg cramps include oral contraceptives, diuretics, nifedipine, ß-agonists, steroids, morphine, cimetidine, penicillamine, statins, and lithium. Some familial cases have been reported with an autosomal-dominant pattern. Muscle membrane overexcitability and abnormalities in calcium metabolism have been suggested but not confirmed.

- Polysomnographic studies show nonperiodic bursts of gastrocnemius electromyographic (EMG) activity.
- Differential diagnosis includes chronic myelopathy, peripheral neuropathy, akathisia, restless legs syndrome, muscular pain–fasciculation syndromes, and disorders of calcium metabolism.
- Treatment involves massage, application of heat, or slow stretching. Patients should be advised about general measures to improve sleep, such as not going to bed until sleepy, ensuring a comfortable environment for sleep, and avoidance of alcohol and caffeine-containing beverages before bed. Cramps can be aborted by making use of reciprocal inhibition reflexes, in which contracting a group of muscles forces relaxation of the antagonistic group.
- Quinine, an alkaloid originally produced from the bark of the cinchona tree, has been used to treat leg cramps since 1940. However, studies examining its benefit have shown mixed results. The Federal Drug Administration ordered the discontinuation of its use for leg cramps in 1995 after concluding the risk of side effects outweighed the benefits. Side effects included potentially fatal hypersensitivity reaction, particularly quinine-induced thrombocytopenia, pancytopenia, hemolytic uremic syndrome, hepatitis, and cinchonism, a condition manifesting as tinnitus, visual disturbances, vertigo, nausea, vomiting, abdominal pain, and deafness.

## Rhythmic-Movement Disorder

A rhythmic movement disorder (RMD) is a common condition that rarely receives much attention. An RMD is present when the infant has repetitive stereotypic movements of large muscle groups around sleep onset. Two thirds of infants at 9 months of age have some form of rhythmic activity. "Head banging" (movement of the head in an anterior-posterior direction) is the most commonly recognized variant; however, many body areas may be involved, including head rolling (lateral movement of the head and neck); body rocking (rocking of the entire body in an antero-posterior direction as the child rises onto his hands and knees); body rolling (rotation of the entire torso); and leg banging or rolling.

- Typically, the onset is prior to one year of age and resolves by 3 years. For some, the body movement may persist into childhood. The relationship with a developmental delay is rare. The condition is more common in males.
- Postulated predisposing factors include environmental stress or lack of environmental stimulation. Some hypothesize that RMD represents a vestibular form of self-stimulation.
- The diagnosis is made by history. One may confirm the diagnosis by having the parents make a videotape of the behavior. Polysomnography is rarely necessary; however, if the movements are atypical, prolonged, or violent, one should consider an overnight polysomnography with an expanded EEG montage and video recording to exclude seizures.
- Management of RMD is supportive. One may consider padding the headboard or having the child wear a protective helmet for violent rhythmic activity.

## Sleep Starts

Sleep starts are sudden brief contractions of the legs or arms that occur at sleep onset. They usually consist of a single asymmetric muscle contraction during the transition from wakefulness to asleep. They are also known as hypnic jerks. The jerks are often associated with at least one of the following: subjective feeling of falling, sensory flash (i.e., a flash of light or a loud bang), or a dream.

- They are benign unless they produce repeated awakenings. Rarely, a person may develop sleep-onset insomnia.
- Prevalence rate is about 70%. Predisposing factors include nicotine use, intense evening exercise, stress, or intake of stimulants especially excessive caffeine.
- One must distinguish sleep starts from the following conditions: epileptic seizures (myoclonus occurs during wakefulness and sleep and is associated with EEG epileptiform discharges); periodic limb movements (movements occur after sleep onset and have a periodicity); fragmentary myoclonus (brief jerks or twitches that are symmetrical and bilateral and occur during all sleep stages); and neonatal sleep myoclonus (marked twitching of the fingers, toes, and face during sleep).
- Polysomnographic monitoring during an episode might demonstrate a brief, high-amplitude muscle potential during the transition from wakefulness to sleep, possibly associated with arousals and tachycardia especially following an intense episode.

## Sleep Talking

Sleep talking or somniloquy is the utterance of sounds or speech during sleep without simultaneous subjective detailed awareness of the event. While it is typically brief, infrequent, and devoid of signs of emotional stress, occasionally it is a nightly occurrence. More frequent cases can involve longer episodes and be infused with anger and hostility. It can be spontaneous, referred to as somniloquy, or induced by conversation with the sleeper.

- Concordance of speech content with recalled mental activity after awakening supports the assertion that utterances reflect ongoing mental activity during sleep.

- The exact prevalence is unknown but is presumed to be very common. Overall, its course is benign and self-limited. It can last from a few days to many years. When present in individuals over 25 years of age, it can be associated with comorbid psychopathologic or medical illness. It may be more common in males than in females but overall is not considered to have a gender preference.

- Precipitating factors include emotional stress, febrile illness, or other sleep disorders (e.g., sleep terrors, confusional arousals, obstructive sleep apnea syndrome, and REM sleep behavior disorder).

- Polysomnographic studies have shown that sleep talking is present in all stages of sleep, but more common in nonrapid eye movement (NREM) stages 1 and 2, and REM sleep. The timing of occurrence can vary if influenced by other sleep disorders. In obstructive sleep apnea, it can occur during an arousal from sleep. In REM sleep behavior disorder, it tends to occur out of REM sleep, whereas in cases of somnambulism, it occurs during arousals out of slow-wave sleep.

- No specific treatment exists. However, recognizing and treating an underlying associated condition that precipitates its occurrence should be helpful, as is the avoidance of stressors.

## KEY POINTS

1. A disorder of arousal is characterized by an incomplete awakening from sleep associated with voluntary movements but no awareness of the latter. These include confusional arousals, sleep terrors, and sleepwalking (somnambulism).

2. Sleep-related movement disorders consist of relatively simple movements that disturb sleep and consist of nocturnal leg cramps, sleep starts, sleep talking, and rhythmic movement disorders.

## BIBLIOGRAPHY

Butler JV, et al. Nocturnal leg cramps in older people. *Postgrad Med J* 2002; 78:596–598.

Frank NC, et al. The use of scheduled awakenings to eliminate childhood sleepwalking. *J Pediatr Psychol* 1997; 22:345–353.

Guilleminault C, et al. Sleepwalking and sleep terrors in prepubertal children: What triggers them? *Pediatrics* 2003; 111: 17–25.

Leung AK, et al. Leg cramps in children: Incidence and clinical characteristics. *J Natl Med Assoc* 1999; 91:329.

Man-Son-Hing M, et al. Quinine for nocturnal leg cramps: A meta-analysis including unpublished data. *J Gen Intern Med* 1998; 13:600–606.

Ohayen MM, et al. Night terrors, sleepwalking, and confusional arousals in the general population: Their frequency and relationship to other sleep and mental disorders. *J Clin Psychiatry* 1999; 60:268–276.

# 27

## REM SLEEP BEHAVIOR DISORDER AND REM SLEEP-RELATED PARASOMNIAS

MAJA TIPPMANN-PEIKERT,[1] TIMOTHY I. MORGENTHALER,[2] BRADLEY F. BOEVE,[1] AND MICHAEL H. SILBER[1]

[1]Mayo Clinic Center for Sleep Medicine and Department of Neurology, Mayo Clinic College of Medicine, Rochester, Minnesota
[2]Mayo Clinic Center for Sleep Medicine and Department of Internal Medicine, Division of Pulmonary and Critical Care Medicine, Mayo Clinic College of Medicine, Rochester, Minnesota

## INTRODUCTION

Rapid eye movement (REM) sleep behavior disorder (RBD) is characterized by the loss of physiologic skeletal muscle atonia during REM sleep in association with excessive motor activity while dreaming. Other REM sleep-related parasomnias include nightmare disorder and recurrent isolated sleep paralysis. These disorders represent a blurring of the boundaries between REM sleep and wakefulness, while others appear to represent exaggerated manifestations of REM sleep-related physiology.

## REM SLEEP BEHAVIOR DISORDER

The prevalence of RBD in the general population is estimated to be between 0.38 and 0.5%. It most commonly affects men (87–90%) with a disease onset in the 6th or 7th decade. RBD can present in an acute form, most often related to drug withdrawal, or more commonly in a chronic form.

### Clinical Features

Dream enactment behavior during REM sleep represents the clinical hallmark of RBD and may consist of vocalizations, including talking, swearing, yelling, laughing, and simple or complex motor behaviors ranging from limb jerks, gesturing, reaching, grabbing, and flailing to punching, kicking, leaping out of bed, and running. Patients appear to be acting out distinctly altered, unpleasant dreams with recurrent themes involving being chased by or fighting off a human or animal attacker. They will often recall the dream content if aroused during or immediately after an episode. The behaviors typically occur during the latter half of the night when most REM sleep occurs. The frequency of abnormal nocturnal behaviors varies from several times nightly to once in several months or years.

- REM sleep behavior disorder most often presents when sleep-related activity is disruptive or has resulted in harm to the patient or bed partner. Self-injury from dream enactment behavior has been reported in 32–77% of patients in different series and may result in ecchymoses, lacerations, fractures, and even subdural hematomas. Assaults on the bed partner occur in about two thirds of cases, and in 16% result in injuries from punching, kicking, pulling hair, and attempted strangulation. The contrast between violent nocturnal behavior and placid or pleasant daytime character has been highlighted by some authors.

- Excessive daytime sleepiness is reported by a significant number of patients in the setting of other coexisting sleep disorders, such as obstructive sleep apnea syndrome. In the absence of daytime symptoms, there is frequently a delay in the diagnosis of RBD of several years or even decades.

### Polysomnographic Findings

The hallmark polysomnographic (PSG) feature in RBD is the loss of normal REM sleep atonia, in the form of persistent elevation of tonic electromyogram (EMG) activity or more commonly excessive amounts of phasic muscle activity. Different muscle groups and limbs are variably involved.

- Most often sleep architecture is normal, unless disturbed by an accompanying medical or sleep disorder, such as in narcolepsy, or Parkinson's disease (PD).

- Patients with neurodegenerative disorders and RBD may occasionally exhibit ambiguous sleep (a pattern that shares features of wakefulness, non-REM (NREM) and REM sleep) and in advanced disease, the electroencephalogram (EEG) of all three states may be indistinguishable, a phenomenon known as *status dissociatus*. Some patients with neurodegenerative disorders may have the incidental polysomnographic finding of REM sleep without atonia (RSWA) but without a history of abnormal dream enactment behavior. Since it is uncertain whether this phenomenon is a subclinical form or prodrome of RBD, it is best denoted as RSWA rather than RBD. When RBD is associated with NREM disorders of arousal, "parasomnia overlap syndrome" may be diagnosed.
- Periodic limb movements of sleep (PLMs) and prominent aperiodic limb movements in NREM sleep are frequently encountered, implicating a generalized dysregulation of the motor system during all sleep stages.

### Differential Diagnosis

When evaluating patients with nocturnal parasomnias, careful attention should be paid to eliciting a history of disruptive, unusual behaviors and to any relationship with dreaming.

- Because acute forms of RBD have been associated with use of medications, a careful drug history is always necessary.

### SUBSTANCES ASSOCIATED WITH ACUTE RBD

| | |
|---|---|
| *Withdrawal* | Alcohol |
| | Amphetamines |
| | Cocaine |
| | Barbiturates |
| | Meprobamate |
| | Pentazocine |
| | Nitrazepam |
| *Medication Use/ Intoxication* | Biperiden |
| | Tricyclic antidepressants |
| | Monoamine oxidase (MAO) inhibitors |
| | Serotonin reuptake inhibitors |
| | Venlafaxine |
| | Caffeine |

- Any symptoms or signs suggestive of a central nervous system disease, especially a neurodegenerative disorder, should be noted. A full neurologic examination is indicated and a neuropsychological evaluation may be of value if cognitive impairment is suspected.
- Polysomnography with additional upper extremity EMG derivations and time-synchronized video recording links episodic nocturnal motor behaviors to REM sleep and documents increased REM

sleep related tonic and/or phasic skeletal muscle activity.
- The differential diagnosis of RBD includes a variety of nocturnal motor behaviors.

### DIFFERENTIAL DIAGNOSIS OF RBD

| | |
|---|---|
| Nocturnal seizures (especially frontal lobe) | Sleep terrors |
| Untreated obstructive sleep apnea syndrome | Nightmares |
| Periodic limb movement disorder of sleep | Rhythmic movement disorder of sleep |
| Sleepwalking | Nocturnal panic attacks |
| Sleep talking | Nocturnal psychogenic dissociative state |
| | Nocturnal rummaging behavior in dementia |

### Diagnostic Criteria

A PSG is needed for the definitive diagnosis of RBD, but probable RBD can be diagnosed on clinical grounds. However, the ability of the clinical history alone to distinguish RBD from other sleep disorders, especially obstructive sleep apnea (OSA), may be low, and thus a PSG should be performed whenever possible. The diagnostic criteria for RBD are:

- Presence of REM sleep without atonia on a PSG reflected by the EMG finding of excessive phasic or tonic muscle activity on submental or limb derivations
- Presence of sleep-related injurious, potentially injurious, or disruptive behaviors either by history or observed during polysomnography
- Absence of EEG epileptiform activity during REM sleep unless RBD can be clearly distinguished from any concurrent REM sleep related seizure disorder
- No other sleep disorder, medical condition, medication use, or substance abuse disorder better explain the behavior

### Comorbidities

Although up to half of patients with RBD present without other neurologic diagnoses, there is a strong relationship to concurrent or eventual development of synucleinopathies such as dementia with Lewy bodies (DLB), multiple system atrophy (MSA), and PD. Since RBD can precede the diagnosis of these diseases by several years, close follow-up is merited.

- About half of the cases of RBD reported in the literature initially present with an associated chronic neurologic illness, most commonly a neurodegenerative disorder. RBD has a strong association with the synucleinopathies MSA, PD, and DLB. RBD is estimated to be present in 15–33% of patients with PD, 50–80% of patients with DLB, and 69–90% of patients with MSA. The positive predictive values for RBD indicating a synucleinopathy in patients with cognitive or Parkinsonian disorders has been estimated at greater than 90%. In addition, 58% of patients with PD and 90–95% of patients with MSA exhibit RSWA. In two series of patients initially diagnosed with idiopathic RBD, 65% developed signs or symptoms of Parkinsonism or dementia at mean follow-up periods of 11.2 and 13.3 years after onset of RBD symptoms. Autopsy studies of 32 patients with RBD revealed concurrent synucleinopathies in 31, only one showed an isolated tauopathy (progressive supranuclear palsy). Furthermore, recent reports of patients with idiopathic RBD describe subclinical abnormalities of olfactory, color vision, motor speed, and cognitive function in a pattern similar to patients with known PD or DLB. These observations suggest that idiopathic RBD may be an early disease manifestation of an underlying synucleinopathy, and that patients with RBD should be followed for the development of neurodegenerative disorders.

- A less frequently identified comorbidity is narcolepsy. The frequency of RBD in narcolepsy has recently been suggested to be 36% in a questionnaire study without polysomnographic confirmation. Both RBD and narcolepsy share disturbances of sleep state boundary control between REM sleep and wakefulness. It is also possible that RBD may manifest in patients with narcolepsy who are treated with tricyclic antidepressants (TCAs) or selective serotonin reuptake inhibitors (SSRIs), both of which may cause REM sleep without atonia and probably clinical RBD.

## Pathophysiology

The pathogenesis of RBD is not entirely clear. Based on the available animal and human lesion and pathologic data as well as the known brainstem structures in humans, a schematic representation underlying RBD in humans is proposed.

- This hypothesis involves structures and networks that are similar to the animal models, with the sublaterodorsal (SLD) nucleus or analogous nucleus with projections to spinal interneurons being the final common pathway that causes active inhibition of skeletal muscle activity in REM sleep. The "indirect route" can also contribute, with SLD lesioning causing reduced excitation of the magnocellular reticular formation (MCRF), thereby causing a net reduced inhibition of spinal motoneurons (either directly or via spinal interneurons). Thus, lesions to the SLD nucleus lead to disinhibition of spinal motoneurons, resulting in increased EMG tone during REM sleep. Whether lesioning or degeneration of the MCRF is sufficient to cause RBD in humans is not yet clear.

## Therapy

Most often RBD can be treated satisfactorily with modifications to the sleep environment and pharmacologic agents, making accurate diagnosis very important.

- Patients with RBD are predisposed to self-injury and violent behavior. Therefore, basic measures to create a safe bedroom environment are of utmost importance and should be undertaken by all patients. These include removal of all furniture from the bedside and placing of padding or mattresses on the floor next to the bed. Some patients have used creative self-confinement devices to tether themselves to the bed in order to avoid injury. Pillow barricades or other barrier devices in the bed may prevent injuries to the bed partner.

- Because the etiology of RBD remains unknown, the therapy to date has been symptomatic. Clonazepam (0.5–2 mg nightly) has been proven safe and effective in controlling the motor behaviors as well as the unpleasant dreams in almost 90% of patients when used as a long-term therapeutic agent. The abuse potential appears negligible and tolerance does not generally develop. There are, however, no randomized controlled double-blind trials to prove the efficacy of the drug. Caution must be exercised if clonazepam is given to elderly, demented, or Parkinsonian patients as side effects include confusion, dizziness, gait unsteadiness, impotence, and daytime sedation. Clonazepam may also worsen OSA, if left untreated. The mechanism of action of clonazepam in RBD is unknown. Clonazepam decreases the amount of phasic muscle activity during REM sleep but tonic EMG activity persists. RBD symptoms typically recur immediately after discontinuation of therapy.

- Recent open-label trials have shown that melatonin (3–12 mg at bedtime) resulted in symptomatic improvement in 26 of 29 patients. Follow-up PSG of patients treated with melatonin showed a decreased percentage of REM sleep without atonia. Although randomized, controlled treatment trials are clearly needed, melatonin may be a valuable drug for treatment of patients who cannot tolerate clonazepam or who experience an incomplete therapeutic response.

## OTHER REM SLEEP PARASOMNIAS

### Nightmare Disorder

Nightmares occur when frightening dream content leads to awakening from REM sleep full dream recall is typical. The lack of associated motor activity, dream enactment behavior, vocalization, confusion, and prominent autonomic activation differentiates nightmare disorder from RBD, sleep terrors, and other disorders characterized by arousals from NREM sleep.

- In adults the prevalence of recurrent nightmares resulting in nightmare disorder is about 4%. Prevalence is higher in children and in adults with psychiatric comorbidities, such as post-traumatic stress disorder or substance abuse. Medications that are known to induce nightmares include levodopa, beta-blockers, SSRIs, TCAs, and acetylcholin-esterase inhibitors.

- Treatment involves the correction of underlying medical or psychiatric conditions and, if necessary, psychotherapy, cognitive–behavioral therapy and hypnosis.

## Recurrent Isolated Sleep Paralysis

Recurrent isolated sleep paralysis represents intrusion of REM sleep atonia into wakefulness leading to complete paralysis of skeletal muscles (except respiratory and extraocular muscles) while the patient is fully conscious. The phenomenon most often occurs in the morning upon awakening from REM sleep, especially when supine, but is rarely seen in the evening during sleep onset. Patients describe the experience as extremely frightening and sometimes experience a sense of dyspnea. The duration of paralysis ranges from seconds to several minutes. External stimuli such as being called or touched by someone may abort an attack, which otherwise resolves spontaneously.

- The lifetime prevalence of at least one episode of sleep paralysis in the general population is estimated to be 6–40%. Recurrent episodes are estimated to occur in 1–10% of the population.
- Treatment of recurrent isolated sleep paralysis is not usually indicated, but tricyclic antidepressants have been reported to be beneficial.

## KEY POINTS

1. A complaint of dream enactment suggests the presence of rapid eye movement (REM) sleep behavior disorder (RBD), but other considerations include parasomnias due to OSA or periodic limb movements of sleep, and non-REM parasomnias such as sleep walking or sleep talking.

2. One third to three quarters of patients with RBD experience self-inflicted injuries, and two thirds inadvertently strike their bed partners during sleep; it is not a benign disorder.

3. Although up to half of patients with RBD present without other neurologic diagnoses, many will eventually develop a neurodegenerative disease with Parkinsonism and/or dementia, which is usually a synucleinopathy such as dementia with Lewy bodies (DLB), multiple system atrophy (MSA), and Parkinson's disease (PD). Since RBD can precede the diagnosis of these diseases by several years, close follow-up is merited.

4. Treatment for RBD includes prudent removal of potentially injurious objects from the bedroom combined with pharmacologic therapy such as clonazepam or melatonin.

## BIBLIOGRAPHY

Bliwise DL, et al. Inter-rater reliability for identification of REM sleep in Parkinson's disease. *Sleep* 2000; 23:671–676.

Boeve BF, et al. Association of REM sleep behavior disorder and neurodegenerative disease may reflect an underlying synucleinopathy. *Mov Disord* 2001; 16:622–630.

Boeve BF, et al. Melatonin for treatment of REM sleep behavior disorder in neurologic disorders: Results in 14 patients. *Sleep Med* 2003a; 4:281–284.

Boeve BF, et al. Synucleinopathy pathology and REM sleep behavior disorder plus dementia or parkinsonism. *Neurology* 2003b; 61:40–45.

Boeve BF, et al. Insights into REM sleep behavior disorder pathophysiology in brainstem-predominant Lewy body disease. *Sleep Med* 2007a; 8:60–64.

Boeve BF, et al. Pathophysiology of REM sleep behaviour disorder and relevance to neurodegenerative disease. *Brain* 2007b; 130: 2770–2780.

Cheyne JA. Situational factors affecting sleep paralysis and associated hallucinations: Position and timing effects. *J Sleep Res* 2002; 11:169–177.

Comella CL, et al. Sleep-related violence, injury, and REM sleep behavior disorder in Parkinson's disease. *Neurology* 1998; 51:526–529.

Fantini ML, et al. Idiopathic REM sleep behavior disorder: Toward a better nosologic definition. *Neurology* 2005; 64:780–786.

Ferini-Strambi L, et al. Neuropsychological assessment in idiopathic REM sleep behavior disorder (RBD): Does the idiopathic form of RBD really exist? *Neurology* 2004; 62:41–45.

Gagnon JF, et al. REM sleep behavior disorder and REM sleep without atonia in Parkinson's disease. *Neurology* 2002; 59:585–589.

Girard TA, Cheyne JA. Timing of spontaneous sleep paralysis episodes. *J Sleep Res* 2006; 15:22–29.

Kunz D, et al. Melatonin as a therapy in REM sleep behavior disorder patients: An open-labeled pilot study on the possible influence of melatonin on REM-sleep regulation. *Mov Disord* 1999; 14:507–511.

Ohayon MM, et al. Violent behavior during sleep. *J Clin Psychiatry* 1997; 58:369–376.

Ohayon MM, et al. Prevalence and pathologic associations of sleep paralysis in the general population. *Neurology* 1999; 52:1194–1200.

Olson EJ, et al. Rapid eye movement sleep behaviour disorder: Demographic, clinical and laboratory findings in 93 cases. *Brain* 2000; 123:331–339.

Plazzi G. REM sleep behavior disorder in Parkinson's disease and other Parkinsonian disorders. *Sleep Med* 2004; 5:195–199.

Plazzi G, et al. REM sleep behavior disorders in multiple system atrophy. *Neurology* 1997; 48:1094–1097.

Postuma RB, et al. Potential early markers of Parkinson's disease in idiopathic rapid-eye-movement sleep behaviour disorder. *Lancet Neurol* 2006; 5:552–553.

Schenck CH, et al. REM sleep behavior disorder: Clinical, developmental, and neuroscience perspectives 16 years after its formal identification in SLEEP. *Sleep* 2002; 25:120–138.

Schenck CH, et al. REM behavior disorder (RBD): Delayed emergence of Parkinsonism and/or dementia in 65% of older men initially diagnosed with idiopathic RBD, and an analysis of the minimum & maximum tonic and/or phasic electromyographic abnormalities found during REM sleep. *Sleep* 2003; 26:A316.

Sforza E, et al. REM sleep behavior disorder: Clinical and physio-pathological findings. *Sleep Med Rev* 1997; 1:57.

Takeuchi N, et al. Melatonin therapy for REM sleep behavior disorder. *Psychiatry Clin Neurosci* 2001; 55:267–269.

Tippman-Peikert M, et al. Idiopathic REM sleep behavior disorder—A follow-up of 39 patients. *Sleep* 2006; 29:A272.

Turner RS. Idiopathic rapid eye movement sleep behavior disorder is a harbinger of dementia with Lewy bodies. *J Geriatr Psychiatry Neurol* 2002; 15:195–199.

Winkelman J, et al. Serotonergic antidepressants are associated with REM sleep without atonia. *Sleep* 2004; 27:317–321.

# 28

## RESTLESS LEGS SYNDROME AND PERIODIC LIMB MOVEMENT DISORDER

PHILIP M. BECKER[1,2] AND CYNTHIA CROWDER[1]
[1]Sleep Medicine Fellowship Program, Department of Psychiatry, University of Texas Southwestern Medical Center at Dallas, Dallas, Texas
[2]Sleep Medicine Associates of Texas, Dallas, Texas

## INTRODUCTION

Restless legs syndrome (RLS) is a common neurologic disorder with sensory and motor components that has both primary and secondary causation. The central nervous system (CNS) pathophysiologic mechanisms that cause RLS remain uncertain.

## CLINICAL FEATURES

As defined by the International Restless Legs Syndrome Study Group and then refined by an National Institute of Health (NIH) Consensus Conference in 2002, RLS is characterized by four core symptoms: an urge or sensation to move the limbs, the urge worsens when at rest, movement improves the urge at least temporarily, and symptoms worsen in the evening or at night.

- The presenting complaint of RLS is often one of sleep-onset or sleep maintenance insomnia that is frequently severe.

## DEMOGRAPHICS

Studies in North America and western Europe that utilized the NIH consensus definition of RLS have consistently reported that approximately 10% of adults experience symptoms of RLS on one or more nights per month. Clinically relevant RLS requiring treatment is estimated to affect 2–5% of the adult population. RLS appears in less than 2% in adults from Asia. Although no study has yet been completed, it is a clinical impression that African-Americans rarely report primary RLS.

- Approximately 60% of adult RLS patients are female. Prior to menopause, women who have had three or more pregnancies have more complaints of RLS than nulliparous women.
- Forty percent of primary RLS patients report onset of some symptoms before age 20 years. Frequency of RLS increases with each decade of life; it is infrequent as a nightly disorder in children under age 10 years and reaches its highest prevalence after age 50 years.

## PERIODIC LIMB MOVEMENTS

Periodic leg movements while awake (PLMW) are present in the sleep–wake transition and represent the most specific and sensitive electromyographic (EMG) evidence in RLS patients. Periodic leg movements of sleep (PLMS) is the polysomnographic finding that defines the severity of restless legs syndrome. Not all RLS patients have PLMS; about 20% of RLS patients have little or no PLMS on a single night of polysomnography (PSG).

## PRIMARY VERSUS SECONDARY RLS

Primary RLS is thought to be a familial/genetic disorder that more commonly presents before age 30 years. Secondary RLS is seen more commonly after age 50 years and arises from various medical conditions, particularly iron deficiency and renal disease.

- Primary RLS is thought to have an autosomal dominant mode of inheritance. Analyses of familial cohorts have identified linkages to chromosome 12q and 14q. However, some studies have not demonstrated these linkages.
- Secondary RLS arises from multiple causes, including reduction of iron stores and renal failure. It is estimated that 35% of patients undergoing renal

*Sleep Medicine Essentials*, edited by Teofilo L. Lee-Chiong
Copyright © 2009 John Wiley & Sons, Inc.

dialysis will have symptoms of RLS. Symptoms commonly resolve after renal transplantation.

- Pregnancy is associated with varying degrees of RLS in 10–30% of expectant mothers. The majority of women report that their RLS resolved quickly after delivery.

- Axonal neuropathies, such as Charcot-Marie-Tooth (CMT) 2, are associated with RLS in up to 37% of patients. RLS symptoms may also be more common in patients with rheumatologic disorders and diabetes, although some investigators dispute these associations.

## CLASSIFICATION OF RLS

|  | Etiology | Symptom Onset |
|---|---|---|
| Primary RLS | Idiopathic<br>Genetic (possibly autosomal<br>dominant) | Before age 30 |
| Secondary RLS | Related to another<br>identifiable cause:<br>Iron deficiency anemia<br>Renal disease<br>Pregnancy<br>Axonal neuropathies<br>Medications:<br>Caffeine, tricyclic<br>antidepressants, serotonin<br>reuptake inhibitors,<br>dopamine blockers<br>(metoclopramide and<br>compazine) | After age 50 |

## ETIOLOGY

The etiology of RLS remains uncertain. Analysis of the substantia nigra in patients with RLS showed signs of iron deficiency with reduction in total iron, reduced H-ferritin, and increased transferring levels.

- A majority of functional imaging studies have found mild reductions of dopamine $D_2$ receptor activity in the basal ganglia or associated brain structures. Dopamine has also been implicated by studies demonstrating that dopamine antagonists exacerbate RLS, and dopaminergic therapy is very successful in managing RLS symptoms. There is interest in areas 10 and 11 of the midbrain, as these rudimentary structures send long dopaminergic projections into the spinal cord and influence gating of peripheral nociceptive input.

## EVALUATION

Restless legs syndrome is a clinical disorder that is principally diagnosed by history. The majority of patients with the four core symptoms of RLS generally do not require polysomnography unless other medical disorders of sleep, such as apnea or narcolepsy, are suspected.

- Patients may have difficulty describing the sensation in their legs. About one-third to one-half of patients report a "creepy, crawly, jumpy, anxious" feeling inside their calves. Fewer describe a painful leg sensation, but pain is generally not incapacitating; movement relieves the sensation, at least temporarily.

- The acronym U-R-G-E can be helpful in remembering the four core symptoms of RLS.

  U = urge or sensation to move the legs
  R = rest or stillness of the legs worsens the urge to move
  G = going is good (at least temporary relief of the urge occurs with movement)
  E = evening or nighttime worsening of symptoms

- Patients will commonly complain about sleep-onset or maintenance difficulties. Reported sleep time of 3–5 h per night is common. Although patients are sleep deprived, RLS often makes it difficult for these patients to nap. If significant sleep-onset delay is reported, the physician should ask the patient if they are ever bothered with "funny feelings in the legs around bedtime."

- When patients report the four core symptoms of RLS (URGE acronym), the physician should determine whether the patient requires a complete blood count, serum chemistry panel, folate, vitamin $B_{12}$, and serum iron/ferritin. Serum ferritin should always be evaluated in women who continue with menstruation, patients with known disorders leading to blood loss, or older patients who report recent development or significant exacerbation of RLS.

- Polysomnography should be considered if other sleep disorders, such as sleep-disordered breathing (including upper airway resistance syndrome), are suspected or when the symptoms of RLS appear in an atypical manner. Although PLMS are found in at least 80% of RLS patients during PSG, the high rate of PLMS of five or more per sleep hour in the general population makes the findings of leg movements during PSG nonspecific and of limited value in arriving at a diagnosis.

- A more specific and sensitive test is the suggested immobilization test (SIT). The SIT is conducted during the one hour before normal sleep. EMG sensors are placed over the anterior tibialis muscles of each leg, and patients are asked to lie in bed making every effort not to move consciously for 1 h. They are asked to rate the level of sensation in their legs on a 10-cm visual analog scale at 5-min intervals. EMG discharges of 2–10 s occurring during wakefulness (PLMW) are then counted. Patients often have to end the SIT after 30–45 min because the intensity of the sensation becomes so distressing that they can no longer lie in bed.

- The use of lower extremity actigraphy has gained interest as a diagnostic tool because the degree of restlessness, sleep disturbance, and PLMS varies significantly from night to night. Actigraphic monitoring can be done with a variety of devices and algorithms, so it is important that the clinician understand the features and limitations of each particular device. Assessment of movement in all directional planes becomes important to assure correlation to body position, sleep disturbance, movement frequency, and movement intensity. Actigraphic studies are most helpful in assessing therapeutic efficacy since it can provide cost-effective, objective evidence of reduction of movements over 3 or more days.

- If patients meet criteria for RLS but also have symptoms of neuropathy, it is appropriate to consider electromyographic and nerve conduction velocity studies of the lower extremities.

## DIFFERENTIAL DIAGNOSIS

Disorders that might be confused with RLS include nocturnal leg cramps and neuropathy. Leg cramps are characterized by painful muscular spasms that awaken the patient from sleep, whereas neuropathy may present as sensation of pins, needles, and numbness. Discerning whether symptoms are present in the morning helps in distinguishing RLS from neuropathy; neuropathy is present on awakening, while the urge to move is rarely noted at this time of day in RLS.

## THERAPY

Goals for treatment need to be defined. Selection of initial treatment is assisted by characterization of the severity and frequency of RLS symptoms into three categories, namely *intermittent/mild*, *daily/moderate*, and *refractory/severe* cases.

### Treatment Goals

The goal is to reduce symptoms to the lowest possible level throughout the 24-h day, while minimizing side effects of pharmacotherapy. Sleep quality should be enhanced with more rapid sleep onset and improved sleep continuity.

### Treatment Classes

Therapeutic classes for the treatment of RLS include benzodiazepine agonists, dopaminergic agents, mineral supplementation, anticonvulsants, and opiates. Only dopaminergic agents have had large-scale, controlled studies in RLS patients using current diagnostic criteria, and there is a lack of well-controlled trials for other therapeutic agents.

**Dopaminergic agents**
Carbidopa/levodopa
Pergolide
Pramipexole
Ropinirole
**Opiate agonists**
Codeine
Hydrocodone
Hydromorphone
Levorphanol
Morphine
Methadone
Oxycodone
Oxymorphone
Propoxyphene

### Treatment of Intermittent/Mild RLS

Patients with mild RLS may benefit from behavioral interventions, including avoidance of substances that overly stimulate the nervous system such as caffeine, chocolate, monosodium glutamate, and decongestants; these substances should be best avoided or minimized after 3:00 PM. Aerobic exercise may be beneficial after conditioning has occurred; when first beginning exercise, some patients report a temporary worsening of their RLS. Many patients have described that counterstimuli, such as knee-high socks, riding a stationary bike, walking on a treadmill, stretching, hot baths, showers, ice packs, massage, or vigorous rubbing, among others, improve their RLS symptoms.

- Antidepressants, particularly selective serotonin reuptake inhibitors, may exacerbate RLS symptoms, while bupropion and trazodone seem to have a lesser propensity to aggravate RLS. Recommendations for mild RLS include pharmacologic therapy when patients have sufficient distress from their urge to move to disrupt sleep and reduce daytime functioning. Some mild patients may have particularly disruptive restlessness occurring only one or two times per month, while other mild patients will report disturbed sleep up to three times per week. If the behavioral interventions above do not offer sufficient relief, the first-line therapy consists of dopaminergic class.

- Therapy will be on an as-needed basis, particularly during situations that usually result in worsening RLS, such as sitting or confinement in a plane, automobile, movie, play, or concert. Initial options include pretreatment with ropinirole 0.25–0.5 mg 1 h before confinement, pramipexole 0.125–0.25 mg 2 h before confinement, or carbidopa/levodopa 25/100 mg 30–60 min before confinement. For patients who are unable to predict when their symptoms of RLS will appear, rapid-acting dopaminergic therapy, such as carbidopa/levodopa 25/100 mg at one-half to one tablet or ropinirole 0.25–0.5 mg may be useful.

- Any of the other treatment classes may also be considered, although they are more commonly utilized for moderate or severe RLS patients.

### Treatment of Moderate/Daily RLS

Patients with moderate RLS generally experience significant symptoms 1–3 h before, or at, bedtime on most nights of the week. Occasionally, patients report falling asleep and then waking 20–60 min later with symptoms of restlessness. There are significant delays in sleep onset as well as intermittent sleep maintenance problems that can lead to daytime fatigue, irritability, and decrease in function.

- The RLS Medical Advisory Board (MAB) recommendation is management by dopamine agonists. The most widely utilized agents are the nonergot agonists, pramipexole and ropinirole.
- The 1-h onset of action of ropinirole makes it easier for patients to remember as bedtime approaches. The longer half-life of pramipexole allows treatment of patients who develop their symptoms 2 h or more before bedtime, often resulting in a dosing of medication at supper and again at bedtime. Treatment is commonly initiated at the lowest tablet size of 0.25 mg of ropinirole or 0.125 mg of pramipexole. Unless nausea or other side effects intervene, the medication can be increased every 2–3 days until relief of the urge to move, sleeplessness, and movement occur. A majority of patients responds to ropinirole dosages of 1.5–2 mg, with a maximum dose of 4 mg. Clinical experience shows a range of therapeutic dosages for pramipexole from 0.125 to 1.5 mg. With dopaminergic therapies, side effects (nausea, achiness, headache, or lightheadedness) have generally been mild to moderate. In the majority of patients the side effects could be managed by a temporary reduction of the dosage before again increasing the dosage in a more gradual manner. For nausea, it is recommended to give the dopaminergic agent with a light meal.
- Gabapentin may be used as initial therapy in moderate RLS, particularly when it is associated with pain. Gabapentin may also be used to enhance sleep onset and maintenance. At common therapeutic dosages, a significant subset of patients complains of excess sedation or other side effects.
- Carbamazepine has demonstrated efficacy in a double blind, placebo-controlled trial from 1984. Other anticonvulsants may be of potential benefit but they have received inadequate study.
- Opiates can be used in the patient with moderate RLS, although it is typical to use them for intermittent exacerbation or in rotation between primary therapy that is complicated by augmentation or other side effects.
- It is common for patients to require more than a single agent. Up to 60% of patients with moderate or severe RLS can be managed with one medication, most commonly pramipexole or ropinirole. Others will need the addition of a sedative/hypnotic agent (e.g., zolpidem 5–10 mg) or gabapentin to enhance sleep. Patients who experience sleep disturbance later in the night might benefit from gabapentin at a dose of 100–900 mg at bedtime. As patients with RLS appear to have a moderately higher prevalence of generalized anxiety, the use of clonazepam 0.5–2 mg 1 h before bedtime can assist sleep onset, maintenance, and daytime anxiety.

### Treatment of Severe/Refractory RLS

Patients with severe RLS experience nearly nightly symptoms with the urge to move often presenting in the afternoon or early evening. Symptoms can be present throughout the entire 24-h day.

- Daytime intensification of the sensation often appears rapidly, and patients are compelled to walk, exercise, or massage/pound their limbs. The lower extremities are most commonly affected, but severe patients are more likely to have involvement of the upper extremities. RLS can affect the entire body.
- Profound insomnia is common. Sleep deprivation and the resulting fatigue can create a cyclical pattern of worsening of RLS.
- Severe RLS does not necessarily require higher dosages of medications or the use of combination therapy, and a significant number of severe RLS patients will respond to a single agent. Split dosing of medications may be required (e.g., ropinirole at a dose of 0.5–2 mg at approximately 6:00 PM and again 1 h before bedtime; or pramipexole 0.25–1 mg in the early evening and again approximately 1–2 h before bedtime).
- Regular monitoring of serum ferritin is indicated since fluctuations of iron stores can result in exacerbation and potentially reduce response to therapeutic intervention.
- Patients with severe/refractory RLS are more likely to require higher total dosages of medications, need combination therapy, develop augmentation on dopaminergic therapy (particularly levodopa), develop augmentation on another dopaminergic agent following augmentation on any dopaminergic agent, require therapy earlier in the day, including the morning, and have more adverse effects such as nausea, vomiting, headaches, myalgia, daytime sleepiness, and orthostatic hypotension because of higher dosages of medications.
- The treatment of severe patients requires the initiation of therapy prior to the onset of symptoms. Ropinirole, pramipexole, or other dopamine agonists should be administered 1–2 h prior to typical time of symptom onset. Titration to the highest effective level that results in the least amount of side effects is recommended. To offer the greatest degree of improvement in sleep and daytime function, combination of various therapeutic classes is often needed. The most common combination therapy is a dopamine agonist with either a hypnotic agent (clonazepam,

temazepam, or zolpidem) or gabapentin to enhance sleep while minimizing carryover sedation. High-potency opiates are particularly important, particularly when augmentation to dopaminergic therapy occurs.

- Selection of high-potency opiates is based on both the onset of action and half-life of the selected agent. Lower potency, short-acting agents such as propoxyphene, codeine, tramadol, hydrocodone, and oxycodone might best be considered for "as-needed" use or for patients with less severe symptoms. Hydromorphone 2–4 mg allows for a fairly rapid onset of action, but its half-life of approximately 4 h may limit its utility. Longer acting, high-potency opiates that include sustained release opiate preparation (oxycodone CR or fentanyl patch), methadone 5–40 mg per day or levorphanol tartrate 2–8 mg per day are often highly efficacious. Patients must be monitored closely for abuse and dependency.
- Opiates are fairly well tolerated, with only occasional problems of daytime sedation, nausea, or constipation. Severe patients treated with opiates are at risk for the development of sleep disordered breathing, particularly upper airway resistance, so that the physician must monitor any complaints of increasing daytime sleepiness and consider PSG testing in the patient who develops new symptoms even as RLS improves.

### Restless Legs Syndrome and Depression

Major depressive disorder is common in patients with RLS. Reports of depression have ranged from 20 to 70% of patients with RLS and PLMD.

- Significant exacerbation of RLS occasionally occurs with tricyclic antidepressants (TCA). Patients appear to better tolerate low dosages of TCAs, such as amitriptyline or imipramine.
- Selective serotonin reuptake inhibitors (SSRIs), such as fluoxetine, paroxetine, sertraline, venlafaxine, citalopram, escitalopram, as well as serotonin modulators, including mirtazapine, buspirone, nefazodone, and trazodone, exacerbate RLS in the majority of patients. In contrast, bupropion does not exacerbate, and may even improve, RLS and PLMS, particularly when it is given early in the day.
- Other patients will report significant dysphoria even though they do not meet clinical criteria for the diagnosis of major depressive disorder. Anxiety occurs more often in RLS patients. The usage of benzodiazepines, particularly clonazepam, or gabapentin may offer significant improvements in mood. Carryover sedation must be monitored when these medications are used during the daytime.

### Side Effects of Dopaminergic Therapy

Side effects of dopaminergic therapy are common. Compared to Parkinson's disease patients, side effects are much less problematic in RLS patients and only infrequently result in discontinuation of therapy. Nausea, vomiting, dizziness, muscle aches, headaches, and occasional sedation may occur. Less commonly, patients report nasal stuffiness, insomnia, constipation, or leg edema.

- In patients treated for Parkinson's disease, excessive daytime sleepiness has been reported from these agents, and there has been concern about the potential for sudden sleep onset. Although less than 10% of RLS patients in clinical trials have reported any degree of sleepiness or lethargy during dopaminergic therapy, continued observation for and precaution about hypersomnia arising from dopamine therapy is recommended.

### Augmentation

The primary limiting factor to long-term therapy with dopaminergic agents is augmentation. Augmentation is defined as the earlier onset of RLS symptoms (at least 2 h before presentation prior to the initiation of therapy). Augmentation is also diagnosed if any two of the following symptoms are present: increased symptoms following increase in medication dosage; decreased symptoms following decrease in medication dosage; spread of symptoms to other body parts; shortening of therapeutic benefit when compared to the start of therapy; or development or worsening of PLMW.

- Various methods have been proposed to manage augmentation. Augmentation is common on levodopa and is best managed by gradually tapering the medication and substituting another therapeutic agent, most commonly ropinirole, pramipexole, or gabapentin. Dopamine agonists are also thought to cause augmentation, although the frequency appears lower than with levodopa and perhaps with less intensity. Other management strategies include dividing the dose and providing the lower divided dose at an earlier time. When these strategies are unsuccessful, the use of high-potency, long-acting opiates such as methadone and levorphanol may prove quite helpful.

### KEY POINTS

1. Restless legs syndrome (RLS) is a common neurologic disorder that occurs during wakefulness and requires the presence of four core symptoms for diagnosis: **U**rge or sensation to move the limbs; **R**est worsens the urge to move; **G**oing (movement) temporarily relieves the urge; and **E**vening or nighttime is associated with worsening symptoms.

2. It has been estimated that symptoms of RLS occur in approximately 10% of the adult population with the higher frequency occurring in the female population. While the exact etiology of RLS remains uncertain, decreased serum and CNS ferritin levels have been shown to correlate with worsening

symptoms. Additional research has also postulated that CNS dopamine metabolism is altered in RLS patients.

3. The diagnosis of RLS is made by clinical history. PSG is not generally required but should be considered if sleep-disordered breathing is suspected or if the patient shows significant daytime sleepiness.

4. The best investigated electrophysiologic study is the suggested immobilization test (SIT) that correlates fairly well with the subjective reports of RLS symptoms.

5. A diagnostic work-up that includes a complete blood count (CBC), serum iron, ferritin, transferrin, folate, and vitamin $B_{12}$ levels should be obtained. Serum ferritin levels less than 50 ng/mL have been shown to exacerbate RLS symptoms. Serum chemistry is also helpful to exclude uremia and diabetes as secondary causes of RLS.

6. Approximately one-third to one-half of patients report symptoms of "creepy, crawly, jumpy, or anxious" feelings inside of either, both or alternating calves. A lesser percentage describes a painful yet nonincapacitating sensation. These symptoms are more prevalent with rest and immobility, resulting in the primary sleep complaint of difficulty with sleep onset and maintenance. Less frequently, other body parts, such as the arms, are involved.

7. Periodic leg movements of sleep are commonly seen on a single night of PSG in 80% of patients with RLS; however, this finding is nonspecific due to the increased rate of PLMS in the aging population and the high degree of nightly variation.

8. Differential diagnosis includes neuropathy, neuroleptic akathisia, claudication, and nocturnal leg cramps.

9. Treatment of RLS is best approached by characterizing the severity and frequency of symptoms. Treatment should be focused on reducing symptoms to the lowest possible level while minimizing the side effects. Caffeine, chocolate, monosodium glutamate, and decongestants should be avoided or limited after 3:00 PM. Iron replacement should be considered with ferritin levels < 30–50 ng/mL.

10. Dopamine agonists such as ropinirole and pramipexole are recommended for the treatment of mild, moderate, or severe RLS. Gabapentin, clonazepam, and mild opiates might also have a role. As severity of RLS increases, patients will benefit from combination therapy of dopamine agonists, sedative/hypnotic medications, gabapentin or other anticonvulsants, and opiates.

11. Although dopaminergic agents offer significant clinical benefit, augmentation of RLS symptoms is the primary limiting factor to long-term therapy. Augmentation is more common with levodopa and is best managed with tapering the medication and substituting another agent such as ropinirole, pramipexole, gabapentin, or clonazepam.

## BIBLIOGRAPHY

Allen RP, et al. Restless legs syndrome: Diagnostic criteria, special considerations, and epidemiology: A report from The RLS Diagnosis and Epidemiology Workshop at the National Institutes of Health. *Sleep Med* 2003a; 4:101–119.

Allen RP, et al. Restless legs syndrome: The efficacy of ropinirole in the treatment of RLS patients suffering from periodic leg movements of sleep [abstr]. *Sleep* 2003b; 26(Suppl):A341.

Becker PM, et al. Encouraging initial response of restless legs syndrome to pramipexole. *Neurology* 1998; 51:1221–1223.

Bonati MT, et al. Autosomal dominant restless legs syndrome maps on chromosome 14q. *Brain* 2003; 126(Pt 6):1485–1492.

Chesson AL, et al. Practice parameters for the treatment of restless legs syndrome and periodic limb movement disorder. An American Academy of Sleep Medicine Report. Standards of Practice Committee of the American Academy of Sleep Medicine. *Sleep* 1999; 22:961–968.

Connor JR, et al. Neuropathological examination suggests impaired brain iron acquisition in restless legs syndrome. *Neurology* 2003; 61(22):304–309.

Earley CJ. Clinical practice. Restless legs syndrome. *N Engl J Med* 2003: 348(21):2103–2109.

Earley CJ, et al. Abnormalities in CSF concentrations of ferritin and transferrin in restless legs syndrome. *Neurology* 2000; 54 (8):1698–1700.

Garcia-Borreguero D, et al. Treatment of restless legs syndrome with gabapentin: A double-blind, cross-over study. *Neurology* 2002; 59(10):1573–1579.

Garcia-Borreguero D, et al. Ropinirole is effective in the treatment of restless legs syndrome (RLS): A double-blind placebo-controlled 12-week study conducted in 10 countries [abstr]. *Neurology* 2003; 60(Suppl 1):A11–A12.

Hening WA, et al. Restless Legs Syndrome Task Force of the Standards of Practice Committee of the American Academy of Sleep Medicine. An update on the dopaminergic treatment of restless legs syndrome and periodic limb movement disorder. *Sleep* 2004; 27(3):560–583.

Manconi M, et al. Restless legs syndrome and pregnancy. *Neurology* 2004; 63(6):1065–1069.

Michaud M, et al. Effects of immobility on sensory and motor symptoms of restless legs syndrome. *Mov Disord* 2002; 17 (1):112–115.

Ondo W, et al. Restless legs syndrome: Clinicoetiologic correlates. *Neurology* 1996; 47(6):1435–1441.

Ondo WG, et al. Clinical correlates of 6-hydroxydopamine injections into A11 dopaminergic neurons in rats: A possible model for restless legs syndrome. *Mov Disord* 2000; 15(1):154–158.

Phillips B, et al. Epidemiology of restless legs syndrome in adults. *Arch Intern Med* 2002; 160:2137–2141.

Rothdach AJ, et al. Prevalence and risk factors of RLS in an elderly population: The MEMO study. *Neurology* 2000; 54:1064–1068.

Saletu M, et al. Acute placebo-controlled sleep laboratory studies with clonazepam. *Eur Neuropsychopharmacol* 2001; 11:153–161.

Silber MH, et al. An algorithm for the management of restless legs syndrome. *Mayo Clin Proc* 2004; 79(7):916–922.

Walters A, et al. Ropinirole versus placebo in the treatment of restless legs syndrome (RLS): A 12-week multicenter double-blind placebo-controlled study conducted in six countries [abstr]. *Sleep* 2003; 26(Suppl):A344.

# 29

## SLEEP IN INFANTS AND CHILDREN

STEPHEN H. SHELDON

Northwestern, University, Feinberg School of Medicine, Sleep Medicine Center Children's Memorial Hospital, Chicago, Illinois

### INTRODUCTION

Sleep occupies a major portion of the lives of newborns, infants, and children. A newborn infant typically sleeps about 70% of every 24 h. In contrast, adults spend 25–30% of their lives sleeping.

- Sleep in normal infants varies significantly from normal sleep in adults. Premature infants frequently reveal a lack of concordance between electrophysiological parameters of sleep and behavioral variables. This may also be true in some term infants. Sleep in infants and children is significantly different than adults and may serve different functions in the developing infant and child.

### SLEEP IN PREMATURE INFANT

Periods of activity and quiescence can be identified in the human fetus by 28–32 weeks gestation. However, clearly definable sleep states cannot be identified in premature neonates between 24 and 26 weeks gestation. By 28–30 weeks postconception, active sleep can be identified by the presence of eye movements, body activity, and irregular respiration. Chin muscle hypotonia is very difficult to evaluate in the fetus and premature infant since there are so few periods of tonic activity before 36 weeks gestation.

- Quiet sleep cannot be clearly identified at this time, and active sleep comprises the vast majority of time the premature infant is asleep. Quiet sleep can be identified by the development of a *tracé discontineau* electroencephalogram (EEG) pattern at about 32 weeks postconception and can be clearly identified by a tracé alternant EEG pattern at approximately 36 weeks gestation. Once quiet sleep can be identified, this state increases steadily and becomes the dominant state [equivalent to nonrapid

eye movement (NREM) sleep] at approximately 3 months of postnatal life.

- Behaviorally, fetal movements can be first identified between 10 and 16 weeks gestation. Rhythmic cycling of activity can be recorded by 20 weeks. At 28–30 weeks, very brief quiet periods begin to appear. By 32 weeks postconception, body movements are absent in 53% of 20-s epochs during 2–3 h sleep recordings. The number of "no-movement epochs" increases to 60% at term.

- Maturational patterns can be demonstrated in EEG recordings of premature infants as early as 24 weeks gestation. Conflicting evidence exists concerning the independence of the maturation of sleep and the EEG with respect to intrauterine stage. Very young premature infants and full-term neonates have similar EEG patterns when compared at the same conceptual age. On the other hand, it has been shown that when the premature infant has reached 40 weeks postconception age, the infant still may not have attained a degree of EEG organization as significant as that of the full-term newborn. Premature infants show spindle development that is about 4 weeks in advance of that seen in full-term infants and a statistical difference between the length of quiet sleep in the term and premature infant has been demonstrated, when measured at the same postconception age. However, extra-uterine development of the premature infant occurs in a somewhat artificial environment. Significant medical problems often coexist and often frequent medical interventions are required.

### TERM INFANTS: BIRTH TO TWO MONTHS

Three distinct sleep states can be identified in the term newborn: active sleep [rapid eye movement (REM)],

*Sleep Medicine Essentials*, edited by Teofilo L. Lee-Chiong
Copyright © 2009 John Wiley & Sons, Inc.

quiet sleep (NREM), and indeterminate sleep. Indeterminate sleep is defined as a state in which criteria for neither REM nor NREM can be identified.

- Fine twitches, grimaces, facial movements, and occasional tremors characterize active sleep. Sucking movements that occur during wakefulness can continue during sleep and are common during active sleep. Intermittent large limb movements, stretching, and vocalizations occur. Bursts of phasic muscle activity and respiratory irregularity are present and can occur in conjunction with phasic eye movements.
- Quiet sleep is characterized by minimal movements. Muscle tone is somewhat decreased from waking levels but is increased above the level seen during active sleep.

## TWO TO TWELVE MONTHS

- During the first 3 months of life, substantial changes occur. Ten to twelve weeks of age appears to be a critical period of reorganization, when infantile sleep behavior and physiology matures. Sleep–wake patterns change as well. At birth, total sleep time is about 16–17 h. Total sleep time gradually decreases, reaching 14–15 h by 16 weeks of age, and 13–14 h by 6–8 months.
- Development of attentive behaviors during wakefulness occurs concomitantly with the development of quiet sleep and sustained sleep patterns. These changes suggest continued development of inhibitory and controlling feedback mechanisms secondary to the increasing complexity of neural networks and neurochemical maturation. By 3 months, a relatively stable distribution of sleep and wake occurs across the 24-h day. There is a remarkably regular alternation of active and quiet sleep. Periodic respiration, common until 3 weeks of age, becomes uncommon after the first 2 months of life.
- During the first 6 months of life, consolidation of sleep during nocturnal hours occurs. Major changes seen are in the duration of sleep periods and when they occur in the 24-h day. At 3 weeks of age, the average length of the longest sleep period is about 3.5 h. By 6 months of age, the longest sleep period averages about 6 consecutive hours.
- Between 3 and 6 weeks, sleep periods lengthen considerably, and by 6 weeks of age, the longest sleep period is no longer randomly distributed throughout the day, but occurs during nocturnal hours. At 3 months, the pattern had become more consistent so that by 12–16 weeks of age the longest sleep period occurs during nighttime and the longest wake period occurs during the daytime. At 6 months of age, the long sleep period immediately follows the longest wake period.

- After about 3 months of age, there is continuing development and daytime sleep becomes consolidated into discrete daytime naps.
- Brief awakenings from sleep are more frequent during the first 2 months of life, than at older ages. In addition, infants 1–2 months of age are more likely to awaken from active sleep than from quiet sleep.
- Significant maturation can be seen in the EEG during this period of development. Tracé alternant pattern of quiet sleep can be first identified at 32–34 weeks gestation. This pattern is most often well developed by 36–38 weeks. Tracé alternant pattern gradually disappears over the first month of life and is replaced by continuous high-voltage slow-wave activity.
- Sleep spindles appear at about 4–8 weeks of age. The shape of these spindles changes impressively early in development. Before 2 months of age, sleep spindles are difficult to differentiate from background EEG activity. Identifiable spindles develop between 2 and 3 months of age. When first present, spindles may be quite long and last 2–4 s. Duration decreases continuously to about an average of 0.5–1 s by the end of the second year. Spindle intervals become greater with increasing age.
- True slow-wave activity appears at approximately 8–12 weeks of age, and by 16–24 weeks of age, sleep becomes differentiated into more mature and distinct NREM sleep states. By 3 months of age, NREM (N) sleep is almost twice that of REM (R) sleep, and by 8 months of age, active sleep occupies about 30% of the total sleep time. Adult percentages are reached between 3 and 5 years of age.
- Sleep onset is characteristically through REM sleep in the newborn infant (i.e., the first REM period typically occurs within the first 15 min after sleep onset). At 3 weeks of age, an infant is likely to have two-thirds of sleep periods beginning with REM sleep. Infants less than 3 months of age reveal REM latencies that are predominantly less than 8 minutes in length. During the first 12 weeks of life, latency from sleep onset to the first REM period gradually changes until sleep onset occurs predominantly through NREM sleep. By 6 months, the percentage of sleep episodes beginning with REM sleep is approximately 18%.
- The ratio of active sleep to quiet sleep is sometimes considered an indicator of maturation. Active sleep time exceeds quiet sleep time during the first months of life. A reversal of this relation is noted in 60% of infants at 3 months and 90% of infants at 6 months of age.
- Specific changes in REM sleep percent occurs during this period of development. During the first 6 months of life there is a marked reduction in the total REM sleep time. This represents a redistribution of sleep stages since only a relative mild decrease in the total sleep time occurs during the

first year. This change may be an important indicator of central nervous system maturation.

## TWO TO FIVE YEARS

In contrast to the rapid evolution that takes place during the first year of life, changes in sleep structure during this period are more gradual. Growth and development are steady. Sleep becomes consolidated into a long nocturnal period of approximately 10 h. During the first 2–3 years, daytime sleep occurs in somewhat short daytime naps. Morning naps are typically given up first, and by the end of the fifth year, sleep is generally consolidated into a single nocturnal period.

- During the latter half of the first year of life, REM sleep averages about 30–35% of the total sleep time. REM sleep and NREM sleep are evenly distributed across the nocturnal sleep period. Small and large body movements associated with REM sleep during infancy become less frequent. REM periods are of approximately uniform length. As the child continues to develop, a gradual change is seen in the uniformity and duration of these REM periods. The first REM period of the night becomes shorter, while succeeding periods longer and associated with more intense phasic activity. There is also a slight lengthening of the overall cycle length. Two- to three-year-old children still show a cycle length of about 60 min, with the first REM period occurring one hour after sleep onset. By 4–5 years of age, the cycle lengthens gradually to 60–90 min.

- Between 3 and 5 years of age, REM percentage gradually decreases from 30 to 35% of the total sleep time to an adult level of 20–25%. There appears to be a close relationship between these changes and the augmented periods of wakefulness during the daytime.

- Typically, children in this age range have approximately 7 cycles during each nocturnal sleep period. Sleep-onset latency averages about 15 min in the younger children, but lengthens to between 15 and 30 min in the older age groups. Slow-wave sleep predominantly occurs during the first third of the night and as much as 2 h may be spent in slow-wave sleep. EEG voltage is also very high during this period. Stage 2 sleep first appears from 3 to 4 min after the child falls asleep, Stage 3 sleep appears about 11 min after sleep onset, and stage 4 sleep first appears about 4 min later.

## FIVE TO TEN YEARS

Growth and development continues to be constant and gradual during middle childhood. Searching, exploration, and increasingly mature thinking behaviorally characterize this time. It is a period of trials and errors.

- Sleep continues to develop into a more mature pattern. Although sleep patterns of children during middle childhood resembles that of older individuals, there is considerable individual variability. There is a certain stability of the pattern for given individuals and a fairly consistent amount of time spent in each sleep stage and the number of sleep stages from night to night. When compared with adult sleep patterns, total sleep time in middle childhood is approximately 2.5 h longer with unequal distribution of the added time to each of the sleep stages. Stages in children of this age group tend to be longer in duration than in adults, but the sleep architecture seems to be as stable.

- Though body movements during sleep decrease in frequency, they are generally more often seen in this age group than in adolescents and young adults. Stage 4 duration decreases from approximately 2 h in the preschool child to 75–80 min in the latter portion of middle childhood. There does appear, however, to be a gender-related difference in slow-wave sleep. Males tend to exhibit a significantly greater percentage of slow-wave sleep than females of comparable age.

- Naps during this period of development are unusual. Consistent daytime napping during middle childhood may represent a pathological process. Prepubescent children are generally very alert throughout the entire day. Mean sleep onset latencies of pre-adolescent (Tanner stage 1) children is often greater than 15 min, which is an extremely alert and vigilant level.

## KEY POINTS

1. Sleep occupies a major portion of the lives of newborns, infants, and children. A newborn infant typically sleeps about 70% of every 24 h.

2. Periods of activity and quiescence can be identified in the human fetus by 28–32 weeks gestation. Clearly definable sleep states cannot be identified in premature neonates between 24 and 26 weeks gestation.

3. Three distinct sleep states can be identified in the term newborn: active sleep (REM equivalent), quiet sleep (NREM equivalent), and indeterminate sleep. Indeterminate sleep is defined as a state in which criteria for neither REM nor NREM can be identified.

4. NREM (N) and REM (R) sleep can be identified polysomnographically after 2 months of age.

5. Sleep becomes consolidated into a long nocturnal period of approximately 10 h between 2 and 5 years of age. During the first 2–3 years, daytime sleep

occurs in somewhat short daytime naps. Morning naps are typically given up first, and by the end of the fifth year, sleep is generally consolidated into a single nocturnal period.

6. Although sleep patterns of children during middle childhood resembles that of older individuals, there is considerable individual variability. When compared with adult sleep patterns, total sleep time in middle childhood is approximately 2.5 h longer with unequal distribution of the added time to each of the sleep stages.

## BIBLIOGRAPHY

Anders T, et al (Eds): *A Manual of Standardized Terminology, Techniques and Criteria for Scoring of States of Sleep and Wakefulness in Newborn Infants.* UCLA, Brain Information Service, NINDS Neurological Information Network, Los Angeles, California, 1971.

Iber C, et al for the American Academy of Sleep Medicine. *The AASM Manual for the Scoring of Sleep and Associated Events: Rules, Terminology and Technical Specification*, 1st ed. American Academy of Sleep Medicine, Westchester, IL, 2007.

# 30

## OBSTRUCTIVE SLEEP APNEA IN CHILDREN

PREETAM BANDLA AND CAROLE L. MARCUS
The Children's Hospital of Philadelphia, University of Pennsylvania, Philadelphia, Pennsylvania

## INTRODUCTION

Obstructive sleep apnea syndrome (OSAS) is common in children. It is characterized by recurrent episodes of partial or complete upper airway obstruction during sleep, resulting in the disruption of normal ventilation and sleep patterns. Its symptoms, polysomnographic findings, pathophysiology, and treatment are significantly different from the condition in adults (Table 30.1).

## EPIDEMIOLOGY

Obstructive sleep apnea syndrome occurs in children of all age groups. It is commonest among preschoolers, due to adenotonsillar hypertrophy. The prevalence of OSAS in children is estimated to be about 2%. It occurs equally between both sexes. This is in contrast to adults, where there is a male preponderance of the disease.

## PATHOPHYSIOLOGY

In children OSAS occurs as a result of a combination of multiple factors. These include abnormal upper airway structure and neuromuscular control as well as other factors such as hormonal and genetic influences.

### Structural Factors

Structural factors play a major role in the pathophysiology of OSAS. Most children with OSAS have some degree of upper airway narrowing as a result of either one or a combination of the following: adenotonsillar hypertrophy, craniofacial anomalies, or excess adipose tissue due to obesity.

- In otherwise normal children, tonsillectomy and adenoidectomy usually leads to a significant improvement in sleep and respiratory abnormalities, suggesting that adenotonsillar hypertrophy is a major contributing factor to childhood OSAS.
- Many congenital syndromes, including Down, Crouzon, achondroplasia, Pierre Robin, Treacher Collins, and Cornelia de Lange syndrome, among others, have associated OSAS as a result of craniofacial anomalies such as midfacial hypoplasia, micro- or retrognathia, macroglossia, and/or obesity or hypotonia that result in narrowing of the upper airway.

### Neuromotor Factors

A number of factors suggest that there are additional neuromotor abnormalities that play a role in the development of OSAS. These are:

1. Children with OSAS only obstruct while asleep and not during wakefulness.
2. OSAS may persist after adenotonsillectomy. In one study, 75% of otherwise normal children with OSAS secondary to adenotonsillar hypertrophy and/or obesity had persistent obstructive sleep apnea postoperatively.
3. OSAS may recur following adenotonsillectomy. Some children with OSAS who had undergone an adenotonsillectomy with resolution of disease have developed recurrence of OSAS during adolescence.
   - Although normal children have a smaller upper airway than adults, their airways are less collapsible; thus, they snore less and have fewer obstructive apneas. This suggests that normal children compensate for a smaller upper airway by an increased ventilatory drive to their upper airway muscles. It is thought that children with OSAS may have abnormal centrally mediated activation of their upper airway muscles, resulting in increased collapsibility of the upper airway.

**Table 30.1  Differences between Childhood and Adult OSAS**

| Characteristics | Children | Adults |
|---|---|---|
| *Clinical* | | |
| Peak age | Preschoolers | Elderly |
| Sex ratio | Equal | Male predominance, postmenopausal females |
| Etiology | Adenotonsillar hypertrophy, obesity, craniofacial anomalies | Obesity |
| Body habitus | Failure to thrive, normal, obese | Obese, normal |
| Excessive daytime Somnolence | Uncommon | Very common |
| Neurobehavioural | Hyperactivity, developmental delay, cognitive impairment | Cognitive impairment, impaired vigilance |
| *Polysomnographic* | | |
| Obstruction | Cyclic obstruction or prolonged obstructive hypoventilation | Cyclic obstruction |
| Sleep architecture | Normal | Decreased delta and REM |
| State with OSAS | Rapid eye movement (REM) | REM or non-REM |
| Cortical arousal | <50% of apneas | At terminatioxn of most apneas |
| *Treatment* | | |
| Surgical | Tonsillectomy and adenoidectomy (majority) | Uvulopharyngoplasty (selected cases) |
| Medical | CPAP (occasionally) | CPAP |

## CLINICAL FEATURES

The clinical features of OSAS include nocturnal symptoms such as snoring, labored breathing, paradoxical respiratory effort, observed apnea, restlessness, sweating, unusual sleep positions (e.g., sleeping sitting up, or hyperextension of the neck) and secondary enuresis.

- Daytime symptoms may include mouth breathing related to adenotonsillar hypertrophy, frequent upper respiratory tract infections, excessive daytime somnolence, morning headaches, fatigue, hyperactivity, aggression, and social withdrawal.
- Children with OSAS may be of normal height and weight, but obesity has been increasingly recognized as a risk factor. Failure to thrive and developmental delay can occur in rare cases of longstanding OSAS. Other physical examination findings may include mouth breathing and nasal voice quality secondary to adeno-tonsillar hypertrophy, retrognathia or micrognathia. Tonsillar hypertrophy is a common physical finding in children with OSAS, although its absence does not exclude the diagnosis.
- A constellation of physical findings including a small steep mandibular plane, a high arched hard palate and an elongated soft palate, retroposition of the mandible, and a long face have been associated with OSAS. The size of the adenoids and tonsils has been shown to correlate with the severity of obstructive apneas on polysomnography; however, there is a large amount of clinical variability, so this cannot be used to establish a diagnosis. Rarely, untreated OSAS resulting in pulmonary hypertension may manifest as a loud pulmonary component of the second heart sound.

## COMPLICATIONS

If left untreated, OSAS can result in serious morbidity from various adverse sequelae that occur as a result of chronic nocturnal hypoxemia, hypercapnia, and sleep disturbance.

- Growth impairment can occur with OSAS and, in severe cases, may result in failure to thrive. Following an adenotonsillectomy, children with OSAS frequently have a growth spurt. This appears to be due to decreased caloric expenditure secondary to decreased work of breathing, and an increase in the secretion of insulin-like growth factor-1.
- Cardiovascular complications such as pulmonary hypertension, cor pulmonale, and heart failure used to be common presentations of OSAS in children, but these are now rare. Treatment of the OSAS reverses cor pulmonale. OSAS in children can result in cardiac remodeling and hypertrophy of both the right and left ventricles, though the exact mechanism of left ventricular hypertrophy is unclear. One study showed that children with OSAS have dysregulation of systemic blood pressure in the form of greater mean blood pressure variability during wakefulness and sleep, a higher night-to-day systolic blood pressure, and smaller nocturnal dipping of the mean blood pressure. The blood pressure dysregulation correlated with the severity of the OSAS. Increased blood pressure variability and decreased nocturnal blood pressure dipping have been shown to be associated with end-organ damage and an increased risk for cardiovascular disease.
- Untreated OSAS may result in neurocognitive deficits, learning problems, behavioral problems, and

Obstructive Hypoventilation

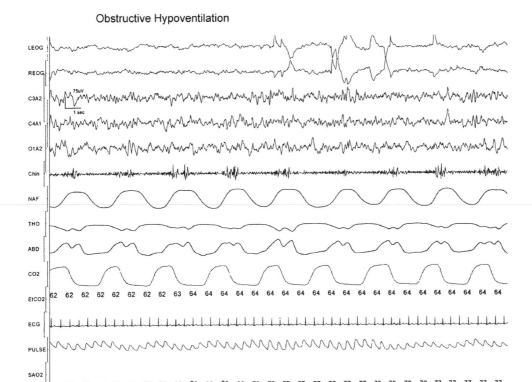

**Figure 30.1** 30-s epoch demonstrating obstructive hypoventilation in a child. Note snoring (on the chin EMG) and paradoxical breathing but no apnea, associated with oxyhemoglobin desaturation and hypercapnia. LEOG, left electrooculogram; REOG, right electrooculogram; EEG leads (C3A2, C4A1, O1A2); Chin, chin electromyogram; NAF, oronasal thermistor; THO, thoracic wall movement; ABD, abdominal wall movement; CO$_2$, end-tidal PCO$_2$ waveform; EtCO2, numerical value of end-tidal PCO$_2$; Pulse, pulse oximeter waveform; S$_a$O$_2$, arterial oxygen saturation.

symptoms mimicking attention deficit hyperactivity disorder. Adenotonsillectomy may improve behavioral, cognitive, and psychiatric indices in children who had OSAS prior to surgery.

## EVALUATION

The gold standard for diagnosing childhood OSAS is polysomnography. This can be performed in infants and children of any age and must be scored and interpreted using pediatric criteria. Polysomnography can differentiate between primary snoring (i.e., snoring not associated with apnea, excessive arousals, or gas exchange abnormalities), and OSAS. Children have a different pattern of upper airway obstruction compared with adults and will often desaturate with relatively short apneas. This is due to a lower functional residual capacity (FRC) and a higher respiratory rate compared to adults. Therefore, obstructive apneas that are 2 breaths in length are scored, as compared to the 10-s duration in adults. Additionally, obstructive hypopneas in children are scored if they are associated with an arousal, awakening, or ≥ 3% desaturation. An apnea hypopnea index of 5, while considered normal in adults is indicative of significant OSA in children. An index of 1.5 is statistically abnormal. Many children have partial upper airway obstruction associated with

hypercapnia and hypoxemia, rather than discrete obstructive apneas. This pattern has been termed "obstructive hypoventilation" (Figure 30.1). Though normative data exist for childhood sleep apnea, it is yet unclear as to the degree of polysomnographic abnormalities (e.g., apnea index) that warrants intervention.

- Screening tests such as nocturnal videotaping, pulse oximetry and nap polysomnograms, although indicative of OSAS when positive, have limited utility because of a high false-negative rate.

## TREATMENT

The vast majority of children with OSAS have significant symptomatic and polysomnographic improvement following tonsillectomy and adenoidectomy. Even children with associated medical conditions such as Down syndrome or obesity tend to improve after adenotonsillectomy, although additional treatment may be needed. This is due to the fact that OSAS results from the relative size and structure of upper airway components, rather than the absolute degree of adenotonsillar hypertrophy. However, some children may have persistent polysomnographic evidence of OSA following adenotonsillectomy, particularly obese children.

- In patients in whom adenotonsillectomy is contra-indicated, or in those patients who continue to be symptomatic following adenotonsillectomy, continuous positive airway pressure (CPAP) delivered via an appropriate mask interface may be used to treat OSAS successfully in infants and children. This can be challenging, especially in very young or developmentally delayed children. Rarely, a tracheostomy may be necessary in very young patients, patients with craniofacial anomalies, or patients who cannot tolerate CPAP or bilevel positive airway pressure following the failure of adenotonsillectomy to resolve symptoms.

- Rarely, supplemental oxygen may be used in certain select patients with OSAS, either as a transitional intervention such as in neonates with mild craniofacial abnormalities who are expected to improve with growth, or in patients where all other therapeutic interventions fail and a tracheostomy is refused. Supplemental oxygen has been shown to improve oxygenation in patients with OSAS, although it does not alter the increased work of breathing or sleep fragmentation. A few individuals develop a marked rise in their $PCO_2$ in response to supplemental oxygen. Therefore, when indicated, supplemental oxygen must be started under controlled circumstances while monitoring $PCO_2$.

## PROGNOSIS

The long-term prognosis and the natural history of childhood OSAS is unknown. It is not known whether children with OSAS will develop OSAS as adults, or whether these are two discrete entities. OSA may recur during adolescence in those who had been successfully treated for childhood OSAS. This suggests that children with OSAS, despite treatment, may be at increased risk for the development of adult OSAS if they acquire additional risk factors such as androgen secretion at puberty, weight gain, or excessive alcohol ingestion.

- Most of the complications of OSAS, including cor pulmonale, growth impairment, and possibly neurobehavioral abnormalities, are reversible after successful treatment.

## KEY POINTS

1. Unlike adults, children with OSAS are usually of normal height and weight, although the dramatic increase in childhood obesity in the United States has resulted in obesity being increasingly recognized as a risk factor.

2. In young children with OSAS, hyperactivity and behavioral problems are more common than daytime sleepiness and fatigue.

3. Adenotonsillar hypertrophy is a common physical finding in children with OSAS, although its absence does not exclude the diagnosis.

4. The gold standard for diagnosing childhood OSAS is polysomnography. History and physical examination are poor at discriminating between primary snoring and OSAS.

5. Screening tests such as nocturnal videotaping, pulse oximetry, and nap polysomnograms have limited utility because of a high false-negative rate.

6. The majority of children with OSAS have significant symptomatic and polysomnographic improvement following a tonsillectomy and adenoidectomy. However, a significant number of children may have persistent polysomnographic evidence of OSA following an adenotonsillectomy.

7. Continuous positive airway pressure can be successfully used in children of all ages for persistent OSAS following adenotonsillectomy, but an intensive behavioral modification program may be needed for young or developmentally delayed children.

## BIBLIOGRAPHY

Amin RS, et al. Left ventricular hypertrophy and abnormal ventricular geometry in children and adolescents with obstructive sleep apnea. *Am J Respir Crit Care Med* 2002; 165:1395–1399.

Amin RS, et al. Twenty-four-hour ambulatory blood pressure in children with sleep-disordered breathing. *Am J Respir Crit Care Med* 2004; 169:950–956.

Brooks LJ, et al. Adenoid size is related to severity but not the number of episodes of obstructive apnea in children. *J Pediatr* 1998; 132:682–686.

American Thoracic Society. Cardiorespiratory sleep studies in children. Establishment of normative data and polysomnographic predictors of morbidity. *Am J Respir Crit Care Med* 1999; 160:1381–1387.

Chervin RD, et al. Sleep-disordered breathing, behavior, and cognition in children before and after adenotonsillectomy. *Pediatrics* 2006; 117:769–778.

Guilleminault C, et al. Morphometric facial changes and obstructive sleep apnea in adolescents. *J Pediatr* 1989; 114:997–999.

Iber C, et al. AASM Manual for the Scoring of Sleep and Associated Events: Rules, Terminology and Technical Specifications 1st ed. 2007.

Marcus CL, et al. Adherence to and effectiveness of positive airway pressure therapy in children with obstructive sleep apnea. *Pediatrics* 2006; 117:442–451.

Marcus CL, et al. Developmental changes in upper airway dynamics. *J Appl Physiol* 2004; 97:98–108.

Marcus CL, et al. Determinants of growth in children with the obstructive sleep apnea syndrome. *J Pediatr* 1994; 125:556–562.

Redline S, et al. Risk factors for sleep-disordered breathing in children. Associations with obesity, race, and respiratory problems. *Am J Respir Crit Care Med* 1999; 159:1527–1532.

Tauman R, et al. Persistence of obstructive sleep apnea syndrome in children after adenotonsillectomy. *J Pediatr.* 2006; 149:803–808.

# 31

## THE SLEEPLESS CHILD

WILLIAM H. MOORCROFT
Northern Colorado Sleep Consultants, Fort Collins, Colorado

## INTRODUCTION

Sleeplessness in children resembles insomnia in adults but has important differences. For both children and adults, the problem may be with one or more of the following: initially getting to sleep, staying asleep, or awakening too early. The result is a negative effect on waking behavior and on medical and psychological status. In children, more than in adults, sleeplessness also affects the entire family and parent–child relationship.

- In the sleepless child, the agents of change are the parents or other caregivers of the poor sleeper. The decision to make a change rests with the parents or caregivers and is somewhat subjective. What is seen as sleeplessness in a child for one caregiver may not be for another.

- Developmental milestones can affect the sleep of children. Teething, crawling, walking, as well as cognitive development can suddenly change a good sleeper into a sleepless one. The development of independence and autonomy in toddlers may increase bedtime resistance. Usually the change is transient, but it may lead to reactions that perpetuate more enduring sleeplessness.

- The most common causes of sleeplessness in children are sleep-onset association disorder, problematic night wakings, early awakenings, nighttime eating/drinking, separation anxiety, parental limit setting, and night fears.

- Other less common causes of insomnia in children include nightmares and bad dreams, delayed sleep phase syndrome, parasomnias, poor sleep hygiene, obstructive sleep apnea, restless legs syndrome, periodic limb movement disorder, and narcolepsy. Paradoxically, insufficient sleep may also be the cause of sleeplessness in children, with hyperarousal occurring in their overtired child.

- Nighttime distractions, such as television, videos, and computer games, have become a major source of sleeplessness in children.

- Finally, sleeplessness can be caused by a medical factor or the treatment of a medical problem; in such cases sleeplessness may develop into an independent behavioral condition that requires direct treatment.

## EARLY CHILDHOOD

Sleeplessness in early childhood is common. The National Sleep Foundation's Sleep in America Annual Poll of 2004 found that 71% of parents reported that their infants woke up and needed help or attention in the prior 2 weeks; 21% stated that this happened more than three times per week.

### Behavioral Insomnia of Childhood, Sleep-Onset Association Type

Sleep-onset association disorder occurs when children are unable to fall asleep by themselves; instead, they regularly need external help, such as being nursed, rocked, or riding in a car. In most cases, this situation is created and maintained by parents who actively help their child get to sleep at bedtime and nap times, although it can occasionally result from separation anxiety, which peaks at 18–24 months of age.

- The most apparent feature of the disorder is problematic night awakenings. The issue is not the awakenings per se, since all young children awaken several times during the night, but whether the child is a "soother" or a "signaler." Most of the time, parents are not aware that soothers awaken during the night because they remain quiet and return to sleep without parental intervention. Signalers, on the other hand, cry and fuss until their parents

*Sleep Medicine Essentials*, edited by Teofilo L. Lee-Chiong
Copyright © 2009 John Wiley & Sons, Inc.

respond to them before they will fall back to sleep; when the child learns to associate some condition, such as parental attention, with sleep onset, they develop difficulty falling asleep or returning to sleep without this condition. There can be night-to-night and week-to-week variability in night awakenings with signaling. Corrections of what happens at bedtime most often also eliminate night waking and nap problems. In those cases where this does not happen, similar corrections can later be applied during the night or for naps.

- Sleep-onset association problems can develop in many ways. Parents are more likely to try to continue to comfort infants who had been colicky; however, this condition can also develop in children who are not colicky. Two other causes are an inadequate amount of sleep, and parents who respond to every sound the child makes at night.

- Treatment is aimed at allowing the child to form a new set of associations for falling asleep without ignoring their genuine needs. Provide a good sleep environment that is conducive to asleep. Put the child to sleep when drowsy but still awake but do not hold or rock him or her thus allowing the child to learn to fall asleep on his or her own. Since children should be able to "sleep through the night" by about 3 months of age, parents should be advised to start putting their child to bed when "drowsy but awake" at about 2–4 months of age.

- Establish and consistently follow a regular schedule of bed and nap times that are consonant with a child's natural schedule. A regular bedtime routine that is quiet, such as reading, and takes place in the space where the child sleeps may be beneficial.

- A transitional object (e.g., a blanket or stuffed animal) that is present at bedtime, nap time, and when the child awakens during the night can be of great help. A pacifier can serve this purpose in infants but is discouraged after about 5–6 months of age since it frequently falls out during the night and the baby cannot retrieve it.

- For children older than 3 years of age, positive reinforcement for bedtime behaviors appropriate to falling asleep can also be helpful, but punishment—overt or subtle—is not helpful.

- Soothing music at bedtime may not be beneficial because the child will associate falling asleep to this music and can have problems sleeping without it following night awakenings or at naptime,

- Once a stable bedtime routine is established, parents should take steps to eliminate sleep-onset dependencies and promote self-soothing. There are several options available to the parent. At one extreme is total extinction ("cry it out" method) whereby the child is put to bed before falling asleep without additional parental intervention (e.g., rocking, nursing, or holding). Typically this will result in loud and prolonged crying when first attempted; however, this response will usually subside over a few days as the child learns to self-sooth. This extinction procedure is a well-established and effective treatment for sleep-onset association problems. It has the advantage of being quick (a few days) and simple. However, many parents cannot endure their child's prolonged crying, feel guilty about it, and eventually give in and comfort the child; giving in is highly counterproductive because it only serves to strengthen the signaling behavior. There is evidence of completely normal psychological development when children are allowed to cry during bedtime as long as they receive love and attention during their waking hours.

- A modification of this procedure is for the caregiver to remain in the room during the extinction. This is more acceptable to some caregivers because they feel that they are not "abandoning" the child but are "doing something" by remaining in the room. This modification has been found to be effective for problems of getting to sleep or night awakenings.

- An alternative approach that is generally more tolerated by parents and generally more widely recommended is called fading, graduated extinction, or "sleep training." Some crying is allowed, but also some soothing. The soothing should be brief and largely verbal in a voice that is slow and quiet. Parents verbally encourage their child to sleep by saying something like, "It's time for you to sleep now." Direct contact should be minimal and short, if at all. This minimal interaction is enough to reassure the child but not to reinforce the signaling. The soothing is gradually reduced in intensity and duration as the child learns to develop self-soothing skills. Checking regularly on the crying child is encouraged, but the interval between checks should be progressively lengthened during a single night and over successive nights. Stop checking when the child is asleep, quiet, or just whimpering a little.

- If a child needs to be nursed to fall asleep, the amount of time nursing the child before sleep is gradually reduced (or if bottle-fed, the amount of liquid in the bottle is gradually reduced). A similar approach can be used for gradually eliminating holding or rocking the child to sleep.

- Fading is thought to have several advantages and is probably efficacious. It can be less trying for the parents. It also is flexible and can be varied to suit individual needs. Fading is thought to be especially good for children experiencing separation anxiety. However, it can take longer to arrive at the goal of making the child self-soothing, and some parents may abandon it too soon. All of the child's caregivers need to be persistent and consistent, and to make appropriate adjustments depending on the response and progress of the child.

- Following successful extinction or fading, an "extinction burst" is a common occurrence. Some time (days or weeks) later, crying at bedtime or following awakening reoccurs, often with great intensity. If not overreacted to, it will usually quickly subside. If it persists, parents may need to repeat some of the extinction or fading techniques.

- Scheduled awakenings have also been proposed to reduce night awakenings in children. The parents wake their child before their child's typical time of self-awakening. Following this early waking, the child usually quickly falls asleep without later awakening. The scheduled wakings are then gradually reduced until they are completely eliminated. This method can be quite disruptive and difficult for parents, yet may be more efficacious than other methods with older children.

- Bed sharing (family bed) has been employed by some parents for sleep-onset association problems. Cosleeping encompasses bed sharing but also more generally refers to a child sharing the same bedroom. Although a controversial sleeping arrangement for young children in Caucasian Western societies, bed sharing is a common practice with some non-Caucasians, especially in non-Western parts of the world. Other than a very slight potential risk of injuring the child, it is an acceptable practice as long as the child and the parents sleep well. Some parents start bed sharing from day one, but others resort to it later out of desperation in response to signaled awakenings by their child. However, it reduces the parents' privacy, can disrupt the parents' sleep, and may be a source of disagreement among caregivers. Bed sharing may only delay confronting the problem of night awakening because at some point the child has to transfer to sleeping in his or her own bed or crib, and may still have difficulty falling asleep on his or her own. However, some children can make the transition without problem. The transition is easiest before 6 months of age and should be done before 3 years of age. The older the child, the greater the likelihood that the transition may be more difficult. The transition process can go more smoothly by putting the child in a bed or crib in his or her own room and having one parent also sleep in the room in a separate bed, a cot, or a mattress on the floor. Over the next several nights, the parent should leave the room, at first briefly, but gradually extending the time away until his or her presence is no longer needed for the child to sleep. Alternatively, the child can first be shifted from the parents' bed to a crib next to their bed, then gradually moving the crib further and further away in the parents' bedroom, and finally into a separate room. In any case, parents should insist that the child sleep in his or her own bed or crib. Regardless of how it is done, limit-setting and positive rewards should be a part of the process. The exact method used and the timing of the exiting depends on the age and personality of the child.

- Finally, a combination of delaying bedtime coupled with positive bedtime routines and/or conditional removal from bed may be beneficial. Bedtime is delayed to a time when the child typically falls asleep. Positive bedtime routines can also be instituted to help the child fall asleep. These can be any set of calm, pleasurable activities that are regularly done immediately prior to bedtime. Any arousing activities or thoughts should be excluded at this time. The child may be removed from the bed if sleep has not begun after a specified period of time.

### Behavioral Insomnia of Childhood, Nighttime Eating/Drinking Type

A nighttime eating/drinking problem occurs when the child, after 2 months of age, frequently and regularly awakens to drink or eat without actually needing nourishment but has learned to expect it. A soaked diaper during the night can be an indicator of this problem.

- Night feedings are not physiologically needed after about 6 months of age, but night awakenings may continue to occur in up to 50% of infants; in most infants, these gradually diminish, but some do not seem to "outgrow" night awakenings to feed and may need behavioral intervention. A nighttime eating/drinking problem is more likely to occur in breast-feeders.

- The most effective treatment for nighttime eating/drinking problem is to gradually lengthen the interval between feedings (fading) over a week or two, and/or gradually reduce the amount of fluid in the bottle. Sudden cessation is not recommended. To prevent the development of a child becoming dependent on night feedings, it is best to wean him or her from night breast-feedings by 6 months or to not put the child to bed with a bottle after this age.

### Sleep Problems at Nap Time

Some children may only have a sleep problem at nap time. This could be a problem with the nap schedule. Insisting that a child nap when she or he is not sleepy or delaying a nap for a long time in a sleepy child are usually unsuccessful. Difficulties with naps may also be due to separation anxiety or poor sleep associations.

- Sleep problems at nap time often resolve when steps are taken to improve the child's sleep onset during his or her main bedtime as long as nap time occurs when the child is usually sleepy. Addressing separation anxiety, if present, is also helpful.

### Separation Anxiety

If separation anxiety is the main source of the child's sleeplessness, parents should increase daytime nurturing but also fade-in multiple brief separations throughout the day. They can do this by occasionally going to another room while singing or whistling so that the child knows the parent, although out-of-sight, is still there.

- Quiet time prior to nap time or bedtime should be encouraged. A large photo of parent(s) can be placed at the child's bedside for reassurance. If the child is awake when she or he is placed down for a nap, the parent should not sneak away but cheerfully say "good night" on the way out. The parent should respond quickly to the child's nighttime calls with "I'm here and everything's okay."

## Early Awakening

Some children have problems with early awakenings. There is no definite definition of an early awakening (awakening before 5 AM is commonly used), and this will vary among different families. The source of the problem may be learned, such as feeding or watching TV upon awakening; allowing a child to join his or her parents in bed in the morning; or other reinforcing events that lead to conditioned awakening. Additional causes include regular morning environmental disturbance, phase advance of the circadian sleep clock, or less need for sleep. Treatment should be directed at modifying underlying cause(s).

## Colic

Infantile colic, typically starting at 2–3 weeks of age, and resolving within a few months, can cause sleeplessness. The sleeplessness may continue beyond this time if the child has learned to expect a lot of attention from parents.

## LATER CHILDHOOD

### Behavioral Insomnia of Childhood, Limit-Setting Type

Insomnia in older children is most commonly due to failure by patents to consistently set or enforce limits during bedtime, nap time, or night awakenings. The problem can manifest itself by outright refusal to go to bed or more subtle "curtain calls." Conflicting parenting styles by various caregivers or the bedroom environment (e.g., loud TV or older siblings who go to bed later) can also be producing this type of insomnia.

- Parents need to be responsible for setting and enforcing a reasonable bedtime. They need to be firm, clear, and consistent, yet calm in denying or ignoring delaying tactics or protests; importantly, they should also avoid scaring the child with punishments or threats. The goal is to teach the child a better way to fall asleep by increasing positive behaviors, rather than simply eliminating negative ones.

- Parents should never *ask* the child to go to bed; rather they should give a gentle, but firm, command or they may be given narrow choices from which to choose. If the child is upset or cries when sent to bed, the parent should do brief (e.g., 1 min) checks in a reassuring but nonstimulating way, gradually lengthening these intervals to several minutes. If the child comes out of his or her bedroom, immediately, but gently, guide the child back to bed. Parents should praise the child the next morning for staying in bed.

- It may be necessary to place a gate in the child's bedroom doorway or close (but not lock) the door when the child gets out of bed, then opening it again when he or she returns to bed. Tell the child that the gate will be removed (or door will be opened) when she or he stops trying to leave the room. Parents should not go into the room; rather, they should stand on the other side of the gate/door out of sight and speak to the child in regular intervals, as necessary, in a calm voice. Gradually lengthen the interval between interventions in about five steps to several minutes.

- When faced with a limit-setting problem, it is critical for the parents to remain consistent. Giving in or letting up will only cause the child to try longer and harder to avoid bedtime in the future and will greatly prolong the process of changing the child's behavior. Parents should also be made aware of the likelihood of an "extinction burst" some days or even weeks after successful training.

### Sleep-Onset Association Disorder

For sleep-onset association disorder in older children, desensitization is an effective treatment strategy. The parent sits in a chair near the bed, but not in or on the bed, until the child falls asleep. After a few successful nights, the chair is gradually moved farther from the bed and toward the door; eventually, the chair is moved out of the door. The door is left open if the child does not get out of bed; the door is briefly closed, but not locked, if the child gets out of bed. Efficacy is increased by telling the child ahead of time what to expect and if the procedure is coupled with positive reinforcement, such as placing stars on a calendar or giving small prizes for staying quietly in bed. Praise the child the next morning for successful evenings. Reminders are provided just before the next bedtime.

### Night Fears

Night fears may also be a cause of sleeplessness in children. The child typically has an aversion to being alone in his or her bedroom at night, especially without a light. A variation is a child who worries that his or her parents may be harmed during the night. Additionally, some children feign being afraid as a delaying tactic.

- Night fears may be seen in toddlers, but incidence peaks between ages of 3–6 years when the child's imaginations and fantasies start to mature. Night fears are common but usually benign. Parents need to respond to their child's genuine night fears with reassurance while being careful not to reinforce the child's fears by overreacting. If the nighttime fear is severe, and persistent, it may be necessary to seek help from a behavioral sleep therapist or psychologist.

### Rumination

Rumination is a common cause of sleep-onset insomnia in older children. Extra attention from a parent and conversation at bedtime are the best remedies; however, it is important, while showing understanding and support, not to encourage excessive worry or emotional turmoil in the child.

# 32

## THE SLEEPY CHILD

Gerald Rosen

Sleep Disorders Center, Hannepin County Medical Center, Minnesota

### INTRODUCTION

Before discussing the sleepy child, it is important to distinguish him or her from the fatigued child. A sleepy child falls asleep at inappropriate times, times that one would reasonably expect the child to remain awake and alert; the fatigued child does not. Fatigue and sleepiness are different, but parents and health care professionals alike often confuse the two.

- Fatigue is used to describe a subjective, nonspecific feeling that has many causes and is difficult to measure.
- Sleepiness is defined as the propensity to fall asleep and can be objectively quantified using the Multiple Sleep Latency Test (MSLT). Children who are sleepy do feel fatigued; but children who are fatigued are not necessarily sleepy, sleepiness being just one of many causes of fatigue.
- Sleepiness is a cumulative symptom, which results from one or more of the following problems: (1) insufficient sleep quantity; (2) poor sleep quality (sleep fragmentation); (3) attempting to remain awake during the circadian sleep time; (4) as a primary neurological symptom; and (5) as a result of the use and/or withdrawal of psychotropic medications. Table 32.1 lists some of the more common causes for each of these problems that are seen in children.

### NORMAL SLEEP IN A CHILD

A "normal" child is very alert during the day, rarely exhibiting daytime sleepiness except at regular nap times. Conversely, when asleep, he or she appears quiet and peaceful. Normally, children transition to wakefulness rapidly at the end of their sleep period and fall asleep quickly at bedtime and nap time.

- Children normally have a high sleep efficiency, an abundance of slow-wave sleep, no obstructive apneas, and few periodic leg movements, respiratory-related or behavioral arousals.

### DEVELOPMENTAL CHANGES IN THE SLEEP OF CHILDREN

Predictable developmental changes occur in children's sleep from birth through adolescence (see Figure 32.1 and Table 32.2).

- At birth, infants sleep up to 19 h per day and have no clear circadian organization of their sleep–wake patterns. A newborn's sleep is described as active [rapid eye movement (REM) sleep precursor]; quiet [non-REM (NREM) sleep precursor]; or indeterminate. Active sleep accounts for about one-half of the infants total sleep time and is the state into which the child transitions to sleep out of wakefulness.
- By 6 months of age children's sleep can be staged using adult sleep stage scoring criteria; they transition into NREM sleep from wake, and are physiologically capable of consolidating 8 h of sleep without a behavioral awakening, which allows for the long awaited developmental milestone of "sleeping through the night." This is actually a misnomer, insofar as everyone, children and adults alike have numerous normal, brief, spontaneous awakenings every night that are not associated with a complete behavioral awakening.
- At 6 months of age most children are sleeping 11–12 h at night and another 3.5 h during the day divided between a morning and an afternoon nap.
- At 1.5 years of age, nighttime sleep remains at about 11–12 h, but daytime naps have decreased to once daily for 1–2 h duration, generally in the afternoon.

*Sleep Medicine Essentials*, edited by Teofilo L. Lee-Chiong
Copyright © 2009 John Wiley & Sons, Inc.

**Table 32.1  Sleep Problems and Their Causes That Lead to Sleepiness in Children**

| Sleep Problem | Causes |
|---|---|
| Insufficient sleep quantity | Acute, chronic |
| Poor sleep quality | Sleep apnea, periodic movements of sleep, seizures |
| Attempting to remain awake during the circadian sleep time | Delayed sleep phase, advanced sleep phase, irregular sleep–wake times, jet lag |
| As a primary neurologic symptom | Narcolepsy with/without cataplexy, idiopathic hypersomnia, myotonic dystrophy, seizures, central nervous system pathology—tumor, trauma, stroke, infection, postinfection, Prader–Willi, Moebius, Smith–Magenis, fragile X, Nieman–Pick syndromes, recurrent hypersomnia |
| As a result of use and/or withdrawal of psychotropic medications | Stimulants, antidepressants, antipsychotics, antihistamines, alcohol, opiates, sedatives, antiepileptics, $\alpha$ agonists, $\beta$ blockers |

- Most children discontinue their daytime naps between 3 and 6 years of age without increasing their nighttime sleep, which remains at about 11 h. There is a gradual decrease in nighttime sleep duration from 11 h to 10 h that occurs between 6 years of age to the beginning of adolescent sexual development.

- Preadolescent children are usually very alert during the day, with mean MSLTs generally above 18 min.

- Adolescents become sleepier during the day at about the time of sexual maturation, at Tanner stage III, and they also have a phase delay of their preferred time of sleep onset. If they are not sleep deprived, the increase in daytime sleepiness during adolescence is modest, with an decrease in mean MSLTs from 18 to 15 min. If they are sleep deprived, the mean MSLTs are often less than 9 min.

- If children are allowed to sleep *ad lib*, in an environment that is appropriate, that does not have excessive light exposure at night, and is conducive to sleep, without an externally imposed schedule, and

they have no primary sleep problems, they generally will establish a regular sleep–wake pattern and a consistent sleep duration that is a reflection of the synchronization of their homeostatic sleep needs and their preferred circadian sleep times.

- Though there is a great deal of intraindividual variation in a children's sleep duration and preferred sleep times, both of these traits tend to be stable over time in an individual child, and these changes occur within the context of the child's stable homeostatic and circadian traits. Children who were short sleepers as toddlers, typically remain short sleepers as they get older; the same is true for children who were long sleepers. As shown in Figure 32.1, children will typically maintain their percentile in sleep duration relative to other children as they get older.

- The preferred circadian timing for sleep and wake is also a relatively stable individual trait. Toddlers who are night owl's, preferring to go to sleep after their parents do, remain night owls as they get older.

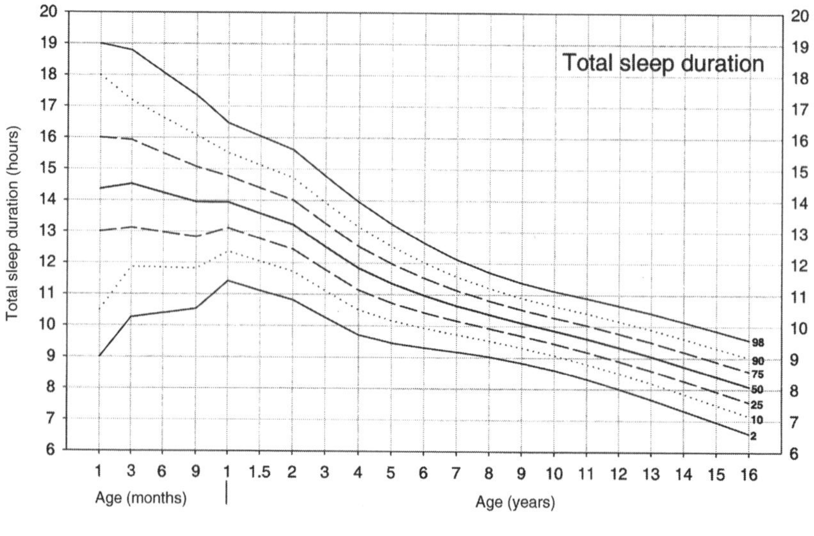

**Figure 32.1**  Percentiles of sleep duration per 24 h from infancy to adolescence based on structured interviews with parents of 493 children enrolled in the Zurich Longitudinal Study. (From Iglowstein I, et al. Sleep duration from infancy to adolescence: Reference values and generational trends. *Pediatrics* 2003;111:302–307; with permission.)

**Table 32.2  Average Sleep Duration Birth–Adolescence**

|  | Average Hours of Sleep/Day | Range (h/day) | Naps |
|---|---|---|---|
| Infants (2–12 months) | 14.5 h | 10–16 h | 3 |
| Toddlers (1–3 years) | 13.5 h | 9–16 h | 2 |
| Preschool (3–5 years) | 11 h | 8–12 h | 1 |
| School age—preadolescent (5–13 years) | 10 h | 8–10 h | 0 |
| Adolescent (delay in sleep phase); (increase in daytime sleepiness) | 9 h | 8–12 h | 0 |

- For a child to have the best and longest sleep possible, the circadian and homeostatic processes must be synchronized. This occurs largely through how we schedule our lives, the amount of time we allow for sleep, and the exposure to light after dusk and at dawn. When the circadian and homeostatic systems are properly synchronized, sleep onset occurs quickly, sleep efficiency is high, arousal in the morning is spontaneous, and the level of daytime alertness is high if there are no other intervening sleep problems.

## EXCESSIVE SLEEPINESS IN CHILDREN

The problems and causes of daytime sleepiness are listed in Table 32.1. In addition to the defining symptom of falling asleep at inappropriate times, children who are sleepy have behavioral symptoms—yawning, eye rubbing, irritability—and cognitive symptoms—slower reaction times, poorer learning. Though most of these symptoms occur concomitantly, there is not a tight correlation among them, and there is a great deal of individual variability in their expression in an individual child. The causes of daytime sleepiness are cumulative, and many children will have more than one cause that is contributing to their daytime symptom of sleepiness. The symptoms of sleepiness are similar regardless of their cause. As described in Table 32.1, children become sleepy if:

- They have had an inadequate amount of sleep (defined as how much sleep they are getting relative to their individual sleep need).
- They have a problem that leads to multiple awakenings that may fragment sleep, such as sleep-disordered breathing, periodic movements of sleep, or sleep-related seizures.
- They attempt to remain awake during their circadian sleep time or have an erratic sleep–wake schedule.
- They have a primary sleep problem such as narcolepsy, with and without cataplexy, or idiopathic hypersomnia.
- They have a primary neurologic disorder such as seizures, brain tumor, central nervous system (CNS) infections/strokes/trauma, idiopathic hypersomnia, myotonic dystrophy, Klein–Levin syndrome, or Prader–Willi syndrome.

- They are taking or withdrawing from a psychotropic drug or alcohol.

## DIAGNOSTIC APPROACH TO THE SLEEPY CHILD

The first step is the evaluation of a child with sleepiness is a complete medical/neurologic/sleep history that, in most cases, will point toward one or more of the causes of excessive daytime sleepiness (EDS) listed in Table 32.1. Since sleepiness is a cumulative symptom, if a child has more than one cause for the EDS, the symptoms will persist until all of the causes are treated. Consequently, it is important to gather a complete sleep history on all children who present with EDS.

- The most common cause of sleepiness in developed countries is chronic sleep insufficiency. It is important to recognize that the amount of sleep an individual requires to be well rested varies from child to child. Sleep insufficiency is present if a child is not getting the amount of sleep they need. It is not defined as a specific amount of sleep at a specific age. Consequently, children who have a long sleep requirement often experience chronic sleep insufficiency and as a consequence are very sleepy, even though they may be getting an average amount of sleep. During adolescence, sleep insufficiency is often associated with a sleep phase delay. Sleep logs are often sufficient to define this problem though occasionally actigraphy is necessary. The characteristic finding in these cases is of chronic sleep curtailment when the child needs to adhere to a defined sleep schedule, with sleep extension when the schedule permits, typically on the weekends. The best way of evaluating whether sleep insufficiency is the cause for daytime sleepiness is to allow the child to sleep *ad lib*, without any scheduling constraints for 2 weeks. A sleep log or actigraphy should be used to document the timing and amount of sleep. If the daytime sleepiness resolves with sleep extension, than the cause is most likely chronic sleep insufficiency. Some children have a very long sleep requirement, up to 12–14 h/day, which if not met results in sleepiness.
- If the sleepiness does not resolve with sleep extension, than a polysomnogram (PSG) is necessary for defining the presence and severity of sleep fragmentation from periodic leg movements of sleep (PLMS), obstructive sleep apnea (OSA), and seizures and/or for

establishing the diagnosis of narcolepsy or idiopathic hypersomnia. A PSG must be obtained before an MSLT. A cautionary note is important in the interpretation of the MSLT. Sleep deprivation and/or withdrawal from psychotropic drugs can mimic the MSLT findings of narcolepsy. In adolescents it is advisable to always obtain at least a sleep log and preferably a 2-week actigraphic recording before the MSLT and a urine drug toxicology screen the night of the PSG.

## NARCOLEPSY

Narcolepsy, with and without cataplexy, affect about 0.02% of the U.S. population. Onset is rare before 5 years of age and typically occurs between the ages of 10–25 years.

- Excessive daytime sleepiness, defined as falling asleep at inappropriate times is usually the first symptom. Cataplexy, hypnagogic hallucinations, and sleep-onset paralysis, are less common at the time of presentation, and a history of these symptoms may be difficult to elicit from young children.
- Narcolepsy will most often manifest itself with the resumption of daytime napping in a child who had previously discontinued their naps, when there is an adequate sleep quantity and no evidence of other sleep problems.
- The PSG and MSLT are important in the diagnosis of narcolepsy in children, but the studies may initially show hypersomnolence with mean MSLTs below 8 min, but without the characteristic two or more REM-onset naps. However, over time with repeat testing, the MSLTs invariably do show the REM sleep abnormalities characteristic of narcolepsy.
- Classical narcolepsy is caused by the loss of hypocretin secreting cells in the lateral hypothalamus. Secondary narcolepsy has the same PSG findings but is seen in children with known neurologic disease. The most common pediatric cause of secondary narcolepsy is hypothalamic injury secondary to a brain tumor.
- The daytime sleepiness of narcolepsy is treated with education of the importance of a regular sleep schedule and getting an adequate amount of sleep, strategic napping, and stimulant medication. If cataplexy is causing significant problems, it can usually be successfully treated with tricyclic antidepressants or selective serotonin reuptake inhibitors.

## IDIOPATHIC HYPERSOMNIA

Idiopathic hypersomnia, with and without a long sleep requirement, is characterized by a constant and severe daytime sleepiness regardless of how much sleep is obtained. Similar to narcolepsy, the onset is typically adolescence to early adulthood. At the time of presentation, many children who ultimately will prove to have narcolepsy will be diagnosed with idiopathic hypersomnia

because of the absence of REM sleep abnormalities on their PSG/MSLT.

- Treatment of idiopathic hypersomnia is the same as for narcolepsy with stimulant medication. Some children with a very long sleep requirement experience severe sleepiness because it may simply not be possible for them to obtain an adequate amount of sleep and to participate in the activities of their lives. This can be a truly disabling condition because modern American society simply does not recognize the necessity of adequate sleep or the consequences of sleep insufficiency. This typically becomes a problem during adolescence when the demands of these children's lives increase.
- The diagnostic evaluation of these children should include a PSG and MSLT, and treatment requires a combination of education of the teens, and their parents; regular sleep scheduling; and often judicious use of stimulant medications.

## SLEEP DISORDERED BREATHING

Sleep disordered breathing is present in 2–5% of children. In adults with OSA, daytime sleepiness is a common symptom. However, sleep disordered breathing is different in children than in adults, and one of the ways it is different is the prevalence of daytime sleepiness.

- Children with OSA will have snoring, and many also have observed apnea and neurocognitive deficits. However, EDS among children with OSA is less clear-cut. Although many children with OSA and their parents will complain of daytime sleepiness, most do not meet the stringent criteria of short mean sleep latencies on the MSLT that has been used to define daytime sleepiness.
- The causes of sleep disordered breathing in children is always multifactorial. It is the final common pathway of processes that affect the size, shape, and dynamics of the pharyngeal airway. The factors contributing to the upper airway obstruction in children with OSA are soft tissue anatomy, most commonly enlarged tonsils and adenoids, as well as obesity and macroglossia, neuromuscular tone, and craniofacial anatomy.
- Although most cases of OSA on children are improved after adenotonsillectomy, nasal continuous positive airway pressure (CPAP) is also an effective treatment option that is appropriate in some children. Recently, dental techniques, including rapid maxillary expansion and dental appliances, have been shown to be effective for the treatment of OSA in children.
- Childhood is a time of growth, learning and development. In order for these processes to occur, the child must be awake, alert, and able to interact with and learn from the environment. Daytime sleepiness impairs the child's ability to do this. The problems that lead to EDS in children can generally

be elucidated by a careful history and eliminated by appropriate treatment. For these reasons, the symptom of EDS in children should be taken seriously and investigated thoroughly.

## KEY POINTS

1. Fatigue and sleepiness are different; a sleepy child falls asleep at inappropriate times, times that one would reasonably expect the child to remain awake and alert; the fatigued child does not.
2. Sleepiness results from one or more of the following factors, namely insufficient sleep quantity, poor sleep quality, circadian sleep–wake misalignment, a primary neurological symptom, and the use and/or withdrawal of psychotropic medications.
3. A "normal" child is very alert during the day, rarely exhibiting daytime sleepiness except at regular nap times.
4. The most common cause of sleepiness in developed countries is chronic sleep insufficiency.
5. Childhood is a time of growth, learning, and development. In order for these processes to occur, the

child must be awake, alert, and able to interact with and learn from the environment. Daytime sleepiness impairs the child's ability to do all these.

## BIBLIOGRAPHY

Carskadon MA, et al. Regulation of sleepiness in adolescents: Updates, insights, and speculation. *Sleep* 2002; 25:606– 614.

Dijk D, et al. Integration of human sleep-wake regulation and circadian rhythmicity. *J Appl Physiol* 2002; 92:852.

Fallone G, et al. Sleepiness in children and adolescents: Clinical implications. *Sleep Med Rev* 2002; 6:287–306.

Goodwin J, et al. Clinical outcomes associated with sleep-disordered breathing in Caucasian and Hispanic children–The Tucson children's assessment of sleep apnea study (TUCSA). *Sleep* 2003; 26:587–591.

Gozal D, et al. Objective sleepiness measures in pediatric obstructive sleep apnea. *Pediatrics* 2001; 108:693–697.

Iglowstein I, et al. Sleep duration from infancy to adolescence: Reference values and generational trends. *Pediatrics* 2003; 111:302–307.

Marcus C, et al. Adherence to and effectiveness of positive airway pressure therapy in children with obstructive sleep apnea. *Pediatrics* 2006; 117:442–451.

# 33

## NORMAL SLEEP IN AGING

LIAT AYALON AND SONIA ANCOLI-ISRAEL
Department of Psychiatry, University of California, San Diego and Veterans Affairs San Diego Healthcare System, San Diego, California

## INTRODUCTION

With aging, sleep, as with other physiologic processes, undergoes increasingly noticeable changes. Many of the changes accompanying aging reflect changes in both homeostatic and circadian processes that occur throughout the life span. It is important to make a distinction between changes that are part of normal aging and changes that might be considered pathologic.

- Sleep disturbances are common in older adults. Chronological age, by itself, seems to explain very little of the observed prevalence of sleep complaints, and much evidence suggests that medical diseases and chronic illness may account for most of the changes in sleep observed in old age.

## SUBJECTIVE REPORTS AND OBJECTIVE FINDINGS

### Subjective Reports

Spending too much time in bed
Spending less time asleep
Increase in number of awakenings
Increase in time to fall asleep
Less satisfaction with sleep
Increase in tiredness during the day
Longer and more frequent naps

### Objective Findings

Decrease in nonrapid eye movement (NREM) stages 3 and 4 sleep
Decrease in rapid eye movement (REM) sleep
Increase in awakenings
Increase in frequency of sleep disorders
Decrease in sleep efficiency
Increase in daytime sleepiness
Increase in number of naps

## CHANGES IN SLEEP ARCHITECTURE WITH AGE

Percentage of slow-wave sleep and REM sleep, as well as REM latency all significantly decrease with age, whereas percentage of stages 1 and 2 sleep significantly increase. Age-related reduction of electroencephalogram (EEG) power in NREM sleep and REM sleep, with frequency-specific changes in brain topography has been described using spectral analysis. Aging is also associated with a decrease in sleep spindle and K-complex density; this may be interpreted as an age-related alteration of thalamocortical regulatory mechanisms.

## OTHER CHANGES IN SLEEP WITH AGE

Compared to younger adults, older adults show a decrease in total sleep time, take longer to fall asleep, and have more nighttime awakenings, resulting in a lower sleep efficiency (i.e., amount of sleep given the amount of time in bed).

- There is a redistribution of sleep around the 24-h day with a decrease in nighttime sleep and an increase in daytime napping. Evening napping in older adults is associated with early morning awakenings and decreased nocturnal sleep duration. Many factors contribute to this decreased ability to sleep, including medical and psychiatric illnesses, medications, primary sleep disorders, and changes in circadian rhythms.

## CIRCADIAN RHYTHMS AND AGING

There is considerable evidence indicating a weaker circadian regulation of sleep and wakefulness with aging. Older adults report increased daytime sleepiness and sleep more than young adults during the daytime. They also show a reduced circadian modulation of REM sleep and spindle frequency.

- Endocrine changes are seen with aging, including diminished melatonin secretion. Sleep-related growth hormone release is also diminished in older adults. Finally, age-related increases in cortisol level at its circadian minimum is involved in impaired sleep, more β activity during sleep, and earlier times of arising.
- The amplitude and phase of the core body temperature rhythm in older adults do not significantly differ from those of younger adults.
- To stay robust, circadian rhythms are entrained by time cues. It seems that both the endogenous pacemaker and the strength of entrainment to time cues are altered in aging. The most significant exogenous time cue is the daily cycle of light and dark, but other factors such as physical activity, the timing of meals, and social interactions have also been shown to be important regulators of endogenous rhythms. In the older adult, there is often a reduction in retinal sensitivity to light and decreased bright light exposure, decreased physical activity, and, at times even, decreased social interactions, all which could contribute to a weaker circadian rhythm.

## AGE-RELATED CIRCADIAN CHANGES

Rhythm amplitude attenuation (sleep–wake, melatonin)
Reduction in nighttime melatonin levels
Increase in cortisol level at its circadian minimum
Diminished sleep-related growth hormone release
Circadian rhythm phase advance (earlier bedtime and wake-up time and advanced temperature rhythm)
Reduction in retinal sensitivity to light
Reduction in bright-light exposure and activity levels

## EFFECTS OF AGE-RELATED NORMAL PHYSIOLOGIC CHANGES ON SLEEP

Although many age-related physiologic changes may affect sleep, two of the most common ones are changes in voiding during the night and menopause.

- *Nocturia* or frequent voluntary voiding of urine during the night and production of an abnormally large volume of urine during sleep (nocturnal polyuria) are common causes of awakening during the night in the elderly. Age-related changes in the circadian rhythm of urine excretion are associated with nocturnal polyuria. In addition, with normal aging, the bladder's ability to store urine decreases. Age-related lower urinary tract problems can affect frequency and urgency. Prostatic hypertrophy in men and decreased urethral resistance in women as a result of hormonal changes are also involved.

- *Menopause* is associated with hormonal, physiologic, and psychological changes that affect sleep and play a pivotal role in modulating both the presence and the degree of sleep disorder. Lower sleep efficiency and multiple arousals during the night are associated with menopausal vasomotor symptoms (hot flashes). Insomnia becomes common during this time and may be partially related to psychological factors such as depression and anxiety. Sleep-disordered breathing is more common in postmenopausal women and may be explained by the change in distribution of body fat and decrease in progesterone that often accompany menopause.

## PHYSIOLOGIC CHANGES THAT MAY AFFECT SLEEP

Nocturia and nocturnal polyuria
Menopause
Physiologic changes of the lung
    Decreased respiratory muscle strength
    Decreased expiratory flow rates
    Diminished chest wall compliance
Changes in soft palate tissue
Increased use of medications
Conditions causing pain
Neurologic disorders
Psychiatric conditions (mood disorders and anxiety)

## AGE-RELATED FACTORS ASSOCIATED WITH SLEEP DISORDERS

### Medical and Psychiatric Conditions

Complaints of difficulty sleeping are often related to the comorbid medical conditions common in the older adult. For example, insomnia (difficulty falling or staying asleep) can be comorbid with conditions causing pain (e.g., arthritis and malignancies), neurologic disorders (e.g., restless legs, Parkinson's disease, stroke, or dementia), or organ system failure (e.g., chronic obstructive pulmonary disease, congestive heart failure, and gastrointestinal disorders). Insomnia is also related to mood disorders and generalized anxiety disorder and may be a diagnostic symptom for major depression.

### Medication Use

Medication use may also contribute to poor sleep. Alerting or stimulating drugs taken late in the day may cause difficulty falling asleep at night.

- Central nervous system (CNS) stimulants, β-blockers, bronchodilators, calcium channel blockers, corticosteroids, decongestants, stimulating antidepressants, stimulating antihistamines, and thyroid hormones are known to contribute to insomnia.

- Sedating drugs, when taken early in the day, may lead to excessive daytime sleepiness and daytime napping behavior, which may contribute to sleep-onset insomnia or may further exacerbate and maintain an existing insomnia.

## Shifts in Circadian Rhythms

It is believed that much of the insomnia resulting from early morning awakenings reflects changes in circadian rhythms. Synchronization of the sleep–wake cycle by both internal and external rhythms is reduced in older adults. Older adults with advanced sleep phase syndrome are usually sleepy early in the evening and awaken too early in the morning. Increase in daytime napping, inactivity and bed rest, reduced outdoor light exposure, as well as greater susceptibility to external arousal may interact to predispose elderly subjects to poor sleep. Psychological factors such as bereavement, retirement, trauma (e.g., Holocaust or war-related captivity), fear of death in sleep, anxiety, and depression are also correlated with increased nocturnal wake time.

## PRIMARY SLEEP DISORDERS

### Sleep Apnea

The prevalence of sleep apnea in the elderly has been shown to be higher than in younger adults. An estimated 25% of community dwelling elderly have an apnea index of 5 or more, and 62% have an apnea hypopnea index (the number of apneas plus hypopneas per hour of sleep) of 10 or more.

- Several factors that are associated with aging may explain, in part, this high prevalence in the elderly, including decreased respiratory muscle strength, decreased expiratory flow rates, diminished chest wall compliance, multiple physiologic changes of the lung, and, possibly, age-associated changes in the biomechanical properties of the tissues of the soft palate.

### Periodic Limb Movements and Restless Legs Syndrome

Periodic limb movements in sleep (PLMS) prevalence increases significantly with age with estimates at 45% in older adults compared to 5–6% in younger adults. Restless legs syndrome (RLS) is often comorbid with PLMS.

- The reasons for high prevalence of these conditions in older adults are not fully understood. PLMS and RLS are often associated with higher incidence of neuropathy, lower ferritin levels, and changes of iron metabolism. It may also be secondary to various rheumatologic conditions that are more common in older age. Additional causally related conditions include chronic obstructive pulmonary disease, asthma, fibromyalgia, diabetes mellitus, cancer, and neurodegenerative disorders, such as Parkinson's disease. There is some evidence for an association

with coffee intake, sleep apnea syndrome, or snoring, stress, and the presence of mental disorders. Some medications (e.g., tricyclic antidepressants, serotonin reuptake inhibitors, and dopamine receptor blocking agents) can worsen PLMS and RLS.

## IMPORTANCE OF GOOD SLEEP IN THE ELDERLY

Older adults are significantly sleepier throughout the day than younger adults, as confirmed by a Multiple Sleep Latency Test (MSLT), an objective test of daytime sleepiness. In a large epidemiologic study, 20% of participants reported being "usually sleepy in the daytime." Daytime sleepiness can be a very debilitating symptom, causing social and occupational difficulties, reduced vigilance, and cognitive deficits, including decreased concentration, slowed response time, and memory and attention difficulties. These symptoms may be particularly serious in older adults who already have mild or moderate cognitive impairment.

- Although very common, daytime sleepiness is not an inevitable part of aging, and many healthy older adults show intact daytime alertness. A main challenge in sleep medicine in the elderly is to recognize age-related changes and distinguish them from primary or secondary sleep disorders, which are treatable.

## KEY POINTS

1. Percentage of slow-wave sleep and percentage of REM sleep decrease with aging, while percentage of stages 1 and 2 sleep increases.
2. Sleep is redistributed around the 24-h day with a decrease in nighttime sleep and an increase in daytime napping.
3. Weaker circadian rhythms in older adults are related to a reduction in retinal sensitivity to light, decreased bright light exposure, and decreased physical activity.
4. Poor sleep in older adults is often related to the comorbid medical conditions (e.g., pain, neurologic disorders, and depression) and medication use (e.g., CNS stimulants, beta-blockers and bronchodilators).
5. Sixty-two percent of community dwelling elderly have an apnea hypopnea index of 10 or more.
6. Prevalence of PLMS increases significantly with aging with estimates of 45% in older adults compared to 5–6% in younger adults.
7. Daytime sleepiness in older adults may cause social and occupational difficulties, reduced vigilance, and cognitive deficits, including decreased concentration, slowed response time, and memory and attention difficulties.

## ACKNOWLEDGMENTS

This work was supported by NIA AG08415, NCI CA112035, CBCRP 11IB-0034, National Sleep Foundation Pickwick Fellowship (LA), GCRC M01 RR00827, and the Research Service of the Veterans Affairs San Diego Healthcare System.

## BIBLIOGRAPHY

Ali A, et al. Nocturia in older people: A review of causes, consequences, assessment and management. *Int J Clin Pract* 2004; 58:366–373.

Ancoli-Israel S. Insomnia in the elderly: A review for the primary care practitioner. *Sleep* 2000; 23:S23–S30.

Ancoli-Israel S, et al. Increased light exposure consolidates sleep and strengthens circadian rhythms in severe Alzheimer's disease patients. *Behav Sleep Med* 2003; 1:22–36.

Ayalon L, et al. Diagnosing and treating sleep disorders in the older adult. *Med Clin North Am* 2004; 88:737–750.

Backhaus J, et al. Sleep disturbances are correlated with decreased morning awakening salivary cortisol. *Psychoneuroendocrinology* 2004; 29:1184–1191.

Merriam GR, et al. Growth hormone-releasing hormone and growth hormone secretagogues in normal aging. *Endocrine* 2003; 22:41–48.

Prinz PN, et al. Sleep impairments in healthy seniors: Roles of stress, cortisol, and interleukin-1 beta. *Chronobiol Int* 2000; 17:391–404.

Soares CN, et al. Sleep disorders in women: Clinical evidence and treatment strategies. *Psychiatr Clin North Am* 2006; 29(4): 1095–1113.

Veldi M, et al. Ageing, soft-palate tone and sleep-related breathing disorders. *Clin Physiol* 2001; 21:358–364.

Whitney CW, et al. Correlates of daytime sleepiness in 4578 elderly persons: The Cardiovascular Health Study. *Sleep* 1998; 21:27–36.

# 34

## ASPECTS OF WOMEN'S SLEEP

HELEN S. DRIVER
Sleep Disorders Laboratory, Kingston General Hospital, Departments of Medicine and Psychology,
Queen's University, Kingston Ontario, Canada

## INTRODUCTION

Women's reproductive cycles vary across their life span, giving an additional rhythm, longer than the daily circadian (24-h) rhythm, which can affect sleep. The complex reproductive changes are associated with varying levels of two steroid hormones in particular—estrogen and progesterone. Through the reproductive years with menstrual cycles there is a constant flux of estrogen and progesterone levels with a pattern that repeats about every 28 days. During pregnancy, the levels of both hormones increase, then fall rapidly after delivery. With menopause, the levels decline; it is the loss of the effects of estrogen and progesterone that may underlie many of the physical and psychological symptoms women experience.

- Subjective complaints of insufficient or nonrestorative sleep affect between 10 and 35% of the general population. Women are 1.4–2 times more likely than men to report insomnia, yet young women also report having a greater sleep need.

- Reproductive status should be considered as a contributor to complaints of poor sleep in women.

## MENSTRUAL CYCLES

During menstrual cycles, prominent changes in reproductive hormones and body temperature occur. The follicular phase is when estrogen is the predominant hormone. After ovulation, the luteal phase lasts 14–16 days and is when concentrations of estrogen and progesterone are high, and body temperature is elevated by about 0.4°C compared to before ovulation. The withdrawal of both estrogen and progesterone precedes menstruation. It is during the late-luteal (premenstrual) phase and the first few days of menstruation that most negative menstrual symptoms are experienced.

- About 70% of women report that their sleep is affected by menstrual symptoms such as bloating, tender breasts, headaches, and cramps on average 2.5 days every month. Even young women without significant menstrual-associated complaints report poorer sleep quality 3–6 days premenstrually and during 4 days of menstruation compared to other times of the menstrual cycle. Mood, discomfort, and pain can affect sleep during this period.

- Sleep across the menstrual cycle is remarkably stable in women with no menstrual-associated complaints. There is a small variation in rapid eye movement (REM) sleep, which tends to decrease in the luteal phase compared to the follicular phase. Although there is no clear-cut difference in sleep architecture, effects on sleep spindles have been observed, with increased electroencephalogram (EEG) power density in the frequency range of sleep spindles (around 14 Hz) during non-REM (NREM) sleep in the luteal compared with the follicular phase. This effect on sleep spindles has been proposed to be an influence of progesterone via the $\gamma$-aminobutyric acid (GABA$_A$) receptor.

## PREMENSTRUAL SYMPTOMS AND PREMENSTRUAL SYNDROME

Many women experience premenstrual disturbances that vary in severity and type of symptom. Approximately 60% of women experience mild symptoms of premenstrual symptoms (PMS), and an estimated 20% have moderate PMS that they feel requires treatment. For 3–8% of women, the cyclical pattern of symptoms is severe and acknowledged as a clinical mood disorder—premenstrual dysphoric disorder (PMDD).

- Common symptoms that occur in the last week of the luteal phase and lessen after the onset of menstruation include irritability/anger, anxiety/tension, depression and mood swings, change in appetite, bloating and weight gain, and fatigue.
- Sleep disturbances include insomnia, hypersomnia, unpleasant dreams, awakenings during the night, failure to wake at the expected time, and tiredness in the morning. However, no significant, reproducible effects on sleep have been found in the few studies with small sample sizes on women with PMS/PMDD.

## PAINFUL MENSTRUAL CONDITIONS— DYSMENORRHEA AND ENDOMETRIOSIS

With both these conditions, pain and discomfort disturb sleep. Women who suffer from dysmenorrhea experience painful uterine cramps that debilitate them during menstruation every month. Women with endometriosis have misplaced tissue, of the same type that lines the inside of the uterus, which grows elsewhere in the abdominal and pelvic area, and follows the menstrual cycle.

- Women with dysmenorrhea complain of poorer sleep quality and higher anxiety during menstruation compared to symptom-free women. Painful menstrual conditions are associated with reduced subjective sleep quality, sleep efficiency, and REM sleep compared with pain-free phases of the menstrual cycle or with controls. In turn, the disturbed sleep may worsen mood and alter the pain threshold.

## POLYCYSTIC OVARY SYNDROME

In polycystic ovary syndrome (PCOS), menstrual cycles are irregular or absent, and the ovaries produce too much of the male sexual hormones (androgens), which causes infertility, facial hair, and weight gain. PCOS affects approximately 5–8% of women in North America, making it the most common endocrine disorder of premenopausal women. Women with PCOS are more likely to develop obstructive sleep apnea (OSA). Increased sleep-disordered breathing (SDB) has been correlated with waist–hip ratio and testosterone in women with PCOS.

## SLEEP-DISORDERED BREATHING AND MENSTRUAL CYCLE

Being female appears to reduce the risk of developing SDB, at least premenopausally. The prevalence of OSA in premenopausal women is low (0.6%). However, compared with earlier clinical reports, the prevalence of OSA in middle-aged women in the general population at ~2% is higher than initially suggested.

- Polysomnographically, women with OSA tend to have a clustering of events during REM sleep, the frequency of which is related to body mass index (BMI). There may also be an association of SDB with menstrual phase. There is an increased propensity to upper airway obstruction during the follicular phase of the menstrual cycle or more protection from SDB in the luteal phase. In premenopausal women with OSA, the severity of SDB was worse during REM sleep during the follicular compared with the luteal phase. There is a reduction in upper airway resistance during sleep in the luteal compared with the follicular phase in healthy women without any sleep complaints. Although the clinical significance of these findings is not yet certain, it is conceivable that in some women OSA may only be manifest in the follicular phase of ovulatory cycles and that variability of OSA severity depending on menstrual phase might alter disease management.

## ORAL CONTRACEPTIVES

Oral contraceptive (OC) pills contain synthetic estrogen and progestin with 21 days of active hormone and the last 7 days of inactive pills. In monophasic pills the same dosage of hormones is provided all through the entire active cycle; triphasic pills give different dosage levels during each week of the month and are designed to more closely duplicate a woman's natural hormonal pattern. These are called combined pills (containing estrogen and progesterone) whereas "minipills" contain progestin only.

- Women taking monophasic oral contraceptives have persistently raised body temperatures, similar to those of naturally cycling women in the luteal phase (likely due to progesterone). While taking the active synthetic progestin and estrogen, women were found to have more stage 2 sleep compared to the inactive placebo phase. When compared to naturally cycling women in the luteal phase, women taking OC had less deep sleep. In contrast to this small effect on sleep in women who had no sleep or menstrual-associated complaints, for some women with premenstrual and menstrual symptoms, regularization of the menstrual cycle with OCs may reduce their symptoms and thereby improve sleep.

## PREGNANCY AND EARLY POSTPARTUM PERIOD

During the first trimester, sleepiness increases due to rising levels of progesterone. Sleep can be disrupted by morning sickness (waking with nausea), increased urinary frequency, and breast tenderness.

- Sleep can improve during the second trimester. Snoring may start, and leg cramps or restless legs syndrome (RLS) may begin. Some women may experience heartburn.

- Sleep is most disrupted during the third trimester. Problems include difficulty getting comfortable (many women will sleep on their side with a pillow between their knees), heartburn, leg cramps, snoring, frequent urination, more time awake, and morning fatigue.
- Polysomnographic studies may demonstrate frequent awakenings that start during the first trimester but that are most evident in the third trimester.
- The greatest degree of maternal sleep disruption occurs during the first month following delivery. Although there is a gradual increase in maternal sleep time over the subsequent 2–4 months with maturing of the infant's circadian rhythm, sleep efficiency continues to be lower than prepregnancy. The decline in sleep efficiency is greater among first-time mothers compared to multiparous women.
- Breast-feeding, compared with bottle-feeding, has been found to influence sleep, with increased slow-wave sleep, possibly due to high prolactin levels.

### Snoring and Obstructive Sleep Apnea

Anatomical changes during pregnancy, such as weight gain, decreased respiratory functional reserve capacity, and rhinitis (due to estrogen), predispose women to developing OSA. Conversely, increased respiratory drive (due to progesterone) and a preference to sleep in a lateral position may offer protection.

- Some women begin to snore during pregnancy. Snoring, with complaints of sleep disruption and/or excessive daytime sleepiness, should be treated very seriously due to a higher risk for developing pre-eclampsia (hypertension, pedal edema, proteinuria, and headaches) and OSA. Snoring and OSA may start or worsen during pregnancy. Recurrent apneas-hypopneas can lead to sleep disruption and hypoxemia that can also adversely affect the fetus.

### Restless Legs Syndrome and Periodic Leg Movements in Sleep

About 15% of women report symptoms of RLS during the first trimester and up to 23% during the third trimester. RLS symptoms generally resolve with childbirth.

- Since iron and/or folate deficiency are known causes of RLS, women who develop RLS during pregnancy should have their iron status checked and should probably be prescribed a multivitamin preparation containing folic acid.

### MENOPAUSE

Between the ages of 45 and 55 years (average of 51 years), production of estrogen and progesterone among women starts to decrease and menstrual cycles become irregular. This transitional, or perimenopausal, period occurs over a few years (about 4–8 years). Only when menstrual periods have stopped for a year is menopause confirmed.

- Eighty percent of women experience hot flashes (i.e., suddenly feeling hot then flushed enough to sweat). Hot flashes can be extremely uncomfortable, and when they occur during sleep, it can lead to night sweats that can soak bedclothes followed by chills as the body cools down. Hot flashes can be associated with sleep disruption. Polysomnography has not consistently found an association between decreased sleep efficiency and hot flashes, and the efficacy of estrogen therapy in relieving hot flashes at night has been variable.
- Other symptoms that can disrupt sleep, either directly or indirectly, include mood changes (mood swings, anxiety, irritability, or depression), vaginal dryness and irritation, urinary problems (more bathroom trips at night), and weight gain.

### Insomnia

Complaints of insomnia are more common in menopausal than in premenopausal women. Insomnia complaints include difficulty falling asleep, repeated awakenings, and waking too early in the morning.

- Insomnia has been associated with hot flashes, palpitations, and mood swings particularly during perimenopause. Additionally, depression, anxiety, and OSA may be significant sleep-disrupting factors.
- Subjective improvements in sleep with hormone replacement therapy (HRT) are reported but have not consistently been shown in laboratory studies.

### Obstructive Sleep Apnea

Menopause increases the risk of breathing disorders during sleep. Hormone-related changes, weight gain with a change in fat distribution, and increased age are all contributing factors.

- Older, overweight women with hypertension, sleep disturbances, depression, or fatigue should be considered high risk for having OSA.
- Women who use HRT have OSA less frequently than postmenopausal women not on HRT. Many other factors need to be considered before recommending HRT to treat OSA in women.
- The focus of therapy should be on using standard therapy such as continuous positive airway pressure (CPAP), an oral appliance (for milder OSA), and weight loss.

### KEY POINTS

1. A woman's changing hormone profile influences her sleep. In general, more disruption can be anticipated

with abrupt changes and the withdrawal of female hormones.

2. Women are at increased risk for developing insomnia in pivotal periods such as pregnancy, childbirth, and especially menopause.

3. Some sleep disorders, such as sleep-disordered breathing and restless legs syndrome, may also be influenced by the reproductive stage.

4. Women with sleep-disordered breathing are more likely to present with depression and complain of fatigue and unrefreshing sleep rather than the more traditionally accepted symptom of excessive daytime sleepiness. They are more likely to have increased upper airway resistance syndrome rather than frank apneas.

## BIBLIOGRAPHY

Baker FC, Driver HS. Circadian rhythms, sleep, and the menstrual cycle. *Sleep Med* 2007; 8(6):613–622.

Baker FC, et al. Sleep and menstrual-related disorders. *Sleep Med Clin* 2008; 3:25–35.

Banno K, et al. The circuitous route to diagnosing sleep disorders in women: Healthcare utilization and benefits of improved awareness for sleep disorders. *Sleep Med Clin* 2008; 3:133–140.

Bixler EO, et al. Prevalence of sleep-disordered breathing in women. Effects of gender. *Am J Respir Crit Care Med* 2001; 163:608–613.

Blyton DM, et al. Lactation is associated with an increase in slow-wave sleep in women. *J Sleep Res* 2002; 11:297–303.

Davidson JR. Insomnia: Therapeutic options for women. *Sleep Med Clin* 2008; 3:109–119.

Driver HS, et al. Menstrual factors in sleep. *Sleep Med Rev* 1998; 2:213–229.

Driver HS, et al. The influence of the menstrual cycle on upper airway resistance and breathing during sleep. *Sleep* 2005; 28 (4):449–456.

Edwards N, et al. Sleep-disordered breathing in pregnancy. *Sleep Med Clin* 2008; 3:81–95.

Edwards N, et al. Haemodynamic responses to obstructive sleep apnoeas in premenopausal women. *J Hypertens* 1999; 17:603–610.

Franklin KA, et al. Snoring, pregnancy-induced hypertension, and growth retardation of the fetus. *Chest* 2000; 117:137–141.

Krystal AD, et al. Sleep in peri-menopausal and post-menopausal women. *Sleep Med Rev* 1998; 2:243–254.

Lee KA. Alterations in sleep during pregnancy and postpartum: A review of 30 years of research. *Sleep Med Rev* 1998; 2:231–242.

Moline ML, et al. Sleep in women across the life cycle from adulthood through menopause. *Sleep Med Rev* 2003; 7:155–178.

Morin CM, et al. Epidemiology of insomnia: Prevalence, self-help treatments, consultations, and determinants of help-seeking behaviors. *Sleep Med* 2006; 7:123–130.

Pien GW, et al. Sleep disorders during pregnancy. *Sleep* 2004; 27:1405–1417.

Polo-Kantola P. Dealing with menopausal sleep disturbances. *Sleep Med Clin* 2008; 3:121–131.

Sloan EP. Sleep disruption during pregnancy. *Sleep Med Clin* 2008; 3:73–80.

Tasali E, et al. Polycystic ovary syndrome and obstructive sleep apnea. *Sleep Med Clin* 2008; 3:37–46.

Ware JC, et al. Influence of sex and age on duration and frequency of sleep apnea events. *Sleep* 2000; 23:165–169.

# 35

## ASTHMA

DAVID A. BEUTHER AND RICHARD J. MARTIN
National Jewish Health and University of Colorado Health Sciences Center, Denver, Colorado

## INTRODUCTION

Nocturnal symptoms in asthma due to the circadian decline in lung function at night are common. Proposed mechanisms of nocturnal worsening of asthma include sleep-related changes in lung volume, bronchial hyperresponsiveness, cortisol and β-adrenergic receptor responsiveness, parasympathetic tone, and airway inflammation. Other nonpulmonary aspects such as reflux and allergic rhinitis may contribute to nocturnal asthma.

## DEMOGRAPHICS

A majority of asthmatics have nocturnal asthma symptoms, and a disproportionate number of deaths from asthma occur at night and in the early morning hours.

- Most deaths from asthma occur between the hours of 6 PM and 3 AM.
- Nocturnal symptoms indicate inadequate asthma control.

## PATHOPHYSIOLOGY

### Circadian Rhythms in Asthma

There is a circadian variation in peak expiratory flow rates, $FEV_1$ (forced expiratory volume in 1 s), and bronchial hyperresponsiveness in asthmatics and normal subjects.

- Peak lung function usually occurs at 4 PM and minimum lung function at approximately 4 AM.
- Cause of this circadian variation is multifactorial. Studies have demonstrated reduced steroid responsiveness at night; circadian changes in epinephrine levels; reduction in beta-receptor density and

function at night; and a genetic polymorphism in the $β_2$-adrenergic receptor that causes accelerated downregulation of the receptor.

- Melatonin, a key hormonal regulator of circadian rhythm, acts as a proinflammatory hormone in nocturnal asthma; its levels are elevated and phase delayed among asthmatics.

### Airway Resistance and Lung Volume During Sleep

Both asthmatics and nonasthmatics experience a significant decrease in lung volume during sleep. A greater decline in lung volume occurs among asthmatics.

- Supine posture might be an additional contributor to the decline in lung function seen in nocturnal asthma. However, lung volume changes may be a result, rather than the cause, of nocturnal asthma.

### Airway Inflammation

Asthma is an inflammatory disorder, and worsening of symptoms at night could be due to an increase in inflammation.

- Cellular inflammation is increased in nocturnal asthmatics, with elevated numbers of total cells, leukocytes, neutrophils, and eosinophils in bronchoalveolar lavage specimens at 4 AM.
- Distal lung inflammation may also play an important role in nocturnal asthma, with significantly greater number of asthma controller cells, $CD4^+$ T-lymphocytes, effector cells, and eosinophils in alveolar tissue.

### Ventilatory Drive During Sleep

Ventilatory drive during sleep is blunted. In normal sleeping subjects, ventilatory drive in response to hypercapnia

*Sleep Medicine Essentials*, edited by Teofilo L. Lee-Chiong
Copyright © 2009 John Wiley & Sons, Inc.

is blunted in all stages of sleep, especially rapid eye movement (REM) sleep. Sleep deprivation can further decrease ventilatory response to hypercapnia. However, it is unclear whether nocturnal asthmatics demonstrate an excessively blunted ventilatory drive during sleep.

### Parasympathetic System

An increase in vagal parasympathetic tone can contribute to an increase in airway resistance.

- Other disorders that may increase vagal tone have been implicated in contributing to nighttime bronchoconstriction, including obstructive sleep apnea, postnasal drip causing laryngeal irritation, and gastroesophageal reflux disease (GERD).

### Airway Secretions

Many patients with asthma also suffer from allergic rhinitis. Rhinitis often becomes more bothersome at night and could worsen asthma through aspiration of secretions or from irritation of the upper airway, leading to reflex bronchoconstriction.

- Asthmatic patients also demonstrate reduced mucociliary clearance that worsens even more during sleep. The cough reflex is also blunted during REM sleep, which could lead to excessive accumulation of secretions, causing airway narrowing.

### Gastroesophageal Reflux

Gastroesophageal reflux has commonly been associated with asthma, but some studies strongly question its significance. The prevalence of GERD in asthma is high. Asthmatics have significantly decreased lower esophageal sphincter pressures, greater esophageal acid exposure times, more frequent episodes of GERD, and longer esophageal acid clearance times.

- Pathophysiology of GERD-related bronchoconstriction likely involves esophageal acid stimulation of vagal receptors, and resultant vagal-mediated bronchoconstriction; another mechanism may be microaspiration of stomach contents.
- However, some studies have shown that direct installation of acid into the lower esophagus during sleep does not predictably cause worsening bronchoconstriction, and that there was no association between reflux, as measured by pH probe at the proximal and distal esophagus, and asthma symptoms or peak expiratory flows.

### Airway Cooling

Core body temperature has a circadian variability, with a decrease of approximately 1°C between 2 and 4 AM. Airway temperature changes are thought to be important in causing exercise-induced bronchospasm. It is possible that decreased body temperature could contribute to worsening

airflow limitation at night, and that this effect may be more prominent in patients who bypass the heated humidification function of the nose and nasopharynx, such as those with severe rhinitis or who demonstrate significant mouth breathing at night.

## CHRONOTHERAPEUTIC TREATMENT APPROACHES

Chronopharmacologic principles, in which drug dosing and schedule are altered to achieve maximum therapy during the night, while attempting to minimize drug toxicities, may offer unique and improved ways to treat nocturnal asthma.

- If corticosteroid administration is timed to the natural peak in production of endogenous corticosteroid production, efficacy may be maximized while minimizing adrenal suppression. Steroid dosing in the early afternoon (3 PM) was superior to dosing in the evening, with greater improvement in peak expiratory flows and airway inflammation. Single daily dosing also minimizes adrenal suppression.
- Long-acting theophylline administered at night may be helpful. Studies suggest that a once-daily dose timed to achieve peak levels in the early morning hours may be superior to achieving a continuous 24-h therapeutic level of theophylline, in maximizing therapeutic efficacy, while minimizing toxic side effects.
- Salmeterol and other long-acting β agonists can be effective in improving nocturnal symptoms.

## TREATMENT OF OTHER CONTRIBUTING CONDITIONS

Other nonpulmonary contributing conditions should be treated as aggressively as possible.

- In the patient with allergic rhinitis, aggressive nasal anti-inflammatory therapy such as topical steroids should be used along with nasal saline rinses to minimize sinus drainage and irritation at night.
- Gastroesophageal reflux disease should be managed aggressively with behavioral modification, weight loss, elevation of the head of the bed, and medical or surgical therapy, if necessary.
- Since there is evidence that airway cooling may worsen nocturnal asthma, an effort should be made to warm and humidify the patient's bedroom air.

## KEY POINTS

1. Circadian rhythms play an important role in asthma.
2. The pathophysiology of nocturnal asthma is complex, with many factors contributing to a worsening of lung inflammation and airflow limitation at night.

3. Other comorbid processes such as rhinitis and GERD can contribute to a worsening of symptoms, but they probably do not represent the primary cause of nocturnal asthma.

4. Nocturnal asthma is primarily an inflammatory disorder, with a mechanism that appears distinct from nonnocturnal asthma, and that involves worsening of both central and peripheral lung inflammation at night.

## BIBLIOGRAPHY

Cuttitta G, et al. Spontaneous gastroesophageal reflux and airway patency during the night in adult asthmatics. *Am J Respir Crit Care Med* 2000; 161:177–181.

Guilleminault C, et al. Morphometric facial changes and obstructive sleep apnea in adolescents. *J Pediatr* 1989; 114:997–999.

Iber C, et al. *AASM Manual for the Scoring of Sleep and Associated Events*: Rules, Terminology and Technical Specifications American Academy of Sleep Medicine. Westchester, IL. 1st ed. 2007.

Irvin CG, et al. Airway-parenchyma uncoupling in nocturnal asthma. *Am J Respir Crit Care Med* 2000; 161:50–56.

Kraft M, et al. Serum cortisol in asthma: Marker of nocturnal worsening of symptoms and lung function? *Chronobiol Int* 1998a; 15(1):85–92.

Kraft M, et al. Expression of epithelial markers in nocturnal asthma. *J Allergy Clin Immunol* 1998b; 102:376–381.

Kraft M, et al. Lymphocyte and eosinophil influx into alveolar tissue in nocturnal asthma. *Am J Respir Crit Care Med* 1999; 159:228–234.

Kraft M, et al. Decreased steroid responsiveness at night in nocturnal asthma. *Am J Respir Crit Care Med* 2001a; 163: 1219–1225.

Kraft M, et al. Distal lung dysfunction at night in nocturnal asthma. *Am J Respir Crit Care Med* 2001b; 163:1551–1556.

Marcus CL, et al. Determinants of growth in children with the obstructive sleep apnea syndrome. *J Pediatr* 1994; 125:556–562.

Marcus CL, et al. Developmental changes in upper airway dynamics. *J Appl Physiol* 2004; 97:98–108.

Marcus CL, et al. Adherence to and effectiveness of positive airway pressure therapy in children with obstructive sleep apnea. *Pediatrics* 2006; 117:442–451.

Redline S, et al. Risk factors for sleep-disordered breathing in children. Associations with obesity, race, and respiratory problems. *Am J Respir Crit Care Med* 1999; 159:1527–1532.

Sutherland ER, et al. Immunomodulatory effects of melatonin in asthma. *Am J Respir Crit Care Med* 2002; 166:1055–1061.

Sutherland ER, et al. Elevated serum melatonin is associated with the nocturnal worsening of asthma. *J Allergy Clin Immunol* 2003; 112:513–517.

Sutherland ER, et al. Altered pituitary-adrenal interaction in nocturnal asthma. *J Allergy Clin Immunol* 2003; 112:52–57.

Tauman R, et al. Persistence of obstructive sleep apnea syndrome in children after adenotonsillectomy. *J Pediatr* 2006; 149: 803–808.

# 36

## CHRONIC OBSTRUCTIVE PULMONARY DISEASE AND SLEEP

WAJAHAT KHALIL AND CONRAD IBER
University of Minnesota, Minneapolis, Minnesota

### INTRODUCTION

Chronic obstructive pulmonary disease (COPD) is a progressive lung condition characterized by chronic airflow limitation that is incompletely reversible. The initiating triggers are heterogeneous, although COPD typically develops in susceptible individuals from abnormal small airway inflammation caused by long-term exposure to inhaled irritants such as tobacco smoke or noxious particles. COPD causes chronic cough and breathlessness, may result in progressive respiratory failure, and is a major cause for mortality and disability.

### PATHOPHYSIOLOGY OF COPD

Lung injury in COPD occurs as a result of oxidant stress from exogenous agents, such as cigarette smoke, and an imbalance between endogenous proteinases and antiproteinases within the lung. Chronic inflammatory changes center in the smaller airways, but the elastic skeleton of the lung and vasculature are also damaged. Patients with airflow obstruction demonstrate an increased number of macrophages, activated neutrophils, and CD8+ lymphocytes within the lung. Permanent pathologic changes occur in both the small airways and gas-exchanging surfaces of the lung tissue. The pathologic changes are heterogeneous, with varying degrees of airway inflammation, mucous hypersecretion, airway remodeling, and alveolar destruction with coalescence into poorly functioning emphysematous areas.

- When there is a predominance of alveolar destruction and coalescence, the pathologic change is termed emphysema. When airway narrowing predominates, the condition is called chronic bronchitis. Chronic bronchitis is also an epidemiologic term used to describe the accompanying symptom complex of daily productive cough of at least 3 months duration in two consecutive years.

- The most common mechanism for the development of COPD is smoking. Air pollution, occupational exposures, noxious gases, and hereditary deficiency of α-1-antitrypsin are also implicated. COPD may also occur as a result of chronic inflammatory airway diseases such as cystic fibrosis.

- The structural changes associated with COPD can result in the development of progressive dyspnea, hypercapnia, and hypoxemia. The worsening of gas exchange is a function of the severity of airway narrowing and alveolar destruction. Increased resistance within the airways also produces increased work of breathing, and incomplete emptying of the lung results in hyperinflation and inefficiency of the respiratory muscles. Dynamic hyperinflation during rapid respiratory rates contributes to the sensation of dyspnea.

- Chronic obstructive pulmonary disease should be distinguished from other causes of chronic respiratory failure due to lung destruction or restriction of lung expansion.

### DEMOGRAPHICS

Chronic obstructive pulmonary disease becomes symptomatic primarily in middle-aged and elderly adults. The prevalence of COPD rises with age. Chronic bronchitis is more frequently diagnosed in females, while emphysema is more commonly diagnosed in men. Symptoms of limiting dyspnea typically become evident in the fifth decade, although patients may have cough earlier; patients may also have symptomatic dyspnea decades earlier if they are smokers with α-1-antitrypsin deficiency, or if they have destructive lung conditions such as cystic

*Sleep Medicine Essentials*, edited by Teofilo L. Lee-Chiong
Copyright © 2009 John Wiley & Sons, Inc.

fibrosis, dysmotile cilia syndrome, panbronchiolitis, or inhalation injuries.

- The Third National Health and Nutrition Examination Survey (NHANES III) recently completed a survey of 20,050 adults in the United States, and identified obstructive lung disease, including asthma, in 8.5% of the population, and spirometric evidence of airflow obstruction in 6.8%.
- In 2000, chronic lower respiratory diseases (largely COPD) were the fourth leading cause of mortality. It is estimated that by the year 2020, COPD will rank fifth as a cause for disability in the United States.
- Chronic obstructive pulmonary disease cannot be presumed on the basis of smoking alone as individual smokers may show variable or no evidence of airflow obstruction. Genetic predisposition may constitute an independent risk in smokers who develop COPD. Progression of lung disease in COPD is accelerated by continued smoking and by a lesser extent by chronic recurring infections.
- Active asthmatic patients are at perhaps a 13-fold increased risk of developing COPD.

## EVALUATION

Diagnosis of COPD is based on the clinical syndrome of cough and dyspnea associated with irreversible airflow obstruction. Diagnostic tests are used to confirm the presence of airflow obstruction or the structural changes of emphysema. Assessment of the severity of airflow obstruction in COPD may be determined by spirometry; whereas diffusion capacity or high-resolution computerized tomographic (HRCT) imaging may provide a better assessment of lung destruction.

- Airflow obstruction is often defined as a ratio of the forced expiratory volume in one second to the forced vital capacity ($FEV_1/FVC$) of $< 0.70$. In COPD, the severity of spirometric obstruction correlates with the development of hypercapnia and mortality.
- The HRCT of the chest is more specific than chest radiographs in defining the presence and severity of emphysema.
- Differential diagnosis of chronic unremitting airflow obstruction includes tracheal narrowing and incompletely treated asthma.

## CONSEQUENCES OF RESPIRATORY FAILURE

Respiratory consequences of COPD include chronic cough, dyspnea, hypoxemia, and hypercapnia.

- The severity of dyspnea and alterations in gas exchange are determined by the extent of the structural changes, ventilatory drive, and fatigue and inefficiency of the respiratory muscles. Respiratory muscle strength may be augmented by ventilatory rest or by training.

- Ventilatory drive is extremely variable and may be genetically determined and modified by narcotics, changes in state, and adaptation to chronic respiratory failure. Patients with high ventilatory drive may experience severe dyspnea and are less likely to have hypercapnia. Patients with low ventilatory drive frequently have less prominent symptoms of dyspnea or signs of respiratory distress, although they may have profound hypercapnia and hypoxemia.
- Chronic obstructive pulmonary disease restrains the ability to ventilate and impairs gas exchange across the lung surface. Acute stressors, such as infection, may not only worsen airflow obstruction and gas exchange but may lead to fatigue of breathing muscles.
- Chronic progression of the disease results in increasing frequency of episodes of respiratory failure and decreasing functional status. The hypercapnia and hypoxemia that accompany respiratory failure may ultimately produce vasoconstrictive pulmonary hypertension and right ventricular failure as well as a sodium avid state with hypervolemia and edema.
- Progressive weight loss is a relatively common complication of respiratory failure in COPD. Loss of lean body mass occurs in approximately 20% of patients and has been ascribed to systemic inflammatory response e.g., tumor necrosis factor-alpha (TNFα), increased energy expenditure both at rest and with activity, and the calorigenic effects of β-adrenergic agents.

## EFFECTS OF SLEEP ON RESPIRATORY FAILURE

Several mechanisms act in concert to promote oxygen desaturation and hypercapnia during sleep compared to wakefulness: (a) decrease in resting lung volume; (b) decrease in ventilatory drive; (c) increase in upper airway obstruction; (d) decrease in compensation for loads; and (e) irregular breathing and ribcage inhibition during rapid eye movement (REM) sleep.

- Ventilatory responsiveness to hypoxemia and hypercapnia are decreased during sleep compared to wakefulness and are most depressed during REM sleep. Upper airway resistance increases during sleep even in the absence of obstructive sleep apnea. As a result of the profound effects of REM sleep on ventilatory responsiveness and respiratory muscles, oxygen desaturation in COPD is most severe during REM sleep.

## SLEEP-ASSOCIATED OXYGEN DESATURATION

The majority of patients with COPD do not have obstructive sleep apnea (OSA), and sleep-associated oxygen desaturation associated with COPD is more often an expression of worsening respiratory failure during sleep. Sleep-associated desaturation may occur in up to 80% of patients with severe COPD.

- Sleep-associated oxygen desaturation is more common in patients with daytime hypercapnia and typically occurs during REM sleep. Nocturnal oxygen desaturation during REM sleep is typically associated with decreasing tidal volume rather than with upper airway obstruction. Intensity of oxygen desaturation may vary over time, with significant night-to-night variation.

- The mechanism of REM oxygen desaturation in COPD is multifactorial. Hypercapnia, reduction in resting lung volume [functional residual capacity (FRC)], and ventilation–perfusion mismatching have all been implicated. Given the disadvantageous position of the diaphragm in hyperinflated COPD patients and the known effects of REM sleep on the overtaxed ribcage muscles, the observed drop in tidal volume during REM would seem predictable. Adaptive mechanisms in respiratory muscle structure, however, may lessen the impact of hyperinflation on ventilatory stability. Rising $CO_2$ in the alveolus displaces oxygen, making hypoventilation an attractive explanation for sleep-associated desaturation.

- The fall in tidal volume and ventilation during sleep would be expected to cause transient hypercapnia. In one study, sleep-associated rise of $PaCO_2$ was related to baseline $PaCO_2$, %REM sleep, and body mass index).

- Not all discrete episodes of sleep-associated desaturation are related to periods of worsening hypoventilation, and ventilation-perfusion mismatching may play a greater role in sleep-associated oxygen desaturation.

- A reduction in lung oxygen stores during sleep may also contribute to sleep-associated oxygen desaturation. The resting lung volume at end expiration (FRC) is lower in the supine than erect position and falls further during sleep. Since most of the oxygen stored in the body is in the FRC, lower resting lung volumes may accentuate desaturation during sleep. Indeed, the most severe oxygen desaturation is seen in COPD patients with the greatest reductions in sleep-associated FRC. In addition to reducing lung oxygen stores, reduction in FRC also contributes to regional airway closure, aggravating ventilation–perfusion mismatching.

- Oxygen desaturation may occur with modest decreases in $PaO_2$ and increases in $PaCO_2$ when the sleep baseline $PaO_2$ is near or below 60 mm Hg, the "shoulder" of the oxyhemoglobin dissociation curve. COPD patients with awake oxygen desaturation are more likely to have nocturnal oxygen desaturation.

## CAUSES OF SLEEP-ASSOCIATED OXYGEN DESATURATION IN COPD

Hypercapnia
    Sleep-associated decreased ventilatory drive
    REM-associated intercostal/accessory muscle inhibition

    Increased upper airway resistance
    Obstructive sleep apnea
Ventilation–perfusion mismatch
    Decreased lung volumes with airway closure
    Decreased resting lung volumes with reduced oxygen stores
Low position on oxyhemoglobin dissociation curve

## CHRONIC OBSTRUCTIVE PULMONARY DISEASE AND OBSTRUCTIVE SLEEP APNEA

Partial upper airway obstruction or discrete obstructive sleep apnea (OSA) episodes are noted in a minority of patients with COPD. In a large prospective study of 265 patients identified with OSA, 11% had concomitant COPD, and this subset had more hypoxemia, hypercapnia, and pulmonary hypertension. Patients with COPD who have concomitant OSA may be particularly vulnerable to developing respiratory failure and secondary hemodynamic complications. Polysomnography is indicated to identify effective positive airway pressures. Ventilatory support with bilevel positive airway pressure (BPAP) should be considered in patients if severe hypercapnia or respiratory distress persists despite correction of upper airway obstruction.

## EFFECT OF COPD ON SLEEP STRUCTURE

Chronic Obstructive Pulmonary Disease increases the frequency of somatic complaints such as cough, wheezing, and breathlessness. Respiratory complaints may contribute to the development of sleep complaints, such as insomnia or excessive sleepiness, as well as changes in sleep structure.

- Increased sleep disruption is common in COPD as evidenced by increased frequency of arousals and sleep stage changes, and decreased total sleep time.

## THERAPY OF COPD

### Oxygen

Mortality in COPD is related to severity of airflow obstruction and associated comorbidities. In one study, sleep-associated oxygen desaturation was a better predictor of mortality than spirometric evidence of airflow obstruction.

- Oxygen administration is the only therapy that has consistently been shown to reduce mortality in COPD. In the landmark Nocturnal Oxygen Therapy Trial, administration of oxygen for at least 12 h a day improved mortality in COPD patients with awake desaturation ($PaO_2 \leq 55$ mm Hg).

- Current consensus recommendations for chronic oxygen supplementation include a $PaO_2 \leq 55$ mm Hg or $SaO_2 \leq 88$%. If there is evidence of cor pulmonale or erythrocytosis, the threshold is raised to a $PaO_2$ of 56 mm Hg or $SaO_2$ of 89%. These criteria for oxygen administration have been adopted by the Centers for Medicare and Medicaid Services for reimbursement for oxygen administration in COPD. Reimbursement for long-term oxygen is also covered for nocturnal desaturation associated with restlessness, insomnia, or cognitive changes.

- Patients with COPD may have sleep-associated desaturation and yet not meet these criteria for oxygen use. In one case series, COPD patients requiring oxygen during sleep to correct nocturnal desaturation had higher daytime $PaCO_2$ and lower $FEV_1$. It is not clear if correcting nocturnal desaturation benefits COPD patients that do not have awake desaturation or heart failure. In one randomized prospective trial of 76 patients with COPD and an awake of $\geq 56$ mm Hg, nocturnal oxygen therapy conferred no benefit in terms of mortality or pulmonary hemodynamics. These negative findings are supported by a recent evidence review.
- Nonetheless, preventing desaturation may confer other benefits not measured in these negative studies. Oxygen administration has been shown to delay the onset of respiratory muscle fatigue and to improve subjective dyspnea. These beneficial effects may be responsible for improvements in arousal frequency and sleep architecture noted in COPD patients who are given oxygen for nocturnal desaturation.

### Bronchodilators

Bronchodilator therapy is indicated for daytime symptoms. Longer acting agents are appropriate if there are nocturnal symptoms of dyspnea or wheezing, but have variable and unpredictable beneficial effects on nocturnal gas exchange and sleep architecture.

### Respiratory Muscle Training

Unlike normal subjects whose resting ventilation is 5–7% of their maximal capacity, patients with severe COPD often exceed maximal sustainable levels of ventilation and, thus, develop respiratory muscle fatigue.

- Respiratory muscle training can produce modest but significant improvements in exercise tolerance and severity of dyspnea. One case series suggested that inspiratory muscle training in COPD patients improves nocturnal gas exchange.

### Ventilatory Stimulants

In one study of hypercapnic COPD patients, ventilatory stimulation with progesterone resulted in an 8-mm-Hg drop in arterial $PaCO_2$ and improvement in alveolar ventilation and oxygen saturation during non-REM sleep, whereas almitrine and acetazolamide produced more modest effects. Ventilatory stimulation can potentially

increase the severity of breathlessness in severely dyspneic patients and may be most appropriate for those with a low ventilatory drive.

### Positive Airway Pressure Therapy

Chronic ventilatory support can substantially improve the sleep-associated hypercapnia and hypoxemia that accompany respiratory failure. Continuous positive airway pressure (CPAP) has been shown to decrease work of breathing in COPD and would be expected to prevent respiratory muscle fatigue; the latter may be responsible for the improvement in daytime respiratory muscle strength and functional status as measured by the 12-min walk associated with nocturnal CPAP therapy.

- Noninvasive BPAP has been shown to reduce mortality in acute respiratory failure complicating COPD.
- Bilevel positive airway pressure has been proposed as a method of improving sleep quality and gas exchange in patients with chronic respiratory failure due COPD. The utility of chronic BPAP in severe COPD has yet to be determined, although selected hypercapnic patients may benefit if effective pressures are demonstrated to improve sleep and/or gas exchange parameters.

### Surgery

Bullectomy and lung reduction surgery have been shown to benefit highly selected patients with emphysema. Lung reduction surgery may be more likely to benefit younger patients with upper lobe predominance. Recently, a prospective randomized controlled trial of 16 patients with severe emphysema and significant air trapping showed that lung volume reduction surgery resulted in improved sleep quality and nocturnal oxygenation.

### KEY POINTS

1. Complaints of insomnia and daytime sleepiness are common in symptomatic patients with COPD. Sleep is often disrupted by arousals and frequent sleep stage changes.
2. Sleep accentuates respiratory failure in COPD, particularly during REM. Oxygen desaturation occurs in about 80% of patients with severe COPD, typically during REM sleep due to low resting arterial oxygen tension, progressive hypercapnia, decreasing lung oxygen stores, and ventilation–perfusion mismatching. A small subset of patients with COPD has obstructive sleep apnea (OSA).
3. Nocturnal oxygen improves survival in COPD patients with awake hypoxemia and should be offered to patients with less severe hypoxemia but with signs of cor pulmonale. Additional management strategies should include bronchodilator therapy for any reversible component of airway obstruction

and treatment of sleep apnea if documented. The role of ventilatory stimulants, surgery, and noninvasive positive pressure ventilation during sleep remains controversial but may be useful for selected patients.

## BIBLIOGRAPHY

Annane D, et al. Mechanisms underlying effects of nocturnal ventilation on daytime blood gases in neuromuscular diseases. *Eur Resp J* 1999; 13:157–162.

Chaouat A, et al. A randomized trial of nocturnal oxygen therapy in chronic obstructive pulmonary disease patients. *Eur Respir J* 1999; 14(5):1002–1008.

Crockett AJ, et al. Domiciliary oxygen for chronic obstructive pulmonary disease. *Cochrane Database Syst Rev* 2000; 4: CD001744.

de Miguel J, et al. Long-term effects of treatment with nasal continuous positive airway pressure on lung function in patients with overlap syndrome. *Sleep Breath* 2002; 6:3–10.

Kimura H, et al. Nocturnal oxyhemoglobin desaturation and prognosis in chronic obstructive pulmonary disease and late sequelae of pulmonary tuberculosis. Respiratory Failure Research Group in Japan. *Intern Med* 1998; 37(4): 354–359.

Klink ME, et al. The relation of sleep complaints to respiratory symptoms in a general population. *Chest* 1994; 105:151–154.

Krachman S, et al. Effects of noninvasive positive pressure ventilation on gas exchange and sleep in COPD patients. *Chest* 1997; 112:623–628.

Krachman SL, et al. Effects of lung volume reduction surgery on sleep quality and nocturnal gas exchange in patients with severe emphysema. *Chest* 2005; 128:3221–3228.

Lightowler JV, et al. Non-invasive positive pressure ventilation to treat respiratory failure resulting from exacerbations of chronic obstructive pulmonary disease: Cochrane systematic review and meta-analysis. *BMJ* 2003; 326:185.

Mannino DM, et al. Obstructive lung disease and low lung function in adults in the United States: Data from the National Health and Nutrition Examination Survey. *Arch Intern Med* 2000; 160:1683–1689.

Marin JM, et al. Ventilatory drive at rest and perception of exertional dyspnea in severe COPD. *Chest* 1999; 115:1293–1300.

McNicholas WT, et al. Long-acting inhaled anticholinergic therapy improves sleeping oxygen saturation in COPD. *Eur Respir J* 2004; 23:825–831.

National Heart, Lung and Blood Institute and World Health Organization. 1998. Global initiative for chronic obstructive lung disease. available: www.goldcopd.com/.

O'Donoghue F, et al. Sleep hypoventilation in hypercapnic chronic obstructive pulmonary disease: Prevalence and associated factors. *Eur Respir J* 2003; 21:977–984.

Peleman R, et al. The cellular composition of induced sputum in chronic obstructive pulmonary disease. *Eur Respir J* 1999; 839–843.

Sanders MH, et al. Sleep and sleep-disordered breathing in adults with predominantly mild obstructive airway disease. *Am J Respir Crit Care Med* 2003; 167:7–14.

Sergi M, et al. Are COPD patients with nocturnal REM sleep-related desaturations more prone to developing chronic respiratory failure requiring long-term oxygen therapy? *Respiration* 2002; 63:117–122.

Silva GE, et al. Asthma as a risk factor for COPD in a longitudinal study. *Chest* 2004; 126:59–65.

Silverman EK, et al. Genomewide linkage analysis of quantitative spirometric phenotypes in severe early-onset chronic obstructive pulmonary disease. *Am J Hum Genet* 2002; 70:1229–1239.

Weiner P, et al. Comparison of specific expiratory, inspiratory, and combined muscle training programs in COPD. *Chest* 2003; 124:1357–1364.

Yamaguchi K, et al. Computed tomographic diagnosis of chronic obstructive pulmonary disease. *Curr Opin Pulmonary Med* 2000; 6:92–98.

# 37

## RESTRICTIVE THORACIC AND NEUROMUSCULAR DISORDERS

CHRISTOPHE PERRIN, CAROLYN D'AMBROSIO, ALEXANDER WHITE, ERIK GARPESTAD, AND NICHOLAS S. HILL
Division of Pulmonary, Critical Care, and Sleep Medicine, Tufts-New England Medical Center,
Tufts University School of Medicine, Boston, Massachusetts

## INTRODUCTION

Thoracic restrictive disorders, that is, chest wall deformities or neuromuscular diseases that restrict lung volumes, predispose to sleep-disordered breathing (SDB), poor sleep quality, and nocturnal hypoventilation. These disorders amplify the reductions in respiratory center output and central chemosensitivity and increase in upper airway resistance that occur during normal sleep. The onset of rapid eye movement (REM) sleep further suppresses the activity of nondiaphragmatic breathing muscles.

- Disorders that impair diaphragm or upper airway muscle function and reduce chest wall compliance enhance the severity of SDB, particularly during REM sleep, worsening gas exchange, and predisposing to sleep fragmentation. The specific manifestations of SDB vary widely in restrictive thoracic disorders, ranging from obstructive respiratory events to frank hypoventilation, depending on the pattern and severity of neuromuscular involvement.

- Polysomnography is the gold standard for evaluation but is not always necessary for clinical decision making or practical to perform. Nocturnal oximetry has some value as a screening tool, as do measures of pulmonary function and respiratory muscle strength.

- Therapy consists of continuous positive airway pressure (CPAP) for patients with mainly obstructive events or noninvasive positive pressure ventilation (NPPV) for hypoventilating patients. NPPV improves nocturnal ventilation and sleep quality, and stabilizes daytime gas exchange, but associated air leaks may contribute to sleep fragmentation. If the patient is an unsuitable candidate for, or fails, NPPV, mechanical ventilation via a tracheostomy should be considered.

## SLEEP AND BREATHING IN NORMAL SUBJECTS

### Control of Breathing During Sleep

Normal sleep affects central respiratory control, airway resistance, and muscular tone and contractility. Sleep onset reduces respiratory center responsiveness to chemical (hypercapnia, hypoxia) and mechanical (lung inflation) stimuli. Deeper stages of sleep, particularly REM, further blunt ventilatory responsiveness. Although the diaphragm is less affected than the accessory muscles, the responsiveness of respiratory muscles to respiratory center output is also reduced.

- Minute ventilation falls during nonrapid eye movement (NREM) sleep, partly related to the diminished ventilatory responsiveness and partly to a drop in metabolic rate that occurs during sleep. Minute ventilation further declines during REM sleep, particularly during phasic REM when muscle tone and inspiratory drive are further suppressed. These physiologic changes are associated with only minor alterations in gas exchange among normal subjects but may contribute to profound hypoventilation and hypoxemia in patients with respiratory insufficiency.

### Airway Resistance During Sleep

Upper airway resistance increases during sleep compared to wakefulness as upper airway tone decreases. In addition, circadian changes in airway caliber slightly increase resistance in the lower airways during sleep, predisposing to upper airway occlusion and obstructive sleep apnea, particularly in individuals with anatomic or physiologic susceptibilities to sleep apnea.

### Rib Cage and Diaphragm Interactions During Sleep

As though pulling on a bucket handle, the diaphragm expands the rib cage during quiet breathing in upright subjects. Because of an alteration in the shape of the diaphragm during NREM sleep, intercostal muscles are recruited in order to maintain rib cage expansion. In contrast, during REM sleep, intercostal muscle activity is markedly reduced by active supraspinal inhibition of alpha motoneuron drive and selective depression of fusimotor function, leaving the diaphragm as the main ventilatory muscle.

### Functional Residual Capacity During Sleep

Functional residual capacity (FRC) falls during sleep in healthy adults during both NREM and REM sleep, but not enough to substantially alter ventilation/perfusion relationships. This decrease is likely related to cephalad displacement of the diaphragm in the supine position, respiratory muscle hypotonia, central pooling of blood, an increase in lung elastance, or some combination of these factors.

### EFFECTS OF THORACIC RESTRICTION ON BREATHING DURING SLEEP

Restrictive thoracic disorders amplify the effects of normal sleep on gas exchange, especially when the diaphragm is weakened. The mild hypoventilation that occurs at the onset of normal sleep is intensified in patients with restrictive physiology. Decreased chest wall compliance increases work of breathing and potentiates hypoventilation when inspiratory muscle tone drops during REM sleep. Abnormal chest wall mechanics also create instability and uncoordinated chest wall motion that, along with anatomic abnormalities of the upper airway, may predispose to obstructive events.

- Restricted patients with daytime hypoxemia may develop life-threatening hypoxemia during sleep because a drop in $PaO_2$ will be associated with a large drop in arterial oxygen saturation if the oxygen tension is already on the steep part of the oxyhemoglobin dissociation curve. Furthermore, abnormalities in rib cage and abdominal mechanical properties predispose to disruption of ventilation-perfusion (V/Q) matching and exacerbate the hypoxemia.
- Hypoxemia and/or hypercapnia related to SDB evoke arousal responses that stimulate ventilation and limit the severity of gas exchange abnormalities. However, these arousals also promote sleep fragmentation that impairs sleep quality and blunts ventilatory responsiveness. The reduced ventilatory responsiveness increases tolerance to hypercapnia and hypoxemia and may contribute to the progression of both daytime and nocturnal hypoventilation by resetting central chemoreceptors. It also has the effect of reducing sleep fragmentation, but at the cost of worsening hypoventilation and further depressing arousal mechanisms. A vicious cycle can ensue with progressive loss of the arousal mechanism, continued sleep fragmentation, and progressive hypercapnia.

### ASSESSMENT OF BREATHING DURING SLEEP IN RESTRICTIVE THORACIC DISORDERS

A high index of suspicion is essential in diagnosing SDB in restrictive thoracic disorders because the associated symptoms are nonspecific and may be insidious in onset. Some patients with neuromuscular disease have minimal symptoms despite significant apneas and severe nocturnal oxygen desaturation. Others may report symptoms that suggest nocturnal hypoventilation, but these may be misinterpreted as part of the progressive deterioration of the underlying neuromuscular disorder. Furthermore, daytime measurements of respiratory function may be poor predictors of nocturnal breathing events. Arterial blood gases and thyroid function should be checked in any patient with pulmonary restriction and symptoms consistent with hypoventilation.

### Common Symptoms of Hypoventilation Syndromes

Morning headaches

Daytime hypersomnolence

Fatigue

Weakness

Difficulty Concentrating

Depression

Enuresis

Dyspnea

- Several observations may help in determining whether more extensive nocturnal monitoring should be done. First, a drop in vital capacity of 25% or more between the upright and supine positions is a more sensitive indicator of diaphragm weakness than upright measurements of vital capacity and total lung capacity alone. The percentage fall in vital capacity from the erect to the supine position correlates with the lowest $SaO_2$ value during REM sleep. Second, maximum inspiratory and expiratory pressures are more sensitive measures to detect respiratory muscle weakness than vital capacity or total lung capacity and indicate significant respiratory muscle weakness when values are < 60% of predicted. Third, patients who have thoracic cage disorders, a vital capacity of < 1–1.5 L and a high angle of curvature (> 120°) are at high risk of developing respiratory failure. Patients with restrictive thoracic disorders who develop these findings should be considered for nocturnal polysomnography (PSG).

## RECOMMENDATIONS FOR POLYSOMNOGRAPHY IN THORACIC RESTRICTIVE DISORDERS

Symptoms of nocturnal hypoventilation[a]
Risk factors for obstructive sleep apnea including snoring, obesity, macroglossia, or retrognathia[a]
Unexplained gas exchange abnormalities [with forced vital capacity (FVC) > 50% predicted][a]
Abnormal nocturnal oximetry[a]
Pressure titration when initiating NPPV[b]
Assessment for failure to respond to NPPV therapy

[a]PSG is not required in patients meeting criteria for reimbursement of noninvasive positive pressure ventilation. These recommendations assume that criteria for NPPV have not been met, so a diagnostic study is necessary.
[b]Pressures determined during PSG to eliminate respiratory events may not be adequate to augment ventilation.

- The most widely used tests of global inspiratory and expiratory muscle strength are the static maximum pressures measured at the mouth maximal inspiratory pressure ($PI_{max}$) and maximal expiratory pressure ($PE_{max}$). These tests have the advantages of being noninvasive, inexpensive, and easy to perform. Normal values have been established for both adults and children. However, they are effort dependent and failure to get a good air seal around the mouthpiece may cause erroneous measurements, especially when the orofacial muscles are weak.

- Transdiaphragmatic pressure, measured using esophageal and gastric manometry balloons, can be used to assess diaphragmatic function, but aspiration is a risk in patients with severe neuromuscular impairment, particularly if bulbar structures are involved. For these reasons, simplified maneuvers or measures that require no subject effort have been proposed as alternative means of measuring respiratory muscle strength. The maximal sniff pressure test is easier to perform than the $PI_{max}$ maneuver for most subjects. Thus, inspiratory muscle strength is often better reflected by maximal sniff pressure (SNIP) than by the $PI_{max}$ maneuver. SNIP is measured through a plug occluding one nostril during sniffs while the other nostril remains patent. Waxed plugs are hand-fashioned around the tip of a polyethylene catheter to eliminate nasal leaks.

- Some form of nocturnal monitoring is recommended in patients with neuromuscular disease with a vital capacity = 55% of predicted. Factors such as obesity increase the likelihood of detecting significant SDB, even at higher lung function levels. Polysomnography is considered the gold standard for identifying SDB, but oximetry, alone or in combination with nocturnal respiratory monitoring, may be useful in screening for SDB. However, the use of oximetry as a screening tool may lead to overestimation of respiratory events when compared with PSG.

## PATTERNS OF SLEEP-DISORDERED BREATHING IN THORACIC CAGE AND SPECIFIC NEUROMUSCULAR DISORDERS

### Thoracic Cage Disorders

Severe chest wall deformity predisposes to the development of respiratory failure and death. Prior chest surgery, especially thoracoplasty used in the past to treat pulmonary tuberculosis, was a common cause of chest wall deformity leading to respiratory failure and cor pulmonale. The current prevalence of respiratory failure associated with chest wall deformity is unknown, but it is undoubtedly much less than in the past because of the advent of successful chemotherapy for tuberculosis and advances in therapies to prevent the development of severe kyphoscoliosis.

- Thoracic cage abnormalities not only alter chest wall mechanics and increase work of breathing, but also disrupt V/Q distribution and reduce the surface area for gas diffusion. Additional factors associated with thoracoplasty are pleural thickening, variable degrees of scoliosis, and impaired inspiratory muscle function related to the distorted chest wall anatomy. In the past, parenchymal destruction resulting from prior tuberculosis predisposed to V/Q maldistribution and airflow obstruction, but this is uncommonly seen today.

- By placing the respiratory muscles at a mechanical disadvantage, chest wall deformity reduces maximal strength and endurance, thereby increasing susceptibility to fatigue. The supine position has an additional negative impact on respiratory muscle function in these patients and predisposes to oxygen desaturation related to hypopneas during REM sleep caused by reduced inspiratory muscle activity.

- Because it is at a considerable mechanical disadvantage, diaphragm function is often impaired in severe kyphoscoliosis, and accessory muscles are recruited to maintain ventilation. During REM sleep, intercostal and accessory muscle activity is reduced by inhibition of neural output from the bulbar reticular formation. This decrease in intercostal muscle tone contributes to hypoventilation during sleep as well as to a further reduction in FRC, exacerbating hypoxemia via disruption of V/Q relationships. Chest wall instability can also occur and leads to paradoxical chest wall motion, further reducing the efficiency of ventilation and also disrupting V/Q relationships.

- Hypoventilation during sleep may have other physiologic consequences. The associated alveolar hypoxia raises pulmonary arterial pressure via hypoxic pulmonary vasoconstriction. If sustained, alveolar hypoxia causes pulmonary vascular remodeling and pulmonary hypertension leading to cor pulmonale. Hypoxemia and hypercapnia associated with hypoventilation also impair respiratory muscle function, increasing fatigability and susceptibility to development of respiratory failure.

## Neuromuscular Diseases

Sleep-disordered breathing is very common in neuromuscular diseases, occurring in an estimated 42% of individuals overall, and becoming more prevalent as the disease progresses. The nature and severity of SDB varies between the different neuromuscular syndromes, depending on the pattern and severity of respiratory muscle involvement. Weakness of the diaphragm and other respiratory muscles, deformities of the rib cage and spine, upper airway muscle involvement, obesity, and craniofacial abnormalities are all associated with neuromuscular disorders, and may contribute to obstructive respiratory events, nocturnal desaturation, and sleep fragmentation. As respiratory muscle function deteriorates, worsening nocturnal hypoventilation leads to oxygen desaturation, and sleep disruption, nonrestorative sleep, daytime sleepiness, impaired concentration, fatigue, lethargy, and, eventually, diurnal hypoventilation, which is the hallmark of respiratory failure.

- The pattern of SDB in patients with neuromuscular disease reflects the distribution of respiratory muscle involvement. If the upper airway or intercostal muscles are weak but diaphragm strength is intact, then obstructive apneas or hypopneas are more likely to occur. When patients have severe diaphragm dysfunction, suppression of intercostal and accessory muscles during REM sleep leads to hypoventilation. In some forms of neuromuscular disease, such as myotonic dystrophy, primary abnormalities in ventilatory control may also contribute to SDB, often complicated by nocturnal or even diurnal hypoventilation.

- Obstructive respiratory events during sleep are common with neuromuscular disorders. Risk factors for obstructive sleep apnea associated with neuromuscular disease include snoring, high body mass index (BMI), or anatomic abnormalities, such as retrognathia or macroglossia. Abnormal sleep events have been reported in patients with Duchenne muscular dystrophy, amyotrophic lateral sclerosis, and myotonic dystrophy. Even in the absence of frank apneas, increased upper airway resistance during REM sleep may contribute to obstructive hypopneas. Weak pharyngeal or laryngeal muscles may not be able to sufficiently stabilize the upper airway during inspiration, predisposing to airway narrowing and increased upper airway resistance.

- The large variability in the reported prevalence of obstructive events during sleep in patients with the same underlying neuromuscular condition and similar respiratory function is related, at least in part, to differences in how these events are diagnosed and recorded. For example, obstructive events are usually defined as continued or increased chest wall movements in association with reduced or absent airflow. In patients with severely weakened inspiratory muscles, however, chest wall motion during obstructive events may be too diminished to be detected, at least by standard plethysmography techniques, causing the events to be misclassified as central. Esophageal manometry is a more sensitive way of detecting diminished inspiratory efforts, but it is not available in most sleep laboratories.

- In addition to obstructive respiratory events, a number of other sleep-related breathing problems are very common in neuromuscular syndromes. Central apneas occur more commonly in certain neuromuscular syndromes, like myotonic dystrophy. The most common form of SDB in patients with neuromuscular disease is nocturnal hypoventilation due to a reduction in tidal volume attributable to inspiratory muscle weakness. Usually worse during REM sleep, it occurs in many neuromuscular syndromes including bilateral diaphragm paralysis, amyotrophic lateral sclerosis, and myotonic dystrophy. Sustained hypoventilation occurs as respiratory muscle weakness progresses. Respiratory failure, the most common cause of death in neuromuscular diseases that involve the respiratory muscles, may occur gradually over a number of years in slowly progressive neuromuscular disorders, or precipitously in more rapidly progressive disorders, particularly when complicated by atelectasis or respiratory infection with retention of secretions. Scoliosis and obesity also accelerate the development of respiratory failure. As with chest wall deformities, cor pulmonale is also a consequence of respiratory failure associated with neuromuscular syndromes.

- Other factors besides SDB may contribute to poor sleep quality and daytime sleepiness in patients with neuromuscular disease. The inability to change positions during sleep causes pain, discomfort, and frequent awakenings during sleep. Problems with clearance of secretions, anxiety, and depression may also impair sleep quality in these patients.

## Strokes

Cerebrovascular accidents predispose to SDB. The prevalence of SDB after a hemispheric stroke is as high as 77% for men and 64% for women. This is associated with disrupted sleep architecture, including shorter durations of slow-wave and REM sleep. This may be related to involvement of upper airway musculature by large strokes. In addition, sleep apnea increases the risk for stroke. The profound hypoxemia occurring during apneic episodes, changes in cerebrovascular tone in association with abrupt swings in blood gases that might predispose to atherosclerosis, and an increased platelet aggregation associated with sleep apnea could predispose to strokes. These associations justify a low threshold for evaluating SDB in patients with strokes, and consideration of CPAP therapy among patients found to have sleep apnea, although no studies have established the effectiveness of such an approach.

## Parkinson's Disease

Up to 65% of patients with Parkinson's disease complain of sleep disorders, related largely to abnormalities of upper airway and respiratory muscles. Muscle rigidity predisposes to upper airway obstruction and chest wall restriction, both of which may contribute to gas exchange disturbances during sleep. Oxygen desaturation and hypoventilation occur commonly during sleep, and up to two-thirds of patients report sleep-related problems in patient surveys. Upper airway muscle abnormalities cause fluttering and irregular, abrupt changes on the flow volume loop. Rhythmic oscillations that correspond to tremors of upper airway muscles are the cause of the fluttering and may increase upper airway resistance. Lower respiratory muscles also function abnormally, with less efficiency and inability to sustain high-resistance loads compared to normal individuals. Obstructive sleep apnea is not thought to be associated with idiopathic Parkinson's disease, but multiple system atrophy, a similar condition that is associated with a number of extrapyramidal findings including Shy-Drager syndrome, is associated with SDB, including nocturnal stridor and central apneas.

### Myotonic Dystrophy

Myotonic dystrophy is associated with various patterns of SDB including obstructive apneas and hypopneas, central apneas, and frank central hypoventilation. Daytime hypersomnolence, nocturnal oxygen desaturation, and diurnal hypoventilation are also common and may not be explained by either SDB or disturbances of sleep architecture. These symptoms have been related to an irregular breathing pattern during wakefulness and light sleep that does not persist during slow-wave sleep, suggesting that there may be a brainstem abnormality affecting respiratory control. Histopathologic studies have shown less neuronal density in the medullary arcuate nucleus of patients with myotonic dystrophy and central hypoventilation than in those without hypoventilation or in controls with other neurologic conditions, supporting the idea that the hypoventilation results from a primary dysfunction of the central nervous system.

### Amyotrophic Lateral Sclerosis

Amyotrophic lateral sclerosis (ALS) has protean effects on breathing during sleep, depending on the pattern of neuromuscular involvement. The upper airway muscles are usually involved, predisposing to obstructive events, although frank obstructive sleep apnea is less common than might be predicted, perhaps because the muscles are too weak to generate inspiratory pressures low enough to collapse the upper airway. Total sleep time is less, and arousals and SDB are more frequent than in age-matched controls, although SDB is relatively mild and without frank apneas. REM-associated hypoventilation also occurs, similar to that seen in non-ALS patients with respiratory muscle weakness. The largest unselected cross-sectional study of sleep in ALS observed a mean of only 11.3 events/h; the principal cause of nocturnal oxygen desaturation was hypoventilation. Surprisingly, bulbar involvement has not been associated with the severity of SDB.

- Diaphragm dysfunction also plays an important role in the respiratory impairment seen in ALS. Patients with diaphragm dysfunction typically recruit other inspiratory muscles to breathe, including the intercostals and accessory muscles, and this recruitment is thought to be a major contributor to dyspnea in ALS. Diaphragm dysfunction increases the likelihood of major sleep-related respiratory abnormalities, particularly during REM sleep, when maintenance of ventilation is critically dependent on diaphragm function. ALS-related diaphragm dysfunction has also been associated with a dramatic reduction in REM sleep and reduced survival. The presence of orthopnea predicts responsiveness to therapy with NPPV in ALS, further underscoring the importance of this connection.

### Spinal Cord Injury

The level of spinal cord injury determines the severity of pulmonary impairment. Patients with C5–6 injuries or lower have intact diaphragm function and, unless encumbered with secretions from a respiratory infection, are able to ventilate without difficulty.

- The importance of obstructive sleep apnea in patients with lesions at C5 or higher has been recognized for some time. Factors that predispose to sleep apnea in such patients include paralyzed intercostal and abdominal muscles, impaired activation of the diaphragm, increased upper airway resistance, sleep in the supine position, antispasmodic medication, traumatized and weakened laryngeal muscles by a previous intubation, and disrupted feedback afferents from rib cage receptors that alter compensatory reflexes to ventilatory loading.

- The sleep apnea syndrome in tetraplegic patients is caused mainly by obstructive events associated with an increase in neck circumference. This is thought to be related to a redistribution of body fat caused by a pathologic insulin sensitivity due to altered sympathetic function following high spinal cord injury. In quadriplegic patients, the enlargement of neck circumference is a better predictor of sleep apnea syndrome than body mass index. Although sleep apneas and hypopneas are usually obstructive in patients with high spinal cord injury, central and mixed apneas may also occur, suggesting that additional central factors may be involved in the pathogenesis of the sleep apnea syndrome in quadriplegia.

### Duchenne Muscular Dystrophy

Sleep-disordered breathing is quite common with Duchenne muscular dystrophy and has traditionally been thought to consist mainly of central apneas. However, some studies on nonambulatory patients have reported that up to 60% of apneas are obstructive. Older patients have more nocturnal hypoxemic periods related to central apneas, or possibly "pseudocentral" apneas that can easily be misclassified as obstructive events because of the difficulty in detecting inspiratory muscle activity. Measurement of transdiaphragmatic pressure during sleep would theoretically resolve the issue, but is difficult for several reasons, including the potential hazard of placing manometry balloons in patients with severe cough impairment, and the profound respiratory muscle weakness that complicates proper positioning of the catheters because the diaphragm may not generate a sufficient pressure difference.

- Hypoventilation could occur in all sleep stages, and those with diaphragmatic dysfunction were especially vulnerable to oxygen desaturation during REM sleep. On the whole, however, sleep architecture is better preserved in Duchenne muscular dystrophy than in subjects with ALS with a similar degree of respiratory function impairment.
- Vital capacity and total lung capacity are poor predictors of sleep hypoventilation in Duchenne muscular dystrophy. In contrast, a forced expiratory volume in 1 s ($FEV_1$) < 40% of the predicted value correlates with sleep hypoxemia, daytime base excess, and $PaCO_2$ elevation. In addition, a base excess of > 4 mmol/L and a $PaCO_2$ > 45 mm Hg are sensitive indicators of sleep-related hypoventilation. Hence, a daytime arterial blood gas and possibly polysomnography are recommended when patients with Duchenne muscular dystrophy have an $FEV1 = 40\%$ of predicted. Awaiting symptomatic evidence of daytime hypoventilation is no longer recommended because sleep-related hypoventilation may long precede diurnal hypoventilation.

## Myasthenia Gravis

Sleep-disordered breathing and nocturnal oxygen desaturation in myasthenia gravis are more pronounced during REM sleep, and the majority of respiratory events are central. As might be anticipated, patients with more advanced disease, as evidenced by a lower total lung capacity and abnormal daytime arterial blood gases, advanced age, and a higher body mass index are the most susceptible to SDB.

## MANAGEMENT OF RESPIRATORY INSUFFICIENCY DURING SLEEP

Respiratory insufficiency caused by restrictive thoracic disorders usually responds well to appropriate therapy, with improvements in functional status and life expectancy. These disorders are characterized by hypoventilation and, as such, oxygen therapy alone is not only usually ineffective but may even be hazardous, often aggravating the severity of $CO_2$ retention. However, the simplest therapy that is likely to be effective should be sought, starting with pharmacological therapy, moving on to CPAP, using noninvasive positive pressure ventilation when ventilatory assistance is indicated, and reserving invasive positive pressure ventilation as a therapy of last resort.

### Pharmacologic Therapy

Pharmacologic therapy should be considered when hypoventilation is worse than can be explained by the severity of pulmonary dysfunction (i.e. $FEV_1$ > 1.2 L), and polysomnography shows evidence of central hypoventilation or apnea but not obstructive respiratory events. However, central stimulants are not recommended for patients with severe ventilatory defects and might even exacerbate dyspnea.

### Continuous Positive Airway Pressure

Continuous positive airway pressure alone is indicated in patients with no more than milld hypoventilation who have polysomnography showing obstructive respiratory events. Obstructive or mixed sleep apneas occurring in the presence of normal or nearly normal daytime pulmonary function in patients with mild neuromuscular disease often respond favorably to CPAP alone. A trial of CPAP is warranted in such patients, but if the condition fails to respond after a reasonable trial or if hypoventilation is more than mild, noninvasive ventilation should be considered.

### Noninvasive Ventilation

In the past, negative pressure ventilation predominated as the noninvasive method of choice for patients with chronic respiratory failure due to restrictive thoracic disorders and neuromuscular diseases. However, negative pressure ventilation has been supplanted by NPPV for a number of reasons. NPPV is more convenient to use, easier to apply, more portable, and, for most patients, at least as comfortable. In addition, neuromuscular disease patients treated with negative pressure ventilation often have sleep fragmented by frequent arousals. Furthermore, episodes of severe oxygen desaturation persist, particularly during REM sleep, associated with obstructive events that may be induced by negative pressure ventilation. Because of its advantages over negative pressure ventilation, NPPV is the noninvasive ventilation (NIV) mode of first choice for patients with restrictive thoracic disorders. Rarely, negative pressure ventilation or another noninvasive approach might be considered for a patient who cannot tolerate NPPV.

### Indications and Contraindications for NPPV

Most clinicians agree that patients should have symptoms attributable to respiratory insufficiency because the desire for symptom relief is a strong incentive to adhere to therapy. The most common symptoms are those associated with nocturnal sleep disruption. Gas exchange criteria are also important, including evidence of daytime ($PaCO_2$ > 45 mm Hg) or nocturnal hypoventilation (sustained oxygen desaturation with $SaO_2$ < 88% for > 5 consecutive minutes).

- Initiation of NPPV is warranted when nocturnal hypoventilation develops and before the onset of daytime hypoventilation, so nocturnal monitoring is indicated when nocturnal hypoventilation is suspected.

- In progressive neuromuscular diseases, NPPV is recommended if symptoms are present with a forced vital capacity $< 50\%$ predicted or $PI_{max} < 60$ cm $H_2O$. With more rapidly progressive neuromuscular syndromes like ALS, orthopnea has been shown to be a strong predictor of NPPV success and should be added to the list of symptoms justifying NPPV initiation.

- *Indications for NPPV in restrictive thoracic disorders*: Symptoms (such as fatigue, dyspnea, morning headache, orthopnea, etc.) and one of the following physiologic criteria:

  (a) $PaCO_2 > 45$ mm Hg

  (b) Nocturnal oximetry demonstrating oxygen saturation $\leq 88\%$ for $> 5$ consecutive minutes

  (c) For progressive neuromuscular disease, maximal inspiratory pressure $< 60$ cm $H_2O$ or FVC $< 50\%$ predicted

- Absolute contraindications to noninvasive ventilation are few but include the inability to fit a mask or cooperate. Relative contraindications include a lack of motivation and a compromised ability to protect the airway because noninvasive ventilation, unlike invasive ventilation, affords no direct access to the airways for suctioning. Thus, invasive ventilation should be considered in patients with severe bulbar involvement, weakness of expiratory muscles, or secretion retention. Invasive mechanical ventilation should also be considered in patients with neuromuscular disease requiring nearly continuous ventilatory support. However, some clinicians advocate noninvasive ventilation even in patients who require continuous ventilatory support to avoid the complications and greater care burdens of ventilation via a tracheostomy.

- *Contraindications to noninvasive ventilation in patients with restrictive thoracic disorders*:

  Relative contraindications

  Weakened cough

  Swallowing dysfunction

  Upper airway obstruction (depends on severity)

  Poorly motivated patient or family

  Inadequate financial resources

  Inadequate family/caregiver support

  Need for continuous ventilatory assistance

  Absolute contraindications

  Anatomic abnormalities that preclude interface fitting

  Inability to cooperate

  Uncontrollable retention of secretions

- Patients with thoracic cage disorders and neuromuscular diseases and their families should be counseled about the options for ventilator support well in advance of the development of respiratory insufficiency so that they are prepared for the possible outcomes. With appropriate counseling and monitoring, respiratory crises leading to unanticipated and sometimes unwanted intubation should be a rare occurrence.

### Invasive Mechanical Ventilation

Invasive positive pressure ventilation is indicated in patients who have contraindications for, or who have failed, noninvasive ventilation and desire aggressive support. It has long been used to treat respiratory failure and prolong survival in patients with restrictive thoracic disorders or neuromuscular diseases, but it has significant disadvantages.

- Invasive mechanical ventilation requires a high level of care, including tracheostomy maintenance and suctioning, and its initiation may necessitate institutionalization for some patients because of inadequate caregiver resources in the home. It is also associated with a number of complications, including possible interference with speech and swallowing, repeated respiratory and soft tissue infections, tracheal stenosis, and tracheomalacia due to excessive cuff pressures.

## TECHNICAL ASPECTS OF ADMINISTERING NONINVASIVE POSITIVE PRESSURE

Continuous positive airway pressure and NPPV are administered using a device that delivers pressurized gas to the lungs through an interface (mask or mouthpiece) affixed to the nose, mouth, or both.

- For long-term outpatient applications, nasal masks are the most widely used interface for administration of CPAP or NPPV. Nasal masks are available from many manufacturers in multiple sizes and shapes. Because skin irritation and ulceration are problems with nasal masks, numerous modifications to reduce pressure on the face and enhance comfort are available, including soft silicon and gel seals that may enhance comfort. Also available to optimize comfort and minimize claustrophobia are "minimasks" that fit over the tip of the nose or nasal "prongs" that consist of small cones inserted directly into the nares. Because of the plethora of commercially available mask types and sizes, custom-molded masks are now rarely used.

- Nasal interfaces are also limited by air leaking through the mouth, a problem that may be ameliorated by chin straps or switching to a full-face (or oronasal) mask that covers both the nose and the mouth. Used more often for acute respiratory failure, full-face masks are available that are specifically designed for long-term noninvasive ventilation. However, nasal masks are likely to remain the preferred interface because they are rated as more comfortable by patients. Also, asphyxiation may be a concern with full-face masks in neuromuscular patients who are unable to remove the mask in the event of ventilator malfunction or power failure. Furthermore, interference with speech, eating, and expectoration, claustrophobic reactions, and the theoretical risk of aspiration and rebreathing are greater with full-face than nasal masks. On the other hand, full-face masks may be preferred in patients who are unable to close their mouths during nasal ventilation, such as those with bulbar dysfunction "Hybrid" masks that combine nasal prongs with a mask over the mouth help to reduce oral air leaking in patients using nasal prongs and may be better tolerated by same patients than standard oronasal masks.

- Mouthpieces held in place by lip seals can be used to provide up to 24 h per day of NPPV. Commercially available mouthpieces are simple to apply and inexpensive. Alternatively, custom-fitted mouthpieces that may enhance comfort and efficacy, and may be strapless, are also available at some centers. On average though, patients adapt more readily to nasal than to mouth interfaces. Mouthpieces can also be attached to gooseneck clamps on wheelchairs to serve as a convenient means of providing daytime noninvasive ventilatory assistance that enhances patient mobility.

## VENTILATORS FOR NPPV

Portable pressure- or volume-limited ventilators or those that offer both modes are available to deliver NPPV.

- Volume-limited ventilators are used in the assist-control mode and set to deliver large tidal volumes (10–15 mL/kg) to compensate for air leaks.
- Portable pressure-limited ventilators cycle between two levels of positive airway pressure using either flow or time triggers (bilevel ventilation). Some also offer spontaneous/timed modes that deliver backup time-cycled inspiratory and expiratory pressures with adjustable inspiratory:expiratory ratios at a preset rate. Backup settings just below spontaneous breathing rates may be desirable to ameliorate nocturnal hypoventilation; patients with advanced neuromuscular disease often allow the ventilator to control their breathing during sleep. The "bilevel" ventilators are best suited for patients requiring part-time ventilatory assistance, such as nocturnal only or intermittently during the daytime. Newer versions of these devices are suitable for patients requiring continuous ventilation, however, as long as adequate alarms and backup batteries have been incorporated.
- Controlled data are lacking to guide selection of ventilator settings, but inspiratory pressures between 12–22 cm $H_2O$ are often used. Higher pressures are sometimes needed for patients with high respiratory impedance, such as those with advanced scoliosis or morbid obesity. Expiratory pressure, usually 3–6 cm $H_2O$, is also applied during pressure-limited ventilation to minimize $CO_2$ rebreathing because many of these ventilators have single-tube ventilator circuits. It is important to remember that if expiratory

pressure is increased, inspiratory pressure must be raised equally to maintain the same level of inspiratory assistance (or pressure support). Patients are usually intolerant of higher pressures initially and must be started at subtherapeutic levels (inspiratory 8–10 cm $H_2O$, expiratory 2–3 cm $H_2O$) in order to facilitate adaptation. Therapeutic pressures can usually be attained within a matter of weeks. It is important to realize that pressures titrated in a sleep laboratory to eliminate respiratory events may not augment ventilation sufficiently and gas exchange must be monitored during adaptation.

- Pressure-limited ventilators are most commonly used for chronic ventilatory support because they are inexpensive, well tolerated, and highly portable. Volume-limited ventilators may be preferred in patients with advanced disease because of their better monitoring capabilities, backup batteries and longer battery lives, and ability to "stack" breaths to assist with coughing. A newer generation of "hybrid" ventilators offers a variety of volume- and pressure-limited modes, sophisticated alarms, and a backup battery but is more expensive than the pressure-limited devices. Newer devices also offer sophisticated monitoring capabilities that can be downloaded via telephones wirelessly.

## EFFECT OF NONINVASIVE AND INVASIVE POSITIVE PRESSURE VENTILATION ON SLEEP

Patients usually report better sleep soon after initiating nocturnal NPPV. This improvement may not be immediate because some patients require days to weeks to successfully adapt to NPPV. Nonetheless, sleep is almost always symptomatically improved by nocturnal NPPV when patients are using the device for at least 4–5 h nightly.

- Although no randomized controlled prospective trials have been performed, several studies have examined gas exchange or sleep quality during temporary withdrawal of noninvasive ventilation from patients with restrictive thoracic diseases who had previously responded favorably to it. In one study, nocturnal hypoventilation worsened during the period of temporary NPPV withdrawal indicating that NPPV ameliorates nocturnal hypoventilation. Another showed that sleep quality deteriorated during the period of withdrawal, including reduced sleep efficiency and total sleep time, supporting the idea that NPPV improves sleep quality. On the other hand, NPPV use is associated with frequent arousals in some patients in association with air leaks through the mouth. Thus, NPPV improves sleep in most patients with restrictive thoracic disorders but may contribute to sleep fragmentation in some. Sleep studies during invasive mechanical ventilation in patients with neuromuscular disease or chest wall deformity are lacking. In a survey of patients who had experienced both noninvasive and invasive forms of ventilation, sleep was rated as better during invasive mechanical ventilation.

## MONITORING NONINVASIVE POSITIVE PRESSURE VENTILATION

Patients should be seen at least every few weeks during initiation of NPPV. Morning headaches and daytime hypersomnolence are usually the first symptoms to respond. Daytime arterial blood gases (or end-tidal $PCO_2$ if there is no parenchymal disease) should be checked and should gradually drop over several weeks as duration of usage increases.

- Resetting of the respiratory center sensitivity to $CO_2$, along with improved respiratory muscle strength or endurance, are thought to explain the improvement in daytime spontaneous ventilation associated with nocturnal ventilatory assistance.

- If $PaCO_2$ doesn't fall into the desired range (40s to 50s) and symptoms fail to respond, inspiratory pressure and duration of NPPV should be increased. Once a plateau is reached, daytime $PaCO_2$ may remain elevated but tends to be stable for long periods of time, depending on the natural history of the underlying disorder. This improvement in gas exchange is usually sufficient to allow patients to be completely free from supplemental oxygen or ventilation during the daytime.

- Improvement of nocturnal hypoventilation occurs promptly once the patient is using NPPV through the night, but some patients require several weeks or more time before they reach this point. Nocturnal oximetry should be done at that time to assess adequacy of nocturnal ventilation as evidenced by maintenance of a saturation of at least 90% overnight (in the absence of supplemental oxygen).

- Follow-up polysomnography is usually reserved for those patients whose ventilatory status fails to improve after an adaptation period and attempts at adjustments in ventilator settings.

## KEY POINTS

1. Sleep is a complex physiologic process that is primarily restorative but also increases vulnerability to disordered breathing that may adversely affect gas exchange or sleep quality.

2. Sleep-disordered breathing is common in restrictive thoracic and neuromuscular diseases. The specific sleep-related abnormalities depend on the distribution, rate of progression, and severity of the chest wall and neuromuscular defects. Hypoxemia and hypoventilation are common during sleep, related to reductions in FRC and blunting of central drive (either primary or secondary to progressive bicarbonate retention). These gas exchange abnormalities lead to arousals, fragmenting sleep, and producing symptoms such as morning headache and daytime hypersomnolence. Sleep quality is adversely affected, as the arousals reduce sleep efficiency, total sleep time, and the percentage of time spent in slow-wave or REM sleep.

3. The therapies of sleep-disordered breathing and hypoventilation in restrictive thoracic disorders include CPAP alone, which may be effective in patients with obstructive sleep apnea. For most, however, NPPV is the therapy of choice. NPPV not only maintains upper airway patency but also actively assists inspiration using positive pressure, augmenting tidal volume and reversing hypoventilation. Invasive mechanical ventilation is used only if the patient is an unsuitable candidate for NPPV, or if NPPV fails and the patient desires aggressive support.

## BIBLIOGRAPHY

Consensus Conference: Clinical indications for noninvasive positive pressure ventilation in chronic respiratory failure due to restrictive lung disease, COPD, and nocturnal hypoventilation—A consensus conference report. *Chest* 1999; 116:521–534.

Dematteis M, et al. Charcot-Marie-Tooth disease and sleep apnea syndrome: A family study. *Lancet* 2001; 357:267–272.

Garcia-Borreguero D, et al. Parkinson's disease and sleep. *Sleep Med Rev* 2003; 7:115–129.

Karlsson AK. Insulin resistance and sympathetic function in high spinal cord injury. *Spinal Cord* 1999; 37:494–500.

Mehta S, et al. Noninvasive ventilation. *Am J Respir Crit Care Med* 2001; 163:540–577.

Meyer TJ, et al. Air leaking through the mouth during nocturnal nasal ventilation: Effect on sleep quality. *Sleep* 1997; 20:561–569.

Ono S, et al. Decrease of neurons in the medullary arcuate nucleus in myotonic dystrophy. *Acta Neuropathol* 2001; 102:89–93.

# 38

## CONGESTIVE HEART FAILURE

INDIRA GURUBHAGAVATULA[1,2] AND EMILIO MAZZA[3]
[1]Division of Sleep Medicine and the Center for Sleep and Respiratory Neurobiology and Division of Pulmonary and Critical Care Medicine, Department of Medicine, Hospital of the University of Pennsylvania, Philadelphia, Pennsylvania
[2]Pulmonary, Critical Care and Sleep Section, Philadelphia VA Medical Center, Philadelphia, Pennsylvania
[3]Allergy and Pulmonary Associates, Trenton, New Jersey

## INTRODUCTION

Congestive heart failure (CHF) is a major public health problem of growing magnitude, with approximately 5 million individuals in the United States carrying the diagnosis of CHF, and an additional 500,000 new cases being identified each year. Perhaps still more concerning is the association between CHF and increased mortality, an outcome that has been linked to overactivity of the sympathetic nervous system. Accordingly, beta-adrenergic antagonists and angiotensin-converting enzyme (ACE) inhibitors have become cornerstones of pharmacologic therapy. With the goal of countering the neurohormonal alterations of CHF, use of these classes of pharmacologic agents has mitigated the risk of mortality associated with this disorder, but only to a limited degree. Despite the use of these agents, nearly 300,000 patients continue to die each year from CHF, and this number continues to grow steadily.

- These limitations in conventional pharmacotherapy have led some to question whether other coexisting conditions might interact with CHF and contribute toward the excess mortality associated with CHF. One such condition is sleep-disordered breathing (SDB), which encompasses two distinct clinical conditions: obstructive sleep apnea (OSA) and central sleep apnea—Cheyne–Stokes respiration (CSA-CSR). As is the case for CHF, SDB affects multiple organ systems, including the respiratory, cardiovascular, and neurohumoral systems, and activates the sympathetic nervous system. Both OSA and CSA-CSR can exist either separately or together, and interact in the same patient with CHF.

## PREVALENCE OF SLEEP-DISORDERED BREATHING IN CONGESTIVE HEART FAILURE

### Obstructive Sleep Apnea

The largest study to date to evaluate the association between OSA and CHF is the Sleep Heart Health Study, a cross-sectional, multicenter evaluation of 6424 state employees who underwent full overnight home polysomnography. This study found that even individuals who had mild degrees of OSA [apnea–hypopnea index (AHI) > 11 events/h] have more than double the risk of CHF, with relative odds of having CHF of 2.38.

- Researchers have found that 11% of ambulatory male patients with stable CHF had AHI = 15 events/h without symptoms of OSA. In a separate cohort, 37% of ambulatory men and women with stable CHF and symptoms of OSA had an AHI = 10 events/h. OSA was found in 35% of CHF patients with diastolic dysfunction and preserved systolic function, with no gender difference in prevalence. In contrast, among healthy, middle-aged individuals, OSA defined by AHI = 5 events/h alone occurs among 24% of men, while OSA defined by AHI = 5 events/h together with symptoms occurs in 4% of men and 2% of women. Thus, the prevalence of OSA in patients with heart failure appears to be greater than that in a general, community-based population.

- Several authors have attempted to elucidate the risk factors for developing OSA in CHF. Male gender is considered a major risk factor. Among men, obesity defined by body mass index (BMI) = 30 kg/m² is also a major risk factor, whereas among women, age = 60 years is significant. Whether the increased risk of OSA in association with advancing age in women is related to changes in body fat distribution, levels of circulating sex hormones, or to some still undefined mechanism remains unclear.

### Central Sleep Apnea

Several studies suggest that CSA-CSR may be even more common than OSA in CHF, ranging from 33 to 40%. Male gender has been identified as a major risk factor, and CSA-CSR is rarely seen in women.

- Additionally, awake $PCO_2$ = 38 mm Hg, presence of atrial fibrillation, and age = 60 years are other risk factors. In contrast to OSA, obesity is not a risk factor for CSA-CSR.

## CARDIOVASCULAR EFFECTS OF SLEEP-DISORDERED BREATHING

### Effects of Obstructive Sleep Apnea

Obstructive sleep apnea may increase blood pressure, impair ventricular function, and increase pulmonary artery pressure. Each of these may, in turn, exacerbate CHF (Figure 38.1). While the mechanisms underlying these effects are likely to be complex and still remain to be elucidated, an important premise is that sympathetic activation associated with OSA is a key factor contributing to these cardiovascular effects, as well as to increased mortality in CHF.

**Hypertension**  Two large, population-based studies have suggested that OSA is an independent risk factor for hypertension, even after controlling for important confounders such as age, gender and obesity. The finding of this association is an important result in the context of CHF because the Framingham Heart Study identified hypertension as the single most common risk factor for CHF. Thus, OSA may be a contributing factor to the development of CHF through its effects on blood pressure.

- While reasons for blood pressure elevation in OSA remain unclear, one plausible mechanism is via activation of the sympathetic nervous system. This activation may be related to intermittent hypoxia, arousals from sleep at apnea termination, or to wide swings in intrathoracic pressure during efforts to inspire against an intermittently closed upper airway. Importantly, this increase in sympathetic tone during sleep persists into wakefulness.
- Sympathetic activation in OSA may indeed be responsible for increased mortality in patients with CHF as well. Some of the most powerful evidence for this comes in the form of several large, randomized trials, in which pharmacologic blockade of the sympathetic nervous system led to significantly improved survival compared with the administration of placebo.

**Reduced Cardiac Output**  OSA exacerbates left ventricular dysfunction in patients with CHF through changes in afterload, preload, and ventricular contractility. How OSA does this is the topic of much investigation, with a central focus being placed on cyclic, intermittent hypoxia. Additional evidence suggests a role for the large, negative drops in intrathoracic pressure during obstructive apnea events.

- Intermittent hypoxia associated with OSA impairs both myocardial contractility and relaxation and increases ventricular afterload by raising mean pulmonary artery pressure, not only during sleep but also even during the day.
- Obstructive sleep apnea patients also experience increasingly negative intrathoracic pressure during obstructive events. This enhances venous return and may result in right ventricular dilation and septal bowing into the left ventricle with resultant decrease in left ventricular end-diastolic volume and preload. This effect can be simulated by the Mueller maneuver, in which a wake subject attempts to inspire against a closed glottis, and the effects on septal bowing may be viewed in real time by echocardiography. The large, negative intrathoracic pressure during obstructive apneas also increases afterload. The combination of raised afterload, lowered contractility, and diminished preload has the overall effect of reducing cardiac output.

**Increased Mortality**  Evidence for an association between OSA in CHF and increase mortality is still in its early stages. Preliminary data suggests an increased release of cardiac peptides in OSA patients during sleep, presumably due to right ventricular dilation. OSA patients have a significant increase in brain natriuretic peptide during sleep compared to individuals without OSA. The importance of this is that elevated levels of brain natriuretic peptide (BNP) are not only a marker for the degree of pulmonary hypertension and both right and left ventricular failure, but may be a predictor of sudden death in patients with chronic CHF.

### Effects of Central Sleep Apnea—Cheyne–Stokes Respiration

Evidence suggests that CSA-CSR, when occurring in the setting of CHF, is associated with increased mortality. One prospective case control study showed that patients with CHF and CSA-CSR had a median survival of 1.9 years, compared to 3.7 years among patients with CHF alone. Another prospective cohort study examined clinically stable CHF patients with a left ventricular ejection fraction = 35% and found that the combination of AHI = 30 events/h and left atrial diameter = 25 cm$^2$ were associated with 2-year mortality of 86%. Importantly, however, patients with CHF in both studies were not receiving beta-blocker therapy, which has now become a standard part of treatment of CHF and which has been shown to reduce the occurrence of CSA-CSR, as well as reduce mortality in CHF. A more recent randomized controlled trial of patients receiving beta-blocker and

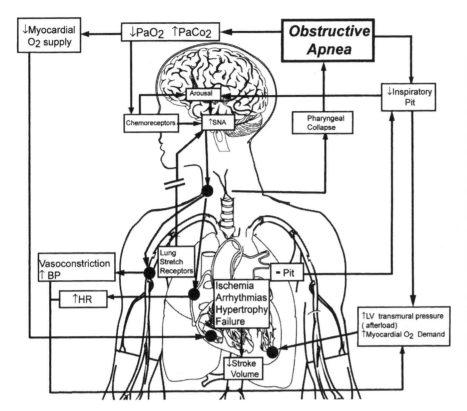

**Figure 38.1** Effects of OSA on the cardio-vascular system. Obstructive apneas increase left ventricular (LV) transmural pressure (i.e., afterload) through the generation of negative intrathoracic pressure ($P_{it}$) and elevations in systemic blood pressure (BP) secondary to hypoxia, arousals from sleep, and increased sympathetic nervous system activity (SNA). Apnea also suppress the sympathetic inhibitory effects of lung stretch receptors, further enhancing SNA. The combination of increased LV afterload and increased heart rate (HR) secondary to increased SNA increases myocardial $O_2$ demand in the face of a reduced myocardial $O_2$ supply. These conditions predispose a patient acutely to cardiac ischemia and arrhythmias, and chronically could contribute to LV hypertrophy and, ultimately, failure. The resultant fall in stroke volume can further augment SNA. (With permission from Bradley TD and Floras JS. Sleep apnea and heart failure: Part 1: Obstructive sleep apnea. Circulation 2003; 107: 1671–1678.

ACE-inhibitor therapy showed that patients with both CHF and CSA-CSR still experienced higher mortality and cardiac transplantation rates compared to patients with CHF alone.

- Whether CSA-CSR actually contributes to mortality risk or is simply a marker of the degree of severity of CHF remains unknown. As for the case of OSA, CSA-CSR is also associated with increased sympathetic activity. However, the degree of risk specifically attributable to CSA-CSR (via, say, intermittent hypoxia) rather than to reduced left ventricular end-diastolic volume (LVEDV) or clinical severity of CHF itself has not been quantified.

- The pathophysiologic effects of CSA-CSR on cardiovascular function are limited in comparison to OSA. Unlike OSA, negative intrathoracic pressure is not generated during central apneas so there is a less direct effect on cardiac afterload and LVEDV. Elevation of LVEDV is more likely a cause rather than an effect of CSA-CSR. This has been demonstrated using pulmonary capillary wedge pressure (PCWP) as a surrogate for LVEDV. When the PCWP is reduced through intensive medical therapy, there is concomitant drop in the AHI. Elevations in PCWP are also associated with hypocapnia, which is a risk factor for occurrence of CSA-CSR.

- A proposed mechanism for CSA-CSR is that elevations in LVEDV raise pulmonary vascular volume, which stimulates pulmonary stretch receptors and increases vagal output, and subsequently increases ventilation. This in turn results in hypocapnia and

induction of apnea. Supporting this is recent data showing that in a subset of CHF patients with CSA-CSR, normalization of ejection fraction through cardiac transplantation results in a reduction of the AHI. In the remaining subset, however, the AHI does not normalize completely despite transplantation, suggesting that additional mechanisms may be at play. One such purported mechanism is increased peripheral chemosensitivity to carbon dioxide; the hypocapnia that occurs in patients with both CHF and CSA-CSR has been associated with a 20 times increased prevalence of ventricular arrhythmia, compared to the prevalence in eucapnic controls.

## TREATMENT OF SLEEP-DISORDERED BREATHING AND EFFECTS ON CONGESTIVE HEART FAILURE

The usual treatment for SDB is continuous positive airway pressure (CPAP) therapy, which acts as a pneumatic splint to prevent airway collapse during sleep and its associated episodic oxygen desaturation. Even among patients with CHF *without* SDB, CPAP has significant beneficial effects, including reduction of LV afterload, increase in cardiac output in patients with elevated PCWP, and in the short term, reduction in cardiac sympathetic output and in myocardial oxygen consumption.

### Obstructive Sleep Apnea

Based on the cardiac effects of CPAP in persons with CHF who do not have SDB, we would expect patients who have both OSA and CHF to experience treatment benefit from CPAP, which exceeds that experienced by patients who have OSA alone. Two recent randomized controlled trials explored the cardiovascular effects of CPAP in CHF patients who also have OSA. In one, patients with systolic dysfunction [Ejection fraction (EF) = 45%] and OSA (AHI = 30 events/h) were randomized to receive medical therapy for CHF plus CPAP therapy for OSA versus medical therapy for CHF alone for 1 month. Patients receiving CPAP experienced a marked reduction in the AHI, which was associated with reduced daytime systolic blood pressure, reduced left ventricular end-systolic dimension, and a significant improvement in left ventricular ejection fraction. In another study, subjects with OSA (AHI = 5 events/h) and CHF (EF = 55%) were randomized to CPAP versus no treatment. After 3 months, in addition to a reduction in AHI, there was also improvement in left ventricular ejection fraction, a reduction in sympathetic activity, and improvement in quality-of-life scores. Thus, CPAP appears to provide significant benefit to patients with CHF and OSA in the short term.

- Since degree of ventricular dysfunction and sympathetic hyperactivity were two markers of reduced survival in the Framingham Heart Study, larger, longer-term studies should assess whether CPAP-associated reduction in sympathetic nervous system activity and improvement in left ventricular function translate into a clear survival benefit.

### Central Sleep Apnea—Cheyne–Stokes Respiration

Improvements in CSA-CSR may occur with treatment of CHF itself, with supplemental oxygen, or with CPAP. In patients with CSA-CSR and CHF, the first consideration is optimal treatment of CHF. In contrast to the case for OSA, intense treatment of CHF itself results in reduction of AHI in CSA.

- Nocturnal oxygen therapy may reduce the AHI by = 50% in eucapnic patients, perhaps because elevated $PaO_2$ may blunt $PCO_2$ sensitivity and prevent the hyperventilation phase of CSA-CSR. In one study, hypocapnia triggers central apneas in CSA-CSR and that inhalation of $CO_2$ but not supplemental $O_2$ reversed central apneas.
- As among patients with OSA, CPAP used in patients with CSA-CSR can improve cardiac function by decreasing afterload or reducing sympathetic activity. Additional evidence also suggests that mitral regurgitant flow and level of circulating atrial natriuretic peptide decrease.

### KEY POINTS

1. Heart failure imposes a major population health burden, and approximately half of patients with CHF experience OSA or CSA-CSR.

2. Obstructive sleep apnea may impair cardiac function and contribute to increased morbidity and mortality in CHF.
3. Instead CSA-CSR may be a marker for poor cardiac function and indicate a worse prognosis and mortality in patients with concomitant heart failure.
4. For both syndromes, CPAP therapy may improve left ventricular dysfunction and reduce sympathetic hyperactivity, each of which otherwise are markers of increased mortality in CHF, according to the results of the Framingham Heart Study. Whether CPAP ultimately improves survival in patients with SDB and CHF must remain a priority for future investigation by well-controlled, sufficiently powered prospective investigations with clearly defined endpoints.

### BIBLIOGRAPHY

Alchanitis M, et al. Daytime pulmonary hypertension in patients with obstructive sleep apnea. *Respiration* 2001; 68: 566–572.

Ancoli-Israel S, et al. The relationship between congestive heart failure, sleep apnea, and mortality in older men. *Chest* 2003; 124:1400–1405.

Berger R, et al. B-type natriuretic peptide predicts sudden death in patients with chronic heart failure. *Circulation* 2002; 105:2369–2379.

Bradley TD. Hemodynamic effects of simulated obstructive apneas in humans with and without heart failure. *Chest* 2001; 119:1827–1835.

Bradley TD, et al. Sleep apnea and heart failure. Part I: Obstructive sleep apnea. *Circulation* 2003a; 107:1671–1678.

Bradley TD, et al. Sleep apnea and heart failure. Part II: Central sleep apnea. *Circulation* 2003b; 107:1822–1826.

Chan J, et al. Prevalence of sleep-disordered breathing in diastolic heart failure. *Chest* 1997; 111:1488–1493.

Franklin KA, et al. Reversal of central sleep apnea with oxygen. *Chest* 1997; 111:163–169.

Hunt HA, et al. ACC/AHA guidelines for the evaluation and management of chronic heart failure in the adult: Executive summary. *Circulation* 2001; 104:2996–3007.

Javaheri S. A mechanism of central sleep apnea in patients with heart failure. *N Engl J Med* 1999; 341:949–954.

Javaheri S, et al. Association of low $PCO_2$ with central sleep apnea and ventricular arrhythmias in ambulatory patients with stable heart failure. *Ann Intern Med* 1998a; 128:204–207.

Javaheri S, et al. Sleep apnea in 81 ambulatory male patients with stable heart failure. Types and their prevalences, consequences, and presentations. *Circulation* 1998b; 97:2154–2159.

Kaneko Y, et al. Cardiovascular effects of continuous positive airway pressure in patients with heart failure and obstructive sleep apnea. *N Engl J Med* 2003; 348:1233–1241.

Kaye DM, et al. Neurochemical evidence of cardiac sympathetic activation and increased central nervous system norepinephrine turnover in severe congestive heart failure. *J Am Coll Cardiol* 1994; 23:570–578.

Kaye DM, et al. Acute effects of continuous positive airway pressure on cardiac sympathetic tone in congestive heart failure. *Circulation* 2001; 103:2336–2338.

Kaye DM, et al. Continuous positive airway pressure decreases myocardial oxygen consumption in heart failure. *Clin Sci* 2004; 106:599–603.

Kita H, et al. The nocturnal secretion of cardiac natriuretic peptides during obstructive sleep apnoea and its response to therapy with nasal continuous positive airway pressure. *J Sleep Res* 1998; 7:199–207.

Kraiczi H, et al. Comparison of atenolol, amlodipine, enalapril, hydrochlorthiazide, and losartan for antihypertensive treatment in patients with obstrcutive sleep apnea. *Am J Respir Crit Care Med* 2000; 161:1423–1428.

Lanfranchi PA, et al. Prognostic value of nocturnal Cheyne-Stokes respiration in chronic heart failure. *Circulation* 1999; 99:1435–1440.

Lanfranchi PA, et al. Sleep-disordered breathing in heart failure: Characteristics and implications. *Resp Physiol Neurobiol* 2003; 136:153–165.

Leuchte HH, et al. Brain natriuretic peptide and exercise capacity in lung fibrosis and pulmonary hypertension. *Am J Respir Crit Care Med* 2004; 170:360–365.

Leung R, et al. Sleep apnea and cardiovascular disease. *Am J Respir Crit Care Med* 2001; 164:2147–2165.

Lorenzi-Filho G, et al. Effects of inhaled carbon dioxide and oxygen on Cheyne-Stokes respiration in patients with heart failure. *Am J Respir Crit Care Med* 1999; 159:1490–1498.

Mansfield DR, et al. The effect of successful heart transplant treatment of heart failure on central sleep apnea. *Chest* 2003; 124:1675–1681.

Mansfield DR, et al. Controlled trial of continuous positive airway pressure in obstructive sleep apnea and heart failure. *Am J Respir Crit Care Med* 2004; 169:361–366.

Merit HF Study Group. Effect of metoprolol CR/XL in chronic heart failure: Metoprolol CR/XL randomized intervention trial in congestive heart failure (MERIT-HF). *Lancet* 1999; 353: 2001–2009.

Nieto FJ, et al. Association of sleep-disordered breathing, sleep apnea, and hypertension in a large community-based study. *JAMA* 2000; 283:1829–1836.

Peppard PE, et al. Prospective study of the association between sleep-disordered breathing and hypertension. *N Engl J Med* 2000; 342:1378–1384.

Sanner BM, et al. Pulmonary hypertension in patients with obstructive sleep apnea syndrome. *Arch Intern Med* 1997; 157:2483–2487.

Shamsuzzaman ASM, et al. Obstructive sleep apnea. Implications for cardiac and vascular disease. *JAMA* 2003; 290:1906–1914.

Sin DD, et al. Risk factors for central and obstructive sleep apnea in 450 men and women with congestive heart failure. *Am J Respir Crit Care Med* 1999; 160:1101–1106.

Sin DD, et al. Effects of continuous positive airway pressure on cardiovascular outcomes in heart failure patients with and without Cheyne-Stokes respiration. *Circulation* 2000; 102:61–66.

Sleep Heart Health Study Research Group. Sleep-disordered breathing and cardiovascular disease. *Am J Respir Crit Care Med* 2001; 163:19–25.

Solin P, et al. Influence of pulmonary capillary wedge pressure on central apnea in heart failure. *Circulation* 1999; 99:1574–1579.

Solin P, et al. Impact of sleep apnea on sympathetic nervous system activity in heart failure. *Chest* 2003; 123:1119–1126.

Tkacova R, et al. Effect of continuous positive airway pressure on mitral regurgitant fraction and atrial natriuretic peptide in patients with heart failure. *J Am Coll Cardiol* 1997a; 30:739–745.

Tkacova R, et al. Left ventricular volume in patients with heart failure and Cheyne-Stokes respiration during sleep. *Am J Respir Crit Care Med* 1997b; 156:1549–1555.

Tkacova R, et al. Overnight shift from obstructive to central sleep apneas in patients with heart failure. Role of $PCO_2$ and circulatory delay. *Circulation* 2001; 103:238–243.

Yan AT, et al. The role of continuous positive airway pressure in the treatment of congestive heart failure. *Chest* 2001; 120:1675–1685.

# 39

## SLEEP AND THE GASTROINTESTINAL TRACT

WILLIAM C. ORR
Lynn Institute for Healthcare Research, Oklahoma City, Oklahoma

## INTRODUCTION

There has been a marked increase in studies describing alterations in gastrointestinal functioning during sleep and the specific applications of these changes to the practice of gastroenterology.

## GASTROESOPHAGEAL REFLUX

Sleep is not associated with notable changes in the lower esophageal sphincter (LES) or in the amplitude of esophageal contractions. In contrast, the upper esophageal sphincter (UES) shows a clear decrease in pressure during nonrapid eye movement (NREM) sleep with an increase in rapid eye movement (REM) sleep to nearly waking levels.

- Gastroesophageal reflux (GER), and its most common symptom heartburn, is a common event postprandially; it is a normal physiologic response to gastric distention that induces a transient relaxation of the LES. Waking reflux is generally postprandial and reflux events are rapidly cleared (i.e., within 1–2 min). Heartburn and regurgitation are also well established as the most common symptoms of esophageal mucosal contact.
- Gastroesophageal reflux occurs during sleep, but its actual occurrence is difficult to estimate by symptoms alone since the sensation of heartburn is a waking conscious experience; reflux events during sleep do not necessarily produce a symptom.
- Sleep-related GER is less common than that occurs in the waking state. However, reflux events during sleep are generally associated with prolongation of acid clearance and longer period of acid contact time. The complications of reflux, which result in discontinuity of the esophageal mucosa, are generally associated with an increase in the percent of recumbent (during sleep) acid contact time.

- Several sleep-related physiologic alterations facilitate the prolongation of acid mucosal contact. There are secretory, motor, and sensory responses that are associated with acid mucosal contact in the human esophagus. Typically, acidification of the distal esophagus will produce a marked increase in the secretion and bicarbonate concentration of saliva. This allows ample buffering potential in order to neutralize the acid lining the distal esophagus. Also, in response to an acidic distal esophagus, there is a marked increase in the rate of swallowing, which allows the delivery of the potent buffer of saliva into the distal esophagus. Finally, acid mucosal contact is associated with a sensation of substernal burning, which is perceived as uncomfortable and/or painful. The combination of these responses typically results in a rapid clearance of the volume of refluxed gastric contents.
- The characteristic responses to acid mucosal contact, which are present in the waking state, are generally absent during sleep. These alterations in response to acid mucosal contact during sleep result in marked prolongation of acid clearance during sleep. Swallowing rate is markedly diminished, and salivary flow is essentially absent. Furthermore, the sensation of heartburn is absent during sleep.
- The prolongation of acid mucosal contact carries significant risks. Since the back diffusion of hydrogen ions into the esophageal mucosa is directly related to the duration of esophageal acid contact time, prolonged episodes of GER would be associated with a greater risk of mucosal damage. An additional risk of prolonged acid mucosal contact relates to the higher risk of the proximal migration and eventual spillover of reflux gastric contents into the tracheobronchial tree.
- In patients with obstructive sleep apnea (OSA), the frequent occurrence of obesity, and the appreciable

*Sleep Medicine Essentials*, edited by Teofilo L. Lee-Chiong
Copyright © 2009 John Wiley & Sons, Inc.

negative intrathoracic pressures associated with upper airway obstruction are certainly risk factors for the occurrence of nighttime GER. Although studies have not indicated a specific relationship between obstructive events and reflux events, patients with OSA tend to have an overall increase in esophageal acid contact time. A reduction in obstructive events, via appropriate continuous positive airway pressure (CPAP) treatment, results in a reduction in heartburn complaints.

## CLINICAL MANIFESTATIONS OF NIGHTTIME GASTROESOPHAGEAL REFLUX DISEASE (GERD)

Patients with nighttime heartburn have a number of complaints related to disturbed sleep. Nighttime heartburn is an independent risk factor for sleep complaints and daytime sleepiness.

- In patients with both daytime and nighttime heartburn, the latter was significantly more bothersome, with more than 50% of individuals complaining that nighttime heartburn awakened them with GERD symptoms, and about 30% were awakened by coughing and choking due to regurgitation.
- About 40% of the patients with nighttime symptoms noted that their heartburn affected their ability to function the next day, and about 60% indicated it affected their mood. The use of sleeping pills was substantially increased in patients with nighttime GERD symptoms.
- Nighttime GER is associated with a number of respiratory symptoms, such as wheezing, chronic cough, and hoarseness. Not uncommonly, patients with GERD-related asthma or chronic cough will not have heartburn as a symptom. Nighttime wheezing is quite common in asthmatics and approximately 41% of asthmatic patients have been shown to have reflux-associated respiratory symptoms.
- The presence of nighttime reflux cannot be ruled out on the basis of a negative history of nighttime heartburn.

## GASTRIC FUNCTION DURING SLEEP

The motor function of the stomach serves to deliver gastric contents into the antrum and ultimately into the duodenum at an appropriate rate and pH.

- Reports of alterations in gastric motility, including motor functioning of the stomach or its ultimate consequence, gastric emptying, during sleep have been contradictory.
- By utilizing surface electrodes placed in periumbilical locations, a three-cycle per minute electrical rhythm can be detected from the surface of the stomach. This electrical rhythm is a product of the endogenous functioning of the enteric nervous

system, and it serves to modulate the contractility of the gastric smooth muscle. The gastric pacemaker activity is influenced by sleep, with a significant decline in the three-cycle per minute gastric electrical activity during NREM sleep, and a significant recovery during REM sleep to levels comparable to the waking state; this suggests that NREM sleep is associated with a marked destabilization of the basic gastric electrical rhythm, and that the cerebral activation of REM sleep appears to result in a stabilization of this basic gastric pacemaker.

## INTESTINAL MOTILITY AND IRRITABLE BOWEL SYNDROME

Sleep disturbances have been noted in patients with functional bowel disorders; conversely, sleep disturbances may contribute to altered gastrointestinal functioning.

- Difficulties in monitoring intestinal activity in humans has somewhat limited the study of intestinal activity during sleep. Studies done to date clearly suggest an inhibition of colonic contractile and myoelectric activity during sleep, as well as diminished colonic tone.
- A decrease in colonic motor activity during sleep and a clear inhibition of the colonic motility index in the transverse, descending, and sigmoid colon is present. A marked increase in activity occurs on awakening or with brief arousals from sleep.
- Ambulatory monitoring of the small intestine in patients with irritable bowel syndrome (IBS) has documented a lack of activity in the small bowel during sleep, and that nighttime motor patterns of the small bowel did not differentiate patient groups from controls.
- There is a relationship between poor sleep and pain in IBS patients. The prevalence of reported sleep complaints may be as high as 25–30% in the population of patients with functional bowel disorders (i.e., IBS and functional dyspepsia). In one study, patients with IBS symptoms alone did not differ from normal controls with regard to the reported incidence of sleep complaints; however, sleep complaints were significantly greater if dyspeptic symptoms were part of the symptom complex.
- Patients with IBS have more sleep complaints, however, compared to normal controls, sleep architecture of patients with functional bowel disorders appears to be quite similar to age- and sex-matched controls.
- The autonomic nervous system appears to be a mediator of visceral pain in patients with functional bowel disorders, and increasing sympathetic tone during REM sleep has been described in patients with IBS. IBS patients who have dyspeptic symptoms did not appear to have this autonomic dysfunction; rather, it was most notable in patients with IBS without dyspeptic symptoms.

## KEY POINTS

1. Sleep-related GER is an important factor not only in the development of esophagitis but also respiratory complications. Although sensory functioning is markedly altered during sleep with regard to most standard sensory functions (i.e., auditory), there appears to be an enhancement of some visceral sensation during sleep that would appear to protect the tracheobronchial tree from the aspiration of refluxed gastric contents during sleep.

2. Sleep is associated with a distinct pattern of GER in which there are less frequent events, but reflux events are typically associated with a marked prolongation of acid clearance.

3. The upper esophageal sphincter pressure decreases during NREM sleep and increases slightly during REM sleep. No changes associated with sleep are noted with either the lower esophageal sphincter or esophageal peristalsis.

4. Gastroesophageal reflux can occur during sleep in spite of the absence of complaints of nighttime heartburn.

5. Patients with functional bowel disorders clearly reveal an increase in sleep complaints compared to normal volunteers. The actual mechanisms of these disturbances remain somewhat obscure, and studies have not demonstrated any consistent abnormalities in actual sleep patterns of these patients. Some studies have shown that autonomic functioning during sleep, particularly REM sleep, can distinguish patients with IBS and dyspeptic symptoms.

## BIBLIOGRAPHY

Bajaj J, et al. Influence of sleep stages on esophago-upper esophageal sphincter contractile reflex and secondary esophageal peristalsis. *Gastroenterology* 2006; 130:17–25.

Elsenbruch S, et al. Disruption of normal gastric myoelectric functioning by sleep. *Sleep* 1999a; 22:453A–458A.

Elsenbruch S, et al. Subjective and objective sleep quality in irritable bowel syndrome. *Am J Gastroenterol* 1999b; 94:2447–2452.

Fass R, et al. Sleep disturbances in clinic patients with functional bowel disorders. *Am J Gastroenterol* 2000; 95:1195–2000.

Gisalson T, et al. Respiratory symptoms and nocturnal gastroesophageal reflux. *Chest* 2002; 121:158–163.

Green BT, et al. Marked improvement in nocturnal gastroesophageal reflux in a large cohort of patients with obstructive sleep apnea treated with continuous positive airway pressure. *Arch Intern Med* 2003; 163:341–345.

Ing AJ, et al. Obstructive sleep apnea and gastroesophageal reflux. *Am J Med* 2000; 108(Suppl 4a):120S–125S.

Orr WC, et al. Proximal migration of esophageal acid perfusions during waking and sleep. *Am J Gastroenterol* 2000; 95(1):37–42.

Robert JJ, et al. Modulation of sleep quality and autonomic functioning by symptoms of depression in women with irritable bowel syndrome. *Dig Dis Sci* 2004; 49(7–8):1250–1258.

Shaker R, et al. Nighttime heartburn is an under-appreciated clinical problem that impacts sleep and daytime function: The results of a Gallup survey conducted on behalf of the American Gastroenterological Association. *Am J Gastroenterol* 2003: 1487–1493.

Sontag SJ. Gastroesophageal reflux disease and asthma. *J Clin Gastroenterol* 2000; 39(Suppl):S9–30.

Thompson JJ, et al. Autonomic functioning during REM sleep differentiates IBS symptom subgroups. *Am J Gastroenterol* 2002; 97:3147–3153.

# 40

## RENAL DISEASE

Kathy P. Parker

Nell Hodgson Woodruff School of Nursing and Department of Neurology, Emory University, Atlanta, Georgia

### INTRODUCTION

End-stage renal disease (ESRD) is a significant health problem in the United States. As of 2007, there were over 400,000 patients with renal failure requiring treatment with dialysis or transplantation, and this number is expected to approach 700,000 by the year 2010. ESRD patients experience significant sleep disturbance. Primary sleep disorders such as sleep apnea (SA), restless legs syndrome (RLS), and periodic limb movement disorder (PLMD), are very common.

### SLEEP COMPLAINTS

Sleep complaints, characterized by difficulty initiating and maintaining sleep, problems with restless, jerking legs, and/or daytime sleepiness, are reported by up to 80% of ESRD patients.

- Sleep problems are among the most disturbing symptoms experienced by ESRD patients and are consistently cited as major sources of stress as well as factors negatively affecting life quality.

#### Demographics

Sleep complaints are more common in elderly ESRD patients. Males are more likely to have sleep complaints than females, and whites may have a higher prevalence of restless sleep than blacks.

#### Risk Factors

Sleep complaints have been associated with caffeine intake, pruritus, bone pain, cigarette use, premature discontinuation of dialysis, anxiety, depression, and stress. Anemia has been associated with complaints of poor sleep with improvement noted after treatment with recombinant erythropoietin. Mild hypercalcemia has also been associated with subjective insomnia. No consistent relationships between subjective sleep complaints and BUN (blood urea nitrogen), creatinine, or Kt/V (a measure of dialysis adequacy) have been detected.

### POLYSOMNOGRAPHIC FEATURES

Sleep of ESRD patients is characterized by decreased total sleep time, reduced sleep efficiency, irregular sleep cycles, and long periods of interspersed waking.

- Large amounts of wake time and numerous arousals are common.
- Increased amounts of nonrapid eye movement (NREM) stages 1 and 2 sleep, and decreased slow-wave sleep (SWS) and rapid eye movement (REM) sleep have been reported.
- Sleep latency and REM sleep latency may be prolonged.

### SLEEP APNEA SYNDROMES

Prevalence rates in ESRD patients are estimated to be approximately 50%, a rate significantly greater than that reported for the general population. Sleep apneas are most commonly obstructive in nature, but central and mixed events have also been observed.

- The type and severity of apneas do not appear to vary substantially with type of dialysis (continuous ambulatory peritoneal dialysis, hemodialysis, or peritoneal dialysis), or between nights "on" versus night "off" treatment. No consistent relationships between apnea indices and biochemical measures, such as BUN, creatinine, hematocrit, waking arterial blood gases, or dialysis adequacy, have been described.

*Sleep Medicine Essentials*, edited by Teofilo L. Lee-Chiong

- The mechanisms underlying the increased prevalence of SA in ESRD patients are not well characterized. Hypocapnia from metabolic acidosis and acidemia may change the apnea–$PaCO_2$ or hydrogen ion threshold and predispose to an unstable breathing pattern. In addition, accumulation of uremic toxins may affect the central nervous system and result in a reduction of airway muscle tone during sleep, discoordination of the diaphragm, or instability of respiratory control. Many patients also have peripheral neuropathy and edema from fluid overload, which makes them more susceptible to upper airway collapse. Anemia, hormone abnormalities, cytokine production during dialysis, and the mechanical effects of peritoneal fluid on diaphragmatic action may all contribute to ventilatory control instability.

- Treatment of SA with continuous positive airway pressure (CPAP) results in stabilization of nocturnal oxygenation, decrease in NREM stage 1 sleep, and increased daytime alertness. However, long-term impact has not been assessed, and improvements in cognition and other aspects of functional status remain to be described. Cure after transplantation has been reported. A decrease in apnea has also been described with the use of bicarbonate versus acetate-based dialysate, and with both slow nocturnal and intensive daily hemodialysis.

## RESTLESS LEGS SYNDROME AND PERIODIC LIMB MOVEMENT DISORDER

Restless legs syndrome is an extremely distressing problem experienced by ESRD patients; up to 80% may experience symptoms. The prevalence of PLMD in ESRD patients, both in association with RLS and as an independent condition, is also high and may approach 70%.

- Higher predialysis urea and creatinine levels have been associated with increased RLS complaints in some, but not all, studies. Higher intact parathyroid hormone (PTH) levels have been observed in association with periodic limb movements while lower PTH levels were noted in those with RLS. Although normalization of hematocrit with recombinant erythropoietin has resulted in a significant reduction in periodic limb movements in a sample of dialysis patients, no specific relationship between RLS symptoms and anemia has been detected.

- Restless legs syndrome severity is unrelated to age, gender, body weight, number of years on dialysis, or median, ulnar, and sural nerve amplitudes.

- Several factors intrinsic to the uremic state may predispose ESRD patients to these disorders. Anemia secondary to decreased production of endogenous erythropoietin and reduced iron stores from dietary restrictions and blood loss during dialysis may be important risk factors. Vitamin deficiencies (particularly water-soluble vitamins such as folate

and $B_{12}$) may occur secondary to poor intake, interference with absorption by drugs or uremia, altered metabolism, and losses to the dialysate. Peripheral neuropathy associated with uremia and/or diabetes and skeleto-muscular abnormalities related to secondary hyperparathyroidism may predispose dialysis patients to RLS/PLMD. Alterations of dopamine (DA) and opioid synthesis/metabolism may also play a role. The beneficial effects of treatment with L-dopa and $DA_2$ agonists in ESRD patients with RLS/PLMD suggest that DA pathways are involved.

- Data regarding the effective treatment of RLS and PLMD in ESRD patients are limited. Reports from three prospective clinical trials of L-dopa cite reduction of RLS symptoms and improved nocturnal sleep, decreased numbers of nocturnal limb movements, and improved subjective quality of life. Although rebound (return) and augmentation (worsening) of symptoms have been reported with L-dopa in other clinical populations, none of these studies mentioned these phenomena. In a double-blind, placebo-controlled, crossover study, treatment with pergolide (a $DA_2$ agonist) resulted in decreased symptoms but had no effect on objective indicators such as numbers of nocturnal limb movements and sleep architecture. Favorable responses to treatment with clonazepam and clonidine in ESRD patients have also been described. Alleviation of RLS symptoms was reported to occur in one patient after renal transplantation.

## EXCESSIVE DAYTIME SLEEPINESS

Excessive daytime sleepiness (EDS) appears highly prevalent and probably underrecognized in ESRD patients.

- The high prevalence of SA, PLMD, and RLS in the dialysis population provides the most parsimonious explanation for EDS. Arousals from sleep and nocturnal sleep disruption related to these conditions have certainly been implicated as important causes of EDS.

- Other factors related to renal disease and/or its treatment may also contribute to EDS. Subclinical uremic encephalopathy commonly present in dialysis patients may play a role; mild elevations of BUN and creatinine in renal failure patients have been associated with both increased slow-wave activity in the waking electroencephalogram (EEG) and abnormalities in cognitive function. Elevations of parathyroid hormone have also been associated with increased waking EEG slow-wave activity in ESRD patients. Low plasma levels of tyrosine (a precursor of norepinephrine and DA, which are neurotransmitters important in neurologic arousal) have also been reported in uremia and may contribute to abnormalities in neurotransmitter synthesis.

- Treatment with dialysis may predispose patients to sleepiness. Abnormal production of interleukin-1 and tumor necrosis factor-alpha (TNFα)-a, which are substances with somnogenic properties, has been demonstrated in response to dialysis. Rapid changes in serum electrolyte, acid–base balance, and serum osmolarity occur and may decrease arousal and alertness. Removal of sleep-promoting substances during treatment has also been suggested as a possible mechanism of sleep fragmentation as well as daytime fatigue and sleepiness. Treatment may disrupt the circadian pattern of sleepiness via inappropriately timed elevations of serum melatonin in response to hemoconcentration, or from changes in the rhythm of body temperature.

- Other factors, including medications commonly prescribed, such as antihypertensives and antidepressants, may also contribute to EDS.

## IMPACT OF SLEEP PROBLEMS

Sleep abnormalities are associated with reduced quality of life and functional status in ESRD patients. In addition, these problems have been related to several other important clinical outcomes, such as the ability to learn and perform home dialysis, quality of family interactions, anxiety and depression, and days of disability.

- An association between obstructive sleep apnea (OSA) and cardiovascular disease has been established in the general population. Because cardiovascular disease is the leading cause of death in the ESRD population, the detection and appropriate management of OSA may have important effects on survival. The nocturnal hypoxemia associated with OSA might also dampen autonomic reflexes and may be linked to the autonomic dysfunction often noted in these patients.
- Both RLS and PLMD have been associated with increased mortality in ESRD.

## KEY POINTS

1. Sleep complaints and primary sleep disorders are very prevalent in ESRD patients and appear to have important adverse affects on their overall health and well-being.
2. Effective assessment and management of these problems has the potential to significantly enhance patient outcomes.

## BIBLIOGRAPHY

Benz RL, et al. A preliminary study of the effects of correction of anemia with recombinant human erythropoietin therapy on sleep, sleep disorders, and daytime sleepiness in hemodialysis patients (The SLEEPO study). *Am J Kidney Dis* 1999; 34:1089–1095.

Hanly P. Sleep apnea and daytime sleepiness in end-stage renal disease. *Semin Dial* 2004; 17:109–114.

Hanly PJ, et al. Daytime sleepiness in patients with CRF: Impact of nocturnal hemodialysis. *Am J Kidney Dis* 2003; 41:403–410.

Kutner NG, et al. Race and restless sleep complaints in older chronic dialysis patients and nondialysis community controls. *J Gerontol Ser B Psychol Sci Social Sci* 2001; 56:P170–175.

Kutner, NG, et al. Association of sleep difficulty with kidney disease quality of life cognitive function score reported by patients who recently started dialysis. *Clin J Am Soc Nephrol* 2007; 2:284–289.

Mucsi I, et al. Sleep disorders and illness intrusiveness in patients on chronic dialysis. *Nephrol Dial Transplant* 2004; 19:1815–1822.

Parker KP. Sleep disturbances in dialysis patients. *Sleep Med Rev* 2003; 7:131–143.

Parker KP, et al. Daytime sleepiness in stable hemodialysis patients. *Am J Kidney Dis* 2003; 41:394–402.

Unruh ML, et al. Restless legs symptoms among incident dialysis patients: Association with lower quality of life and shorter survival. *Am J Kidney Dis* 2004; 43:900–909.

# 41

## ENDOCRINE AND METABOLIC DISORDERS AND SLEEP

ALEXANDROS N. VGONTZAS AND SLOBODANKA PEJOVIC
Penn State College of Medicine, Department of Psychiatry, Hershey, Pennsylvania

GEORGE P. CHROUSOS
Pediatric and Reproductive Endocrinology Branch, National Institutes of Health, Bethesda, Maryland

## OBESITY

Obesity is a very common metabolic disorder caused by a combination of environmental, constitutional, and genetic factors. It is also frequently associated with sleep disorders, and a large proportion of patients evaluated in sleep disorder clinics are obese.

### Obesity and Obstructive Sleep Apnea

Obesity is highly prevalent in western industrialized countries, and the prevalence of excess weight, overweight, and obesity has increased significantly in the last 2 decades in the United States. About 65% of American adults are overweight [body mass index (BMI) $\geq$ 25], while 30% are obese with a BMI $\geq$ 30 (with 33% women and 27% men affected). Among children aged 6–19 years, 16% are overweight (BMI $\geq$ 95th percentile of the sex- specific BMI-for-age growth chart). There is an association between obesity and obstructive sleep apnea (OSA); the onset of OSA frequently follows a marked increase in body weight. Conversely, the development of OSA seems to result in further weight gain, which, in a vicious cycle, leads to further deterioration of OSA.

- The prevalence of OSA in clinical populations appears to be as high as 40% for morbidly obese men (BMI > 39) and 3% for premenopausal morbidly obese women. Another 5–8% demonstrate features of sleep apnea that warrant further follow-up. The best clinical predictors of OSA in obese populations are the severity of snoring, subjectively reported nocturnal breath cessation, and sleep attacks during the day. Severely or morbidly obese middle-aged men have an extremely high risk for OSA and should be routinely referred for a sleep evaluation to rule out this condition. Physicians assessing severely or morbidly obese women should include a detailed sleep history.

- Among obese patients with OSA, central obesity is the predominant pattern in body fat distribution; it is intra-abdominal (visceral) fat and not generalized obesity that predisposes to the development of OSA. Increased visceral adiposity is associated with several metabolic abnormalities, including insulin resistance, dyslipidemia, DM type II, hypertension, and cardiovascular problems. Visceral adiposity also appears to play a strong role in the pathogenesis of OSA and hypertension.

- Weight reduction in obese patients with OSA is associated with an improvement in sleep-disordered breathing (SDB), although the effects on daytime sleepiness are inconsistent. Most obese people are unable to achieve significant weight loss and, even then, the results are inconsistent. It is possible that the critical factor in determining a successful outcome with weight management is reduction of visceral fat rather than of total weight.

- In the Wisconsin Sleep Cohort Study it was shown that 7 h or more of exercise per week compared with 0 h of exercise per week was associated with a significant reduction of apnea–hypoapnea index independent of BMI, age, gender, and other covariates. Also, a recent study found that among obese sleep apneics, lack of regular exercise (only in men), depression, and degree of apnea are significant predictors of EDS. Exercise improves insulin resistance and visceral adiposity independently of body weight, and this mechanism can positively affect nighttime and daytime symptoms of OSA. Reduction of visceral fat has been also associated with exercise or the use of medications (e.g., insulin sensitizing agent, glucosidase inhibitor).

### Obesity, Sleep Disturbance, and Daytime Sleepiness

Obesity that is not associated with OSA is frequently a cause of sleep disruption and excessive daytime sleepiness (EDS) and fatigue. Obese patients, both men and women, without any SDB demonstrate a significant degree of nocturnal sleep disturbance compared with nonobese controls. Specifically, wake time after sleep onset, number of awakenings, and percentage of stage 1 sleep are significantly higher in obese patients than in controls, while percentage of rapid eye movement (REM) sleep is significantly lower.

- Obesity is associated with a bimodal sleep pattern (i.e., some obese patients report a short sleep duration, whereas others report a long sleep duration). It has been suggested that those that sleep longer are morbidly obese.
- A short sleep duration is associated with increased appetite and a disturbance of satiety hormones (decreased leptin levels and increased ghrelin levels). In children, a short sleep duration is a risk factor for obesity.
- In a large study of general random sample from the Penn State Cohort, it was found that approximately 47% of obese subjects report poor sleep and emotional stress, whereas the remaining 53% sleep well and are not emotionally distressed. In another study of 73 morbidly obese patients, using objective sleep measures, decreased sleep efficiency was associated with significantly higher levels of stress. In both studies chronic emotional stress was determined by the Multiple Minnesota Personality Inventory (MMPI). These data suggest that short sleep duration in obese patients is associated with emotional stress and complaints of poor sleep.
- It appears that obesity is associated with EDS independent of OSA and age. One study noted that obese patients without OSA were sleepier during the day (shorter sleep latencies; decreased wake time after sleep onset, and total wake time; and higher percentage of sleep time) compared with controls. Several recent epidemiologic studies have reported that obesity, independent of sleep apnea, is a strong risk factor for sleepiness and fatigue.
- The Prader–Willi syndrome, a rare genetic disorder characterized by mental retardation, neonatal hypotonia, extreme hyperphagia, and obesity, is frequently associated with SDB, daytime sleepiness, and early onset of REM sleep. EDS and early REM sleep appear to be independent of SDB and obesity.

### Obesity, Sleep Apnea, Sleepiness, and Cytokines

The proinflammatory cytokines, tumor necrosis factor-alpha (TNFα) and interleukin (IL)-6, may play a role in mediating sleepiness in patients with OSA and obesity. In controlled studies, it has been shown that men with OSA have higher plasma concentrations of the inflammatory, fatigue-causing cytokines TNFα and IL-6 than

nonapneic obese men, who had intermediate values; lean men had the lowest values.

- Body mass index correlates positively to plasma levels of TNFα and IL-6.
- When etanercept, a medication that neutralizes TNFα was administered in obese apneic men, there was a significant reduction of sleepiness as measured by Multiple Sleep Latency Test (MSLT) and a slight, but significant reduction, of the apnea/hypopnea index, suggesting that the reduction of sleepiness was not related to improvement of OSA but to the neutralizing effect of TNFα and IL-6.

## DIABETES AND INSULIN RESISTANCE

Knowledge on the association between diabetes mellitus (DM) and sleep disturbances is limited.

### Diabetes, Sleep, and Excessive Sleepiness

Studies have shown that DM is associated with more frequent complaints of difficulty initiating sleep, difficulty maintaining sleep, and EDS compared to controls, and that both short and long sleep duration predict the development of type II DM. DM is a risk factor for EDS independent of OSA, BMI, and age.

- Polysomnography of diabetic patients demonstrates increased duration of wakefulness, high number of awakenings, and fragmented sleep. The exact cause of sleep disruption is not well understood; in one study, it was shown that sleep disruption was mediated by physical complications of the disease, such as pain and nocturia, and not by obesity or emotional adjustment. In children, sleep disruption is not associated with nocturnal hypoglycemia.
- There is an increased prevalence of OSA and SDB in patients with type II DM. One study reported that 70% of obese diabetics have moderate or severe OSA. DM is the second most common medical condition (after hypertension) associated with OSA. It appears that OSA is more prevalent in diabetic patients with, than in those without, autonomic neuropathy.
- Two large prospective studies, the one from Sweden and the other from the United States (Nurses' Health Study Cohort) showed that regular snoring is associated with a two- to seven-fold risk for type II DM over a 10-year period.
- Diabetes mellitus and reduced glucose tolerance are also common in patients with narcolepsy.
- Proinflammatory cytokines are elevated in disorders of EDS, including narcolepsy, and hypercytokinemia is associated with metabolic dysregulation.
- In a sample of patients with type II diabetes sleep duration and quality were significant predictors of HbA1c, a key marker of glycemic control. In a recent study in young healthy adults, all-night selective

suppression of slow-wave sleep (SWS), without any change in total sleep time, resulted in marked decreases in insulin sensitivity without adequate compensatory increase in insulin release, leading to reduced glucose tolerance and increased diabetes risk. Also, SWS suppression reduced delta spectral power, the dominant electroencephalographic (EEG) frequency range in SWS, and left other EEG frequency bands unchanged. The magnitude of the decrease in insulin sensitivity was strongly correlated with the magnitude of the reduction in SWS.

## INSULIN RESISTANCE AND SLEEP APNEA

Insulin resistance is defined as the impaired ability of insulin (either endogenous or exogenous) to lower blood glucose. Insulin resistance is very prevalent in the general population (about 25%) and is strongly associated with central obesity.

- In one well-controlled study, subjects with OSA had significantly higher levels of fasting plasma insulin and glucose levels compared to their obese controls. Also, the OSA group demonstrated a higher degree of visceral, but not subcutaneous, fat compared to their obese controls. It was suggested that visceral obesity/insulin resistance determined by both genetic and constitutional/environmental factors may be the principal culprits of OSA, progressively leading to worsening metabolic syndrome. Another study showed that the age distributions of metabolic syndrome and symptomatic OSA (i.e., EDS and hypertension) are similar.
- The association between OSA and insulin resistance is present even in nonobese subjects. Insulin resistance is present even in mild forms of OSA. In the Sleep Heart Health Study, SDB was found to be independently associated with glucose intolerance and insulin resistance.
- Women with polycystic ovarian syndrome (PCOS), in whom insulin resistance is a primary pathophysiologic abnormality, have a much higher prevalence of OSA and EDS, and insulin resistance is a better predictor of OSA than BMI or testosterone levels.
- In summary, studies support the conclusion that OSA in obese patients is a manifestation of a metabolic abnormality.

## REPRODUCTION

### Male Sex Hormones, Sleep, and Sleep Apnea

Men have more disturbed sleep with greater number of awakenings, and poorer quantity (total sleep time) and quality (SWS and REM sleep) of sleep, compared to women. Men tend to lose SWS faster and have lower power density on sleep EEG in delta and theta frequency.

- The male gender is a risk factor for OSA. Exogenous administration of testosterone in men induced OSA. Also, circulating testosterone levels are associated with upper airway collapsibility in patients with OSA. Men taking testosterone for sexual dysfunction or for "andropause" should be monitored during the course of therapy for the development of OSA. Interestingly, agents lowering androgen levels do not improve SDB or awake ventilatory drive.
- In women, OSA has been induced by exogenous administration of testosterone, and resolves after removal of testosterone-producing tumors.
- Testosterone levels appear to be low in men with OSA and increase following treatment of OSA using continuous positive airway pressure (CPAP) therapy. Despite the fall in plasma total and free testosterone levels, there is no increase in basal plasma gonadotropin [luteinizing hormone (LH) or follicle stimulating hormone (FSH)] levels. The mechanism for the decreased testosterone levels in OSA is not well understood; however, it appears that hypoxia and sleep fragmentation may be the principal contributory factors.
- Middle-aged men with a complaint of sexual dysfunction and low testosterone levels should be assessed thoroughly for the presence of OSA before the institution of hormone replacement therapy.

### Female Sex Hormones, Sleep Apnea, and Insomnia

In contrast to the male sex hormones, female sex hormones appear to be protective of OSA.

- Women experience an increase in ventilatory drive during the luteal phase of the menstrual cycle when progesterone levels are at their highest. Oral progesterone has been associated with slight, but definite, improvement in ventilatory indices during sleep in both male and female patients with OSA.
- From clinical and epidemiologic studies, OSA appears to be rather infrequent before menopause, whereas its prevalence reaches almost the prevalence in men matched for age and BMI postmenopausally. The prevalence of OSA in premenopausal women is about 0.6%, and premenopausal women with OSA are almost exclusively obese. The prevalence of OSA in postmenopausal women without hormone replacement therapy (HRT) is significantly higher than the prevalence in postmenopausal women undergoing HRT, in whom the prevalence of OSA is 0.5%.
- Two recent studies, the Sleep Heart Health Study and the Wisconsin Cohort, confirmed the adverse effects of menopause and the protective role of gonadal hormones in OSA. The Women's Initiative Hormone Trial reported that estrogen plus progestin decreased diabetes and insulin resistance in postmenopausal women, which might be a mechanism by which HRT protects women from OSA.

- Although HRT appears to protect women from the development of OSA and its potential cardiovascular sequelae, studies assessing the effects of female hormones after the development of OSA are inconsistent; it is plausible that female hormones are protective of OSA but are ineffective once apnea has developed.

- Polycystic ovary syndrome is the most common endocrine disorder of premenopausal women and is characterized by chronic hyperandrogenic oligo/anovulation and oligo/amenorrhea. Premenopausal women with PCOS are at a much higher risk for development of OSA and EDS. Also, daytime sleepiness is reported frequently by women with PCOS even after ruling out sleep apnea. In one clinical sample, PCOS patients were 30 times more likely to suffer from SDB than controls, and OSA was present even in nonobese patients. OSA in PCOS women is independent of obesity. The use of oral contraceptives seems to protect PCOS women from the development of SDB, which is consistent with the protective role of HRT in postmenopausal women. Given that PCOS is associated with insulin resistance and central obesity, it is possible that visceral obesity and insulin resistance, determined both by genetic and developmental/environmental factors, are the bases for the pathogenetic mechanisms leading to OSA.

- Insomnia is more prevalent in women compared to men, and depression, a major risk factor for insomnia, is twice as prevalent in women compared to men. The increased prevalence of insomnia in women aged 45–54 years has been attributed to menopause. A recent objective study in a large general population sample found that while sleep latency among premenopausal women and postmenopausal women on HRT did not differ, it was significantly increased among postmenopausal women without HRT. Furthermore, postmenopausal women without HRT were less likely to have slow wave sleep compared to those with HRT. Conclusively, hormonal changes during menopause appear to correlate with increased sleep latency, and decreased slow-wave sleep, which presumably may lead to the increased insomnia complaint in this age group.

## HYPOTHALAMIC–PITUITARY–ADRENAL AXIS

The hypothalamic–pituitary–adrenal (HPA) axis is a major component of the stress system whose function is to preserve homeostasis. Corticotropin-releasing hormone (CRH), which is produced and released from the parvocellular neurons of the paraventricular nucleus in the hypothalamus, is the key regulator of the HPA axis. The release of CRH is followed by the enhanced secretion of adrenocorticotropic hormone (ACTH) from the anterior pituitary and cortisol from the adrenal cortex.

### Hypothalamic–Pituitary–Adrenal Axis and Sleep Disturbance

Administration of both CRH and cortisol lead to arousal and sleeplessness in humans and animals. Conversely, sleep, particularly deep sleep, has an inhibitory effect on the stress system of which the HPA axis is a major component.

- Chronic, persistent insomnia is associated with 24-h hypercortisolemia, which correlated with polysomnographic (PSG) indices of the severity of the disorder. Cortisol is elevated in primary insomnia with objectively documented sleep disturbance during the evening and nighttime. These findings suggest that chronic activation of the HPA axis in patients with insomnia places them at risk not only for mental disorders (e.g., chronic anxiety and depression), but also for significant medical morbidity associated with such activation (i.e., hypertension, visceral obesity with its associated metabolic syndrome, and osteoporosis among others). A large epidemiologic study has recently demonstrated an association between insomnia and hypertension.

- In another study, it was shown that bolus intravenous administration of CRH during the first sleep cycle in middle-aged, healthy men was associated with significant sleep disturbance consisting of increased wakefulness and decreased slow-wave sleep compared to young healthy men; thus, changes in sleep physiology associated with aging may play a significant role in the marked increase in the prevalence of insomnia in middle-age people.

- Exogenously administered corticosteroids and/or their excessive endogenous release have adverse effects on sleep. Sleeplessness is one of the most frequent side effects of the administration of glucocorticoids, and sleep disturbances are frequent in conditions associated with endogenous hypercortisolemia, such as melancholic depression.

### Hypothalamic–Pituitary–Adrenal Axis and Sleep Apnea

The sequence of events in OSA—breathing cessation, nocturnal hypoxia, continuous brief arousals, and sleep fragmentation—could activate both the systemic sympathetic/adrenomedullary and the HPA axis limbs of the stress system. Plasma and urinary catecholamines measured during the nighttime, and surge of sympathetic nerve activity determined by microneurography, are elevated in patients with OSA compared with obese controls.

- However, the limited existing literature has failed to detect any differences in plasma cortisol levels between sleep apneics and controls. A recent study found cortisol levels slightly higher in obese apneic patients, compared with obese controls, and both groups had lower plasma levels of cortisol compared with nonobese controls. In the sleep apneic patients, CPAP lowered significantly diastolic and mean blood pressure and tended to reduce cortisol levels. In another study, CRH administration resulted in a higher corticotrophin response in both obese apneic and nonapneic groups compared with nonobese controls, whereas there were no differences of cortisol response to CRH. These results suggest that in nondistressed obese individuals, HPA axis activity is rather low because of hyposecretion of hypothalamic CRH, whereas apnea causes a mild activation of the axis that is corrected with the use of CPAP.

### Adrenal Function, Fatigue, Sleepiness, and Sleep Apnea

Patients with Cushing syndrome frequently complain of daytime fatigue and sleepiness.

- In one controlled study, Cushing syndrome is associated with an increased frequency of sleep apnea, with 32% of patients having at least mild sleep apnea, and about 18% having significant sleep apnea [i.e., apnea–hypopnea index (AHI) > 17.5 events per hour]. Patients with sleep apnea were not more obese or had different craniofacial features compared to those without sleep apnea.
- Visceral obesity, which is prominent in Cushing syndrome, predisposes the development of OSA. Even in the absence of OSA, Cushing syndrome is associated with increased sleep fragmentation, increased wakefulness and nonrapid eye movement (NREM) stage 1 sleep, and decreased delta sleep.
- Adrenal insufficiency or Addison disease is associated with chronic fatigue. Patients with untreated adrenal insufficiency demonstrate increased sleep fragmentation, increased REM sleep latency, and decreased amount of REM sleep; these sleep abnormalities were reversed following treatment with replacement doses of hydrocortisone.
- In normal individuals, exogenous glucocorticoids have been found to reduce REM sleep. It has been suggested that the inhibitory role of glucocorticoids on REM sleep in normal individuals along with their permissive role in Addison patients demonstrate that some cortisol is needed for REM sleep, whereas excess cortisol inhibits REM sleep.
- Fatigue and EDS are prominent in patients with secondary adrenal insufficiency; elevated TNFα and IL-6 levels may be the mediators of EDS and fatigue associated with primary or secondary adrenal insufficiency.

## GROWTH HORMONE DISORDERS: ACROMEGALY, SLEEP APNEA, AND SLEEPINESS

Acromegaly is a condition of excess growth hormone in adults characterized by the insidious development of coarsening facial features, bony growth, and soft tissue swelling. It is usually secondary to a growth hormone-producing pituitary adenoma.

- Obstructive sleep apnea is frequent in acromegaly, with a prevalence ranging from 40–91%. The etiology of SDB in acromegaly is believed to be associated, at least in part, with macroglossia and craniofacial changes.
- Central sleep apnea has also been observed frequently in patients with acromegaly.
- Hypertension is common in acromegalic patients with OSA. In one study, over 50% of patients with both acromegaly and OSA has hypertension.
- Mild growth hormone deficiency has been described in patients with OSA and appears to be secondary to sleep fragmentation or obesity associated with OSA. Treatment of OSA improves growth hormone and insulin-like growth factor 1 (IGF-1) levels.
- Pituitary surgery is the treatment of choice for acromegalic patients. OSA may persist following treatment of acromegaly by pituitary surgery. Nonsurgical methods, such as administration of octreotide, a somatostatin analog, are potentially useful in reducing growth hormone levels and in improving OSA.
- Excessive daytime sleepiness may also be present in patients with acromegaly independent of the presence of OSA. The mechanisms for EDS are not well understood but may be due to growth hormone excess, cerebral irradiation, or acromegalic myopathy.

## THYROID FUNCTION

### Hypothyroidism, Sleep, and Sleep Apnea

Studies have reported that OSA may have a prevalence as high as 50% in hypothyroid patients. However, these studies did not control well for the male gender and the presence of obesity. More recent studies, which assessed the prevalence of undiagnosed hypothyroidism in patients referred for evaluation of OSA, report a lower prevalence of clinical hypothyroidism (1.2–3.1%). Subclinical hypothyroidism appears to be more frequent (about 11%) in obese patients referred to a sleep clinic for SDB. No studies have reported the prevalence of hypothyroidism in patients with EDS and fatigue.

- Thyroid screening does not appear to be appropriate for patients with suspected or confirmed OSA in the absence of signs or symptoms consistent with hypothyroidism.
- "Euthyroid sick syndrome" is a syndrome associated with mild suppression of thyroid function resulting from chronic illness, which resolves with the appropriate treatment of the primary condition. A mild suppression of thyroid function (e.g., slightly suppressed thyroid stimulating hormone (TSH), and mildly suppressed $T_3$ and $T_4$) in patients with OSA consistent with the euthyroid sick syndrome has been described.

- The results of thyroid hormone replacement on OSA and hypothyroidism are inconsistent. While improvement of OSA after the institution of thyroid hormone replacement has been described, it appears that, at least in the initial phase of treatment, both thyroid hormone replacement and treatment of OSA (e.g., CPAP therapy) should be instituted. Patients should be followed clinically and polysomnographically to assess whether thyroid hormone replacement has abolished OSA as well.
- Rapid restoration of the euthyroid state in hypothyroid patients may be associated with significant cardiovascular morbidity and mortality, particularly in the elderly or those with cardiovascular disease. These risks appear to be increased in the presence of undiagnosed OSA.
- Patients with hypothyroidism experience EDS and fatigue not associated with SDB, and a significant reduction of slow-wave sleep, which is reversible with treatment. Reduced REM sleep and REM density have been reported in children with congenital and acquired hypothyroidism.

### Hyperthyroidism

Hyperthyroid patients complain of insomnia and impairment in mood. Hyperthyroidism is associated with a significant increase of slow-wave sleep, which normalizes after treatment.

### KEY POINTS

1. Obesity is strongly associated with OSA, and frequently causes sleep disruption and EDS independently of OSA.
2. Both sleep disturbances and EDS are common complaints of patients with diabetes mellitus.
3. Insulin resistance appears to be both a cause and a consequence of OSA.
4. Administration of testosterone worsens OSA, whereas female hormones are protective of OSA.
5. Primary insomnia is characterized by a chronic activation of hypothalamic-pituitary-adrenal axis.
6. Sleep problems, including OSA, and fatigue are not uncommon in patients with acromegaly and disorders of the adrenal and thyroid glands.

### BIBLIOGRAPHY

Al-Delaimy WK, et al. Snoring as a risk factor for type II diabetes mellitus: A prospective study. *Am J Epidemiol* 2002; 155:387–393.

Ayas NT, et al. A prospective study of self-reported sleep duration and incident diabetes in women. *Diabetes Care* 2003; 26:380–384.

Bierwolf C, et al. Slow wave sleep drives inhibition of pituitary-adrenal secretion in humans. *Neuroendocrinology* 1997; 9:479–484.

Bixler EO, et al. Effects of age on sleep apnea in men: I. Prevalence and severity. *Am J Respir Crit Care Med* 1998; 157:144–148.

Bixler EO, et al. Association of hypertension and sleep-disordered breathing. *Arch Intern Med* 2000; 160:2289–2295.

Bixler EO, et al. Prevalence of sleep-disordered breathing in women. *Am J Respir Crit Care Med* 2001; 162:1–6.

Bixler EO, et al. Insomnia in central Pennsylvania. *J Psychosom Res* 2002; 53:589–592.

Bixler EO, et al. Normal sleep and sleep stage patterns: Effects of age, BMI and gender. *Sleep* 2003; 26(Suppl):A61–A62.

Bixler EO, et al. Excessive daytime sleepiness in a general population sample: The role of sleep apnea, age, obesity, diabetes, and depression. *J Clin Endocrinol Metab* 2005; 90:4510–4515.

Bixler EO, et al. Women sleep objectively better than men and the sleep of young women is more resilient to external stressors: Effects of age and menopause. *J Sleep Res* 2008 (in press).

Bratel T, et al. Pituitary reactivity, androgens and catecholamines in obstructive sleep apnoea. Effects of continuous positive airway pressure treatment (CPAP). *Respir Med* 1999; 93:1–7.

Buckley TM, et al. On the interactions of the hypothalamic-pituitary-adrenal (HPA) axis and sleep: Normal HPA axis activity and circadian rhythm, exemplary sleep disorders. *J Clin Endocrinol Metab* 2005; 90:3106–3114.

Carrier J, et al. The effects of age and gender on sleep EEG power spectral density in the middle years of life (ages 20–60 years old). *Psychophysiology* 2001; 38:232–242.

Cooper BG, et al. Hormonal and metabolic profiles in subjects with obstructive sleep apnea syndrome and the acute effects of nasal continuous positive airway pressure (CPAP) treatment. *Sleep* 1995; 18:172–179.

Dunaif A. Insulin resistance and the polycystic ovary syndrome: Mechanism and implications for pathogenesis. *Endocr Rev* 1997; 18:774–800.

Ehlers CL, et al. Slow-wave sleep: Do young adult men and women age differently? *J Sleep Res* 1997; 6:211–215.

Elmasry A, et al. The role of habitual snoring and obesity in the development of diabetes: A 10-year follow-up study in a male population. *J Int Med* 2000; 248:13–20.

Entzian P, et al. Obstructive sleep apnea syndrome and circadian rhythms of hormones and cytokines. *Am J Respir Crit Care Med* 1996; 153:1080–1086.

Ficker JH, et al. Obstructive sleep apnoea and diabetes mellitus: The role of cardiovascular autonomic neuropathy. *Eur Respir J* 1998; 11(1):14–19.

Fletcher EC, et al. Urinary catecholamines before and after tracheostomy in patients with obstructive sleep apnea and hypertension. *Sleep* 1987; 10:35–44.

Fogel RB, et al. Increased prevalence of obstructive sleep apnea syndrome in obese women with polycystic ovary syndrome. *J Clin Endocrinol Metab* 2001; 86:1175–1178.

García-Borreguero D, et al. Glucocorticoid replacement is permissive for rapid eye movement sleep and sleep consolidation in patients with adrenal insufficiency. *J Clin Endocrinol Metab* 2000; 85:4201–4206.

Garvey WT, et al. Clinical implications of the insulin resistance syndrome. *Clin Cornerstone* 1998; 1(3):13–28.

Gopal M, et al. The role of obesity in the increased prevalence of obstructive sleep apnea syndrome in patients with polycystic ovarian syndrome. *Sleep Med* 2004; 3:401–404.

Grunstein RR, et al. Acute withdrawal of nasal CPAP in obstructive sleep apnea does not cause a rise in stress hormones. *Sleep* 1996; 19:774–782.

Grunstein RR, et al. Neuroendocrine dysfunction in sleep apnea: reversal by continuous positive airway pressure therapy. *J Clin Endocrinol Metab* 1989; 68:352–358.

Gupta NK, et al. Is obesity associated with poor sleep quality in adolescents? *Am J Hum Biol* 2002; 14:762–768.

Hasler G, et al. The association between short sleep duration and obesity in young adults: A 13-year prospective study. *Sleep* 2004; 27:661–666.

Hayashi M, et al. Sleep development in children with congenital and acquired hypothyroidism. *Brain Dev* 1997; 19:43–49.

Hedley AA, et al. Prevalence of overweight and obesity among US children, adolescents, and adults, 1999–2002. *JAMA* 2004; 291:2847–2850.

Hochban W, et al. Obstructive sleep apnea in acromegaly: The role of craniofacial changes. *Eur Respir J* 1999; 14:196–202.

Huang YR, et al. Study on quality of sleep and mental health in patients with hyperthyroidism. *Chung Hua Hu Li Tsa Chih* 1997; 32:435–439.

Hume KI, et al. A field study of age and gender differences in habitual adult sleep. *J Sleep Res* 1998; 7:85–94.

Ip Mary SM, et al. Obstructive sleep apnea syndrome: An experience in Chinese adults in Hong Kong. *Chin Med J (Engl)* 1998; 111(3):257–260.

Ip MS, et al. Obstructive sleep apnea is independently associated with insulin resistance. *Am J Respir Crit Care Med* 2002; 165:670–676.

Kapur VK, et al. Association of hypothyroidism and obstructive sleep apnea. *Am J Respir Crit Care Med* 1998; 158:1379–1383.

Knutson KL, et al. Role of sleep duration and quality in the risk and severity of type 2 diabetes mellitus. *Arch Intern Med* 2006; 166:1768–1774.

Lamond N, et al. Factors predicting sleep disruption in Type II diabetes. *Sleep* 2000; 23:415–416.

Latta F, et al. Sex differences in delta and alpha EEG activities in healthy older adults. *Sleep* 2005; 28:1525–1534.

Liu PY, et al. The short-term effects of high-dose testosterone on sleep, breathing, and function in older man. *J Clin Endocrinol Metab* 2003; 88:3605–3613.

Margolis KL, et al. Effect of oestrogen plus progestin on the incidence of diabetes in postmenopausal women: Results from the Women's Health Initiative Hormone Trial. *Diabetologia* 2004; 47:1175–1187.

Matyka KA, et al. Alterations in sleep physiology in young children with insulin-dependent diabetes mellitus: Relationship to nocturnal hypoglycemia. *J Pediatr* 2000; 137(20):233–238.

Meston N, et al. Endocrine effects of nasal continuous positive airway pressure in male patients with obstructive sleep apnoea. *J Intern Med* 2003; 254:447–454.

Moe KE, et al. Estrogen replacement therapy moderates the sleep disruption associated with nocturnal blood sampling. *Sleep* 2001; 24:886–894.

Papanicolaou DA, et al. The pathophysiologic roles of interleukin-6 in human disease. *Ann Intern Med* 1998; 128:127–137.

Park YW, et al. The metabolic syndrome: Prevalence and associated risk factor findings in the US population from the Third National Health and Nutrition Examination Survey, 1988–1994. *Arch Intern Med* 2003; 163:427–436.

Pasquali R, et al. Effect of long-term treatment with metformin added to hypocaloric diet on body composition, fat distribution, and androgen and insulin levels in abdominally obese women with and without the polycystic ovary syndrome. *J Clin Endocrinol Metab* 2000; 85:2767–2774.

Peppard PE, et al. Exercise and sleep-disordered breathing: An association independent of body habitus. *Sleep* 2004; 27:480–484.

Punjabi NM, et al. Sleep-disordered breathing and insulin resistance in middle-aged and overweight men. *Am J Respir Crit Care Med* 2002; 165:677–682.

Punjabi NM, et al. Sleep-disordered breathing, glucose intolerance, and insulin resistance: The Sleep Heart Health Study. *Am J Epidemiol* 2004; 160:521–530.

Rasheid S, et al. Gastric bypass is an effective treatment for obstructive sleep apnea in patients with clinically significant obesity. *Obes Surg* 2003; 13:58–61.

Reaven GM. Insulin resistance and human disease: A short story. *J Basic Clin Physiol Pharmacol* 1998; 9:387–406.

Redline S, et al. Sleep stage distributions in the sleep heart health study (SHHS) cohort. *Sleep* 1998; 21(Suppl):210.

Resta O, et al. Sleep-related breathing disorders, loud snoring and excessive daytime sleepiness in obese subjects. *Int J Obes Relat Metab Disord* 2001; 25:669–675.

Resta O, et al. Low sleep quality and daytime sleepiness in obese patients without obstructive sleep apnoea syndrome. *J Intern Med* 2003; 253:536–543.

Resta O, et al. High prevalence of previously unknown subclinical hypothyroidism in obese patients referred to a sleep clinic for sleep disordered breathing. *Nutr Metab Cardiovasc Dis* 2004; 14:248–253.

Rodenbeck A, et al. Interactions between evening and nocturnal cortisol secretion and sleep parameters in patients with severe chronic primary insomnia. *Neurosci Lett* 2002; 324:159–163.

Rodenbeck A, et al. The sleep-improving effects of doxepin are paralleled by a normalized plasma cortisol secretion in primary insomnia. A placebo-controlled, double-blind, randomized, cross-over study followed by an open treatment over 3 weeks. *Psychopharmacology* 2003; 170:423–428.

Sekine M, et al. A dose-response relationship between short sleeping hours and childhood obesity: Results of the Toyama Birth Cohort Study. *Child Care Health Dev* 2002; 28:163–170.

Shahar E, et al. Hormone replacement therapy and sleep-disordered breathing. *Am J Respir Crit Care Med* 2002; 167:1186–1192.

Shinohara E, et al. Visceral fat accumulation as an important risk factor for obstructive sleep apnea syndrome in obese subjects. *J Intern Med* 1997; 241:11–18.

Spath-Schwalbe E, et al. Sleep disruption alters nocturnal ACTH and cortisol secretory patterns. *Biol Psychiatry* 1991; 29:575–584.

Spiegel K, et al. Impact of sleep debt on metabolic and endocrine function. *Lancet* 1999; 354:1435–1439.

Spiegel K, et al. Brief communication: Sleep curtailment in healthy young men is associated with decreased leptin levels, elevated ghrelin levels, and increased hunger and appetite. *Ann Intern Med* 2004; 141:846–856.

Taheri S, et al. Short sleep duration is associated with reduced leptin, elevated ghrelin, and increased body mass index. *PLoS Med* 2004; 1:e62.

Tasali E, et al. Relationships between sleep disordered breathing and glucose metabolism in polycystic ovary syndrome. *J Clin Endocrine Metab* 2006; 91:36–42.

Tasali E, et al. Slow-wave sleep and the risk of type 2 diabetes in humans. *Proc Natl Acad Sci USA* 2008; 105:1044–1049.

Valencia-Flores M, et al. Effect of bariatric surgery on obstructive sleep apnea and hypopnea syndrome, electrocardiogram, and pulmonary arterial pressure. *Obes Surg* 2004; 14:755–762.

Vgontzas AN, et al. Elevation of plasma cytokines in disorders of excessive daytime sleepiness: Role of sleep disturbance and obesity. *J Clin Endocrinol Metab* 1997; 82:1313–1316.

Vgontzas AN, et al. Obesity without sleep apnea is associated with daytime sleepiness. *Arch Intern Med* 1998; 158:1333–1337.

Vgontzas AN, et al. Sleep and its disorders. *Annu Rev Med* 1999a; 50:387–400.

Vgontzas AN, et al. Sleep deprivation effects on the activity of the hypothalamic-pituitary-adrenal and growth axes: Potential clinical implications. *Clin Endocrinol (Oxf)* 1999b; 51:205–215.

Vgontzas AN, et al. Sleep apnea and daytime sleepiness and fatigue: Relation to visceral obesity, insulin resistance, and hypercytokinemia. *J Clin Endocrinol Metab* 2000; 85:1151–1158.

Vgontzas AN, et al. Middle-aged men show higher sensitivity of their sleep to the arousing effects of corticotropin-releasing hormone than young men: Clinical implications. *J Clin Endocrinol Metab* 2001a; 86:1489–1495.

Vgontzas AN, et al. Polycystic ovary syndrome is associated with obstructive sleep apnea and daytime sleepiness: Role of insulin resistance. *J Clin Endocrinol Metab* 2001b; 86:517–520.

Vgontzas AN, et al. Chronic insomnia is associated with nyctohemeral activation of the hypothalamic-pituitary-adrenal axis: Clinical implications. *J Clin Endocrinol Metab* 2001c; 86:3787–3794.

Vgontzas AN, et al. Adverse effects of modest sleep restriction on sleepiness, performance, and inflammatory cytokines. *J Clin Endocrinol Metab* 2004a; 89:2119–2126.

Vgontzas AN, et al. Marked decrease in sleepiness in patients with sleep apnea by etanercept, a tumor necrosis factor-alpha antagonist. *J Clin Endocrinol Metab* 2004b; 89:4409–4413.

Vgontzas AN, et al. 24-hour sleep patterns may be a useful marker in phenotypic subtyping of obesity. *Sleep* 2006; 29:A314.

Vgontzas AN, et al. Hypothalamic-pituitary-adrenal axis activity in obese men with and without sleep apnea: Effects of continuous positive airway pressure therapy. *J Clin Endocrinol Metab* 2007; 92:4199–4207.

Vgontzas AN, et al. Short sleep duration and obesity: The role of emotional stress and sleep disturbances. *Int J Obes (Lond)* 2008; 32: 801–809.

von Kries R, et al. Reduced risk for overweight and obesity in 5- and 6-y-old children by duration of sleep—A cross-sectional study. *Int J Obes Relat Metab Disord* 2002; 26:710–716.

Vorona RD, et al. Overweight and obese patients in a primary care population report less sleep than patients with a normal body mass index. *Arch Intern Med* 2005; 165:25–30.

Waradckar NV, et al. Influence of treatment on muscle sympathetic nerve activity in sleep apnea. *Am J Respir Crit Care Med* 1996; 153:1333–1338.

Young T, et al. Menopausal status and sleep-disordered breathing in the Wisconsin Sleep Cohort Study. *Am J Respir Crit Care Med* 2003a; 167:1181–1185.

Young T, et al. Objective and subjective sleep quality in premenopausal, perimenopausal, and postmenopausal women in the Wisconsin Sleep Cohort Study. *Sleep* 2003b; 26:667–672.

# 42

## IMMUNITY AND SLEEP

James M. Krueger and Jeannine A. Majde
Washington State University, Pullman, Washington

### INTRODUCTION

Dynamic changes in sleep occur over the course of an infectious disease. These changes in sleep are part of the microbe-induced acute-phase response and are mediated by cytokines. Cytokines are a large group of proteins made in substantial amounts by activated immune cells; they are also found in the brain and are involved in physiologic and pathologic sleep regulation.

- Sleep loss affects parameters of host defenses even in the absence of infectious challenge. For instance, sleep loss reduces immunization-induced antibody titers as well as many other immune parameters, such as natural killer-cell activity.

- Whether sleep or sleep loss affects microbial-associated morbidity or mortality remains unanswered. Sleepiness is frequently experienced during acute infections and other inflammatory diseases. Fatigue, sleepiness, and social withdrawal associated with the onset of an illness are considered part of the acute-phase response to an infectious challenge, along with fever.

### ENCEPHALITIS LETHARGICA AND SLEEP

In 1930 von Economo described how encephalitic lesions of the hypothalamus result in permanent changes in sleep of the affected individual. The patient slept less if the lesion was in the anterior hypothalamus, whereas the patient slept more if the lesion was in the posterior hypothalamus. This work resulted in the concept that sleep was actively regulated. Von Economo's encephalitis lethargica, first reported in 1916 and still seen clinically, is currently thought to be an autoimmune disease induced by streptococcal infections rather than a viral infection, as previously thought.

### MICROBIAL CHALLENGE: WHAT DOES IT DO TO SLEEP?

The first systematic study of sleep over the course of an infectious disease dealt with Gram-positive bacterial septicemia in rabbits. Within a few hours of the intravenous injection of live *Staphylococcus aureus*, the animals begin to exhibit more nonrapid eye movement (NREM) sleep and less rapid eye movement (REM) sleep, a sleep profile that is characteristic of acute infections. After a period of about 20 h, the rabbits enter into a period of prolonged reduction of NREM and REM sleep. During this biphasic sleep response, other facets of the acute-phase response become evident, including fever, fibrinogenemia, and neutrophilia.

- In subsequent studies using other bacteria and other routes of administration, this biphasic sleep response of initial NREM sleep enhancement followed by sleep disruption was also evident. However, the specific time course of sleep responses is dependent on the ability of the infectious agent to invade the host, dose of inoculum, time of day, and route of administration. For instance, after intravenous administration of the nonpathogenic Gram-negative bacterium, *Escherichia coli*, there is a very rapid increase in NREM sleep, but this enhancement only lasts for 4–6 h. In contrast, intranasal injection of another Gram-negative bacterium that is pathogenic for rabbits, *Pasteurella multocida*, induced more prolonged changes in sleep.

- The mechanisms by which bacteria induce changes in sleep involve macrophage processing of bacteria. Macrophages ingest and digest bacteria and, in the process, release chemically distinct molecules derived from the bacterial cell walls such as muramyl peptides from peptidoglycan and lipopolysaccharide. These molecules can initiate sleep profiles characteristic of

*Sleep Medicine Essentials*, edited by Teofilo L. Lee-Chiong
Copyright © 2009 John Wiley & Sons, Inc.

infections in the absence of living bacteria, although the duration of their action is shorter.

- Microbial components are detected by a family of pathogen recognition receptors [primarily Toll-like receptors (TLR) and NOD-like receptors (NLR)] that initiate the production of the intercellular signaling molecules called cytokines. Cytokines are produced by virtually all cells, particularly immunocytes, such as macrophages, and central nervous system cells, such as neurons and glia. Over a hundred cytokines have been described, both proinflammatory (binding class I receptors) and anti-inflammatory (binding class II receptors), and operate in extremely complex networks to initiate inflammation and acquired immunity. Some class I cytokine receptors share homologies with receptors for classical endocrine hormones such as prolactin and growth hormone.

- Cytokines within the brain are involved in sleep regulation, while cytokines within the peripheral immune system can induce cytokines in the brain through action at circumventricular organs, vagal afferents, and endothelial transporters, thus causing an acute-phase response to extraneural inflammatory events, such as infections.

- Viral infections also induce cytokines and affect sleep. Some viruses may cause brain lesions and give rise to changes in sleep during infections, resulting from either direct damage to the brain or virus-induced cytokine responses.

- Enhanced NREM sleep during the early stages of human immunodeficiency (HIV) infections, before acquired immune deficiency syndrome (AIDS) onset, has been described. Sleep is disrupted after AIDS onset. Rabies, another central nervous system (CNS) viral disease, is also associated with disrupted sleep.

- Viruses are implicated in a wide range of other disorders that involve sleep disruption, such as sudden infant death syndrome, chronic fatigue syndrome, and infectious mononucleosis. However, direct involvement of the viruses in sleep disruption in these various disorders has yet to be demonstrated.

- In viral diseases that involve CNS damage, it is difficult to distinguish whether the effects of the virus on sleep result from virus-induced lesions or other mechanisms. In humans, low doses of influenza that localize to the upper respiratory system induce excess behavioral sleep without other facets of the acute-phase response, such as fever.

- In animal studies, large doses of live influenza virus (but not killed virus) given intravenously to rabbits induce a short-term fever and sleep response similar to that induced by E. coli. Influenza virus does not completely replicate in rabbits, accounting for its short-term effects. However, there are indications that partial viral replication occurs, with the production of the replication intermediate double-stranded dsRNA (ribonucleic acid). dsRNA is probably a primary inducer of the viral acute-phase response through its induction of cytokines.

- Influenza virus replicates completely in the mouse and can cause lethal pneumonitis. This disease is associated with excess NREM sleep and reduced REM sleep that become more marked as the disease progresses. The mice also become severely hypothermic and lose up to 20% of their body weight. Infected mice deficient in the gene for the growth hormone releasing hormone receptor have suppressed NREM sleep compared to controls. On the other hand, mice deficient in the gene for neuronal nitric oxide synthetase show more suppression of REM in response to influenza, while mice deficient in the gene for inducible nitric oxide synthetase show increased REM sleep and reduced NREM sleep compared to controls. Mice deficient in the receptor for type I interferon (IFN), a cytokine known for its antiviral activity, show a marked suppression of spontaneous REM sleep; these mice also show altered expression of certain neuropeptides in their hypothalamus that may mediate the suppression of REM sleep. When infected with low-dose influenza or challenged with dsRNA, these mice show earlier and more intense NREM sleep. REM sleep did not change in response to dsRNA challenge, but was suppressed below baseline in IFN receptor-deficient mice infected with influenza. It, thus, appears that a product of growth hormone releasing hormone (possibly not growth hormone itself), nitric oxide made by inducible nitric oxide synthetase, and type I IFNs are involved in NREM sleep regulation during infection, while nitric oxide made by neuronal nitric oxide synthetase appears to be involved in influenza-induced REM suppression. Type I IFNs are important in spontaneous REM sleep regulation as well as influenza-induced REM sleep regulation.

## SLEEP LOSS AND EFFECTS ON THE IMMUNE SYSTEM

A few studies have examined the consequences of sleep deprivation on the immune response to vaccinations in healthy individuals. Sleep deprivation for only one night substantially impairs the antibody response to hepatitis A vaccine. Chronic but less profound sleep deprivation substantially slows the response to influenza vaccine, although the subjects eventually achieve antibody levels similar to controls.

- Studies of the immune effects of acute sleep deprivation in animals have given inconsistent results. More profound chronic sleep loss in rats (total deprivation for 2–3 weeks) results in sepsis and death of the animals, probably as a consequence of bacterial translocation from the intestine; controls that obtain about 80% of normal sleep survive. These findings suggest an impairment of the innate immune system that normally prevents the escape of normal intestinal flora into the draining lymph nodes.

- While such chronic studies cannot be performed ethically in human subjects, studies in military trainees subjected to prolonged sleep deprivation (in addition to the other stresses of training) experience profound endocrine and immune changes and, in general, more frequent and severe infections. Shift workers, who experience poor sleep quality, also experience more infections. How much of this effect is sleep related vs. stress related cannot be determined.

- Examination of specific immune parameters following sleep deprivation indicate that antigen uptake, lymphocyte mitogenesis, phagocytosis, circulating immune complexes, circulating immunoglobulin, secondary antibody responses, natural killer cells, and T lymphocyte populations are altered. Studies of cytokine production in cultured lymphocytes from sleep-deprived subjects show increased IFN, tumor necrosis factor (TNF), and interleukin (IL) 1β production. Circulating cytokines display circadian variation and associations with different sleep stages; IL1 levels peak at the onset of NREM sleep, and TNF levels vary with electroencephalographic (EEG) slow waves. In sleep-deprived subjects, a trend toward increased circulating IL1 is seen. In sleep apnea, which is associated with sleep deprivation as well as hypoxia, increased TNF levels are seen.

## SLEEP AND IMMUNE RESPONSE MODIFIERS

Research concerning the biochemical regulation of sleep had its origins in the early 1900s when it was observed that the transfer of cerebrospinal fluid from sleep-deprived animals to controls enhances sleep in the recipients. Since that time several sleep regulatory substances (SRSs) have been identified.

- In order for a substance to be classified as an (Table 42.1) SRS, the molecule should meet the following criteria: The candidate SRS should enhance sleep; its inhibition should inhibit spontaneous sleep; its levels should vary in the brain with sleep propensity; it should act on sleep regulatory circuits to affect sleep; and its levels should vary with pathologies that affect sleep. The molecules that have thus far met these criteria include two cytokines, IL1 and TNF, which are also immune response mediators.

- Administration of either TNF or IL1, whether they are given centrally or systemically, alters NREM sleep. NREM sleep is enhanced at low doses. Slightly higher doses result in more NREM sleep, accompanied by a reduction of REM sleep. Even higher doses inhibit both NREM and REM sleep. These effects are also dependent on the time of day, in that some doses inhibit sleep at one time of the

day, while they enhance sleep at another time of the day. Somnogenic doses of either TNF or IL1 also enhance the amplitudes of EEG slow waves during NREM sleep. Enhanced EEG slow-wave activity is thought to be indicative of deeper sleep since it is also observed after sleep loss when the stimulus threshold needed to awake an individual is higher. Other aspects of physiologic sleep persist in TNF- or IL1-treated animals, that is, sleep remains episodic and easily reversible.

- Inhibition of either IL1 or TNF using antibodies, soluble receptors, or inhibitory cytokines (such as the endogenous IL1 receptor antagonist) diminishes spontaneous sleep. These inhibitors also inhibit the sleep rebound that follows sleep deprivation.

- Brain levels of TNF and IL1 vary with the time of day. In rats, TNF mRNA (messenger RNA) and TNF protein levels are higher in the cortex and hypothalamus during the daytime when sleep propensity is highest. In contrast, if animals are sleep deprived, levels of these cytokines in brain increase as does sleep propensity.

- Circulating levels of TNF vary with pathologies such as obstructive sleep apnea, preeclampsia, systemic infections, and insomnia, all of which are associated with changes in sleepiness. Further, infectious challenge is also associated with an upregulation of cytokines and sleepiness. Finally, bacterial cell wall products, such as muramyl peptides and viral dsRNA, also enhance cytokine production (e.g., IL1 and TNF). Collectively, these data strongly implicate these cytokines in physiologic sleep as well as in the sleep responses associated with pathology.

- Both TNF and IL1 act on sleep regulatory circuits to affect sleep. Microinjection of TNF, for example, into the preoptic area of the anterior hypothalamus enhances NREM sleep. In contrast, the injection of the TNF-soluble receptor into this area reduces spontaneous sleep. In this same area, IL1 inhibits wake-active neurons while it enhances sleep-active neurons. Such data suggest that these cytokines are acting on sleep regulatory circuits to induce sleep. However, other evidence suggests they may act elsewhere as well to enhance sleep. Microinjection of either TNF or IL1 directly onto the cortex unilaterally enhances EEG slow-wave power during NREM sleep on the side injected but not on the opposite side of the brain. Further, similar localized injections of either the TNF-soluble receptor or the IL1-soluble receptor inhibit sleep deprivation-induced increases in EEG slow-wave power during

**Table 42.1  Sleep Regulatory Substances**

| NREM Sleep | REM Sleep | Wakefulness |
|---|---|---|
| Growth hormone releasing hormone | Vasoactive intestinal polypeptide | Corticotrophin releasing hormone |
| TNFα (tumor necrosis factor α) | Prolactin | Hypocretin |
| IL1β (interleukin-1β) | Nitric oxide | Noradrenalin |
| Adenosine | Acetylcholine | Serotonin |
| Prostaglandin $D_2$ | | Acetylcholine |

NREM sleep on the side receiving the soluble receptor but not on the other side of the brain. Such state-dependent changes in EEG power suggest that these cytokines can act locally within the cortex to promote functional state changes in small regions of the brain. These changes may also provide a mechanism by which sleep is targeted to specific areas of brain depending upon their prior wakefulness activity.

- Many other cytokines have the capacity to either enhance (e.g., fibroblast growth factor, nerve growth factor, IL2, IL6, IL8, IL15, and IL18) or inhibit (e.g., IL4, IL10, IL13, and insulinlike growth factor) sleep. However, although these molecules may indeed be part of a physiologic network of molecules involved in sleep regulation, insufficient information is available to classify them as SRSs. SRSs are also part of the regulatory mechanism by which the brain keeps track of past sleep–wake activity for prolonged periods of time, and thereby provide a mechanism for sleep homeostasis.

## DOES SLEEP HELP IN COMBATING INFECTIOUS DISEASE?

This question is difficult to address experimentally because it is impossible to isolate sleep per se as an independent variable. If one deprives an animal or person of sleep, many physiologic systems change, including body temperature, food intake, certain hormones, and many immune response parameters. Thus, any change in the host's response to infectious challenge occurring during sleep loss may be secondary to these other changes. Nevertheless, the limited evidence to date suggests that there is an association between sleep and morbidity and mortality. For instance, animals that sleep more during the first few hours after an infectious challenge have a higher probability of survival than those that do not.

## KEY POINTS

1. Changes in sleep are part of the microbe-induced acute-phase response and are mediated by cytokines.

2. Sleep loss affects parameters of host defenses even in the absence of infectious challenges.

3. Whether sleep or sleep loss affects microbial-associated morbidity or mortality remains unanswered.

## ACKNOWLEDGMENTS

This work was supported in part by the National Institutes of Health, Grant numbers NS25378, NS27250, NS31453, and HD36520.

## BIBLIOGRAPHY

Akira S, et al. Recognition of pathogen-associated molecular patterns by TLR family. *Immunol Lett* 2003; 85:85–95.

Alt JA, et al. Alterations in EEG activity and sleep after influenza viral infection in GHRH receptor-deficient mice. *J Appl Physiol* 2003; 95:460–468.

Chen L, et al. Influenza virus-induced sleep responses in mice with targeted disruptions in neuronal or inducible nitric oxide synthases. *J Appl Physiol* 2004; 97:17–28.

Dale RC, et al. Encephalitis lethargica syndrome: 20 new cases and evidence of basal ganglia autoimmunity. *Brain* 2003; 127:21–33.

Gadina M, et al. Signaling by type I and II cytokine receptors: Ten years after. *Curr Opin Immunol* 2001; 13:363–373.

Krueger JM, et al. Sleep function. *Front Biosci* 2003; 8:520–550.

Lange T, et al. Sleep enhances the human antibody response to hepatitis A vaccination. *Psychosom Med* 2003; 65:831–835.

Larson SJ, et al. Behavioral effects of cytokines. *Brain Behav Immun* 2001; 15:371–387.

Majde JA. Viral double-stranded RNA, cytokines and the flu. *J Interferon Cytok Res* 2000; 20:259–272.

Obal Jr F, et al. Biochemical regulation of sleep. *Front Biosci* 2003; 8:511–519.

Spiegel K, et al. Effect of sleep deprivation on responses to immunization. *JAMA* 2002; 288:1471–1472.

Traynor TR, et al. Intratracheal double-stranded RNA plus interferon-gamma: A model for analysis of the acute phase response to respiratory viral infections. *Life Sci* 2004; 74:2563–2576.

Von Economo C. Sleep as a problem of localization. *J Nerv Ment Dis* 1930; 71:249–259.

Yoshida H, et al. Asymmetries in slow wave sleep EEG induced by local application of TNFα. *Brain Res* 2004; 1009:129–136.

# 43

## DEMENTIA

Michael V. Vitiello
Department of Psychiatry and Behavioral Sciences, University of Washington, Seattle Washington

## INTRODUCTION

Alzheimer disease (AD) is a progressive neurodegenerative disorder that accounts for approximately two thirds of all dementias worldwide. It is estimated that between 2 and 4 million older adults have AD in the United States; this number is likely to quadruple over the next 50 years. Both normal aging and AD are associated with disturbances in the daily sleep–wake cycle, although the disturbances in AD are typically much more severe. Within the AD population itself, significant sleep disturbances are quite common, affecting as much as half of community- and clinic-based samples.

- The same neurodegenerative mechanisms that produce the evolving cognitive deficits seen in AD are potential causes of the sleep disruption seen in this population. Nevertheless, sleep can be disrupted for many other reasons as well. The likely major causes of sleep disruption in aging and dementia include: (1) physiologic changes that arise as part of normal, "nonpathological" aging; (2) sleep problems due to comorbid physical or mental health conditions and their treatments; (3) primary sleep disorders; (4) poor "sleep hygiene" or sleep-related habits, which can include patterns of daytime napping that becomes maladaptive; or (5) some combination of these factors.
- For AD patients, sleep disturbance is an additional burden to the compromised function and quality of life directly attributable to dementia. For AD caregivers, disturbances in the patients' sleep and nighttime behavior, particularly reduced nighttime sleep time, increased nighttime wakefulness, and wandering that commonly require considerable caregiver attention, with subsequent chronic sleep loss for the caregivers themselves, are a significant source of physical and psychological burden and are often cited as one of the principal reasons for a family's decision to institutionalize a demented person.

## BIOLOGIC BASES OF SLEEP DISTURBANCES

Sleep disturbances that accompany early-stage or mild dementia may appear as exacerbations of the sleep changes found with "normal" aging, rather than unique disease-related phenomena. There is often an increased frequency and duration of awakenings, decreased slow-wave sleep and rapid eye movement (REM) sleep, and more daytime napping. Damage to neuronal pathways that initiate and maintain sleep is the most likely cause of the acceleration of these age-related sleep changes. These compromised neural structures include the suprachiasmatic nucleus (SCN) of the hypothalamus and the neuronal pathways originating in subcortical regions that also regulate arousal and sleep–wake cycles, including the cholinergic basal forebrain nuclei, serotonergic raphe nuclei, dopaminergic nigrostriatal and pallidostriatal pathways, noradrenergic locus ceruleus, and the cortical regions that generate electroencephalogram (EEG) slow-wave activity during sleep. At least some of the sleep disruption seen in AD may be an inherent trait, likely linked to apolipoprotein E (APOE) status, such that AD patients positive for the APOE epsilon 4 allele show greater sleep disruption over time.

- Sleep disturbance grows more severe with increasing severity of AD. It is typically during the moderate or intermediate stages of the disease when other behavioral disturbances most commonly occur. Breakdown of the basic circadian sleep–wake rhythm of dementia patients can be severe, and in extreme cases may lead to an extremely fragmented sleep–wake pattern or nearly complete day–night sleep pattern reversals. In end-stage AD, patients may appear to sleep throughout most of the day and night, awakening only for brief periods. However, both the course and the individual differences of these sleep disturbances remain uncertain.

- Current treatment for the cognitive deficits of AD includes acetylcholinesterase inhibitors and *N*-methyl-D-aspartate (NMDA) receptor antagonists, both of which target deficiencies in the cholinergic neurotransmitter system and offer limited symptomatic relief. However, recent evidence suggests these drugs may further disrupt the sleep of some AD patients.

## INTERACTION BETWEEN BIOLOGIC CHANGES AND ENVIRONMENTAL FACTORS

Environmental factors that promote circadian dysregulation in dementia patients living in institutionalized settings include light, noise, activity schedules, and the needs of the staff.

- Ambient light levels are typically too low in many congregate care facilities to support natural-light-dependent internal rhythms, and noisy conditions, especially during the night, are both common and inimical to sleep.
- The staffing schedules and timing of specific activities in many facilities caring for demented persons may be driven less by the needs of the patients than by compliance with federal and state requirements governing nursing home operations. Regulatory requirements, in general, fail to incorporate many of the positive evidence-based practices found to be beneficial for demented residents, focusing more attention on feeding and bathing schedules, injury prevention, and detection of medical problems than on sleep and other issues related to quality of life.

## OTHER CAUSES OF SLEEP DISTURBANCE

Little is known about the risk factors, causes, incidence, and persistence of sleep disturbances in AD patients.

### Physical Illness

Many elderly persons, whether demented or cognitively intact, have medical conditions that disrupt sleep. Medical conditions especially likely to disrupt sleep are congestive heart failure, chronic obstructive pulmonary disease, Parkinson's disease, gastroesophageal reflux disease, arthritis, and nocturia. Medically ill older adults admitted to acute-care hospitals are particularly vulnerable to sleep disruption, which appear to be created as much by the various treatments and procedures, unfamiliar routines, and environmental conditions, as by the pain, anxiety, and discomfort associated with their underlying medical condition.

- Many prescription medications, over-the-counter agents, and social drugs (e.g., caffeine, nicotine, and alcohol) can disrupt sleep. In AD, such potential drug effects should always be considered when sleep

is disturbed, as are the multiple pharmacokinetic or pharmacodynamic interactions of medications that can affect brain function and sleep rhythms. Other possible pharmacologic causes of sleep disturbance include high-potency diuretics, or central nervous system (CNS) stimulants (e.g., caffeine, amphetamines, methylphenidate, and modafinil) used too late in the day.

### Concurrent or Complicating Neuropsychiatric Disorders

Sleep in the elderly may also be affected by psychiatric morbidity. Psychiatric disorders, particularly major depression, are not only associated with disturbed sleep but can also greatly impact both self-report and objective ratings of sleep quantity and quality.

- Depressive symptoms are common in older adults, especially among persons who are medically ill, bereaved, or cognitively impaired, but are by no means always associated with disrupted sleep. In AD patients seen in clinical psychiatric settings, rates of major depression as high as 86% have been reported (the majority of studies report rates of 17–29%).
- Depression should always be evaluated as a possible contributor to the sleep disturbance encountered in demented individuals. Pharmacologic treatment of mood or behavioral disorders associated with sleep disturbance in AD frequently improves sleep patterns. In psychotic or severely agitated or aggressive patients, antipsychotics are frequently the drugs of choice; atypical antipsychotic agents with low potential for causing extrapyramidal signs and symptoms are preferred.

### Primary Sleep Disorders

Sleep quality may be impaired by primary sleep disorders, some of which may be seen with increasing prevalence with age, such as sleep-disordered breathing (sleep apnea), restless legs syndrome, and REM sleep behavior disorder (RBD). These conditions may interact with the dementia syndrome to further worsen sleep quality as well as cognitive and functional abilities. It might be expected that the incidence of the primary sleep disorders would increase in demented patients relative to age-matched controls because of the CNS dysfunction underlying these disorders; however, studies comparing the rates of sleep apnea in dementia patients and aged controls have not found consistent differences.

- It has been estimated that 24–62% of community-dwelling older adults have sleep-related breathing disturbances, although the true clinical implications of these observations are unclear. Obstructive sleep apnea (OSA) should be considered in the differential diagnosis when older adults report poor sleep and when cognitive impairment is first discovered. Some studies have shown that sleep apnea is associated with increased morning confusion in AD patients. For most cases of clinically significant OSA, continuous positive airway pressure (CPAP) remains the treatment of choice. However, adherence to CPAP can be problematic, particularly in demented patients who may be unable to understand the value of treatment, or to learn to use or tolerate it, and confusion may lead to removal of the device during the night.

- Seen most frequently in older men, RBD may be an initial manifestation of Parkinsonism.

## SYMPTOMATIC TREATMENT OF INSOMNIA

When insomnia is not caused by, or fails to respond to treatment for, another medical or psychiatric condition, pharmacologic treatment with hypnotic agents may be considered as symptomatic therapy. Controversies regarding the use of hypnotic medications in demented patients revolve around issues of efficacy and potential toxicity; there is evidence that sedative-hypnotics as a class may be inappropriately prescribed or overprescribed for demented patients.

- The use of prescription drugs does not necessarily improve subjective and objective ratings of sleep quality in community-dwelling or institutionalized older patients. No controlled clinical trials have evaluated the efficacy or toxicity of benzodiazepines, nonbenzodiazepine imidazopyridine hypnotics (e.g., zolpidem or zaleplon), or melatonin receptor agonist (e.g., ramelteon) in demented patients.
- The hazards of excessive sedation in patients with dementia, including greater impairment in cognition, gait incoordination and imbalance, and increased risk of falls, have been poorly studied.
- Melatonin has been shown to be ineffective in improving sleep quality in severely sleep-disturbed AD patients.

## NONPHARMACOLOGIC THERAPY OF SLEEP DISTURBANCE

In situations where a sleep disturbance is not wholly the result of age-related sleep change, a primary sleep disorder, a specific medical or psychiatric disorder, or a complication of dementia, sleep may become chronically disrupted through the development of poor sleep habits, conditioned emotional responses, or disruptive environmental conditions. These problematic habits and responses interfere with normal regulatory sleep mechanisms and may serve as inhibitors to sleep.

- A number of behavioral and environmental modification strategies, including sleep hygiene, sleep compression, relaxation training, stimulus control, and multicomponent cognitive–behavioral therapy have proven effective for enhancing sleep in older adults without dementing diseases, and some of their components can be helpful in demented patients. Light and exercise may also have beneficial impact on sleep quality in both the healthy elderly and demented patients, possibly through enhancement of the patient's underlying circadian rhythms.
- Overall, nonpharmacologic treatments can improve sleep quality and reduce sleeping medication use in older adults, including AD patients. Behaviorally based intervention incorporating sleep hygiene education, exercise, and light exposure can be successfully implemented in AD patients. Similarly, individualized social activity intervention results in improved sleep–wake patterns in institutionalized AD patients.

## KEY POINTS

1. Sleep disturbances can occur in Alzheimer patients, not only as a result of AD-related neurodegenerative changes but also from a variety of other causes.
2. Sleep disturbance typically increases with increasing severity of AD.
3. Accurate evaluation of sleep disturbance in demented patients should include assessment of potential contributing factors such as associated medical disorders, current drug treatments, psychopathologies, primary sleep disorders, and behavioral and environmental conditions.
4. Effective treatment of sleep disturbance in AD patients has the potential to reduce the distress caused by these disturbances on both the AD patient and his or her caregiver, and to postpone institutionalization that commonly results from these sleep disturbances.
5. Use of prescription hypnotic drugs does not necessarily improve subjective and objective ratings of sleep quality in community-dwelling or institutionalized older patients.
6. Nonpharmacologic treatments can improve sleep quality and reduce hypnotic medication use in older adults, including those suffering from dementia.

## ACKNOWLEDGEMENTS

This work was supported by Public Health Service Grants: AG025515, MH072736 and NR04101.

## BIBLIOGRAPHY

Department of Health and Human Services (DHHS). National Heart, Lung, and Blood Institute. 2003 National Sleep Disorders Research Plan. NIH Publication No.03-5209. DHHS, Washington, DC, July 2003.

Alessi CA, Schnelle JF. Approches to sleep disorders in the nursing home setting. *Sleep Med Rev* 2000; 4(1):45–56.

Buysse DJ. Rational pharmacotherapy for insomnia: Time for a new paradigm. *Sleep Med Rev* 2000; 4(6):521–527.

Davis B, Sadik K. Circadian cholinergic rhythms: Implications for cholinesterase inhibitor therapy. *Dement Geriatr Cogn Disord* 2006; 21(2):120–129.

Harper DG, et al. Dementia severity and Lewy bodies affect circadian rhythms in Alzheimer disease. *Neurobiol Aging* 2004; 25(6):771–781.

Luijpen MW, et al. Non-pharmacological interventions in cognitively impaired and demented patients—A comparison with cholinesterase inhibitors. *Rev Neurosci* 2003; 14(4):343–368.

McCurry SM, Ancoli-Israel S. Sleep dysfunction in Alzheimer's Disease and other dementias. *Curr Treat Options Neurol* 2003a; 5(3):261–272.

McCurry SM, et al. Anxiety and nighttime behavioral disturbances. Awakenings in patients with Alzheimer's disease. *J Gerontol Nurs* 2004; 30(1):12–20.

McCurry SM, et al. Nighttime insomnia treatment and education for Alzheimer's Disease (NITE-AD): A randomized controlled trial. *J Am Geriatr Soc* 2005; 53(5):793–802.

McCurry SM, et al. Sleep disturbances in caregivers of persons with dementia: Contributing factors and treatment implications. *Sleep Med Rev* 2007; 11(2):143–153.

McCurry SM, et al. Training caregivers to change the sleep hygiene practices of patients with dementia: The NITE-AD Project. *J Am Geriatr Soc* 2003b; 51(10):1455–1460.

McCurry SM, et al. Treatment of sleep disturbance in Alzheimer's Disease. *Sleep Med Rev* 2000; 4(6):603–628.

Richards KC, et al. Effect of individualized social activity on sleep in nursing home residents with dementia. *J Am Geriatr Soc* 2005; 53(9):1510–1517.

Singer C, et al. Alzheimer's Disease Cooperative Study. A multicenter, placebo-controlled trial of melatonin for sleep disturbance in Alzheimer's disease. *Sleep* 2003; 26(7):893–901.

Swaab DF, et al. Therapeutic strategies for Alzheimer disease: Focus on neuronal reactivation of metabolically impaired neurons. *Alzheimer Dis Assoc Disord* 2003; 17 (Suppl 4): S114–122.

Tariot PN, et al. Pharmacologic therapy for behavioral symptoms of Alzheimer's disease. *Clin Geriatr Med* 2001; 17(2):359–376.

Teri L, et al. Nonpharmacologic treatment of behavioral disturbance in dementia. *Med Clin North Am* 2002; 86(3):641–656.

Van Someren EJ. Circadian and sleep disturbances in the elderly. *Exp Gerontol* 2000; 35(9–10):1229–1237.

Vitiello MV. Effective treatment of sleep disturbances in older adults. *Clin Cornerstone* 2000; 2(5):16–27.

Vitiello MV, Borson S. Sleep disturbances in patients with Alzheimer's Disease: Epidemiology, pathophysiology and management. *CNS Drugs* 2001; 15(10):777–796.

Vitiello MV, et al. Sleep complaints co-segregate with illness older adults: Clinical research informed by and informing epidemiological studies of sleep. *Psychosom Res* 2002; 53(1):555–559.

Yesavage JA, et al. Development of diagnostic criteria for defining sleep disturbance in Alzheimer's Disease. *J Geriatr Psychiatry Neurol* 2003; 16(3):131–139.

Yesavage JA, et al. Sleep/wake disruption in Alzheimer's disease: APOE status and longitudinal course. *J Geriatr Psychiatry Neurol* 2004; 17(1):20–24.

Yesavage JA, et al. Sleep/wake cycle disturbance in Alzheimer's disease: How much is due to an inherent trait? *Int Psychogeriatr* 2002; 14(1):73–81.

# 44

## NEURODEGENERATIVE DISORDERS

DAVID G. HARPER

McLean Hospital and Harvard Medical School, Belmont, Massachusetts

## INTRODUCTION

The mechanism(s) of sleep disturbance in neurodegenerative illnesses is complex and often multifactorial. The impact of homeostatic vs. circadian disruption, environmental vs. neurodegenerative etiologies, and the role played by aging across the continuum of age-associated sleep and circadian changes all need to be accounted for to understand the etiology of sleep disturbance associated with a particular neurodegenerative illness.

## CAUSES OF SLEEP DISTURBANCE

Normal human behavior is temporally divided into organized patterns of nocturnal sleep and diurnal alertness by the interaction of two discrete physiologic mechanisms, namely circadian and homeostatic processes. Both of these processes have neuroanatomic substrates in regions of the brain affected by Alzheimer disease (AD) and other neurodegenerative illnesses.

- The circadian, oscillatory rhythm is generated by the suprachiasmatic nuclei (SCN) of the hypothalamus and promotes alertness as a function of time of day, thereby consolidating wakefulness during the diurnal period.
- Opposing this alerting rhythm is a homeostatic process that builds need for sleep as a function of the duration of prior wakefulness. The areas of the brain involved in homeostatic regulation are located in structures of the basal forebrain and hypothalamus, including the ascending reticular system, ventrolateral preoptic area (VLPO), nucleus basalis of Meynart, and thalamus. The interaction between these two processes creates an oscillating pattern of sleep and wakefulness that is responsive to perturbation based on external demands.
- Patients with neurodegenerative illnesses frequently live in environments lacking stimulation and the cues essential for maintaining healthy sleep–wake rhythms. Therefore, it is frequently difficult to determine whether a sleep or rhythm disturbance experienced by an individual is a consequence of the neurodegenerative illness, the environment, or some combination of both factors.
- Most neurodegenerative illnesses are age associated, with incidences that increase dramatically as patients grow older. Sleep changes that occur as a result of normal aging may be mingled with changes resulting from more pathologic forms of aging seen with neurodegenerative illnesses. Taken together, these issues yield an intricate matrix of causal factors any one of which could be responsible for the significant disturbance in the continuity and quantity of sleep in patients with neurodegenerative dementia. Identifying the correct etiologic factors is imperative in choosing correct treatment since many of the pharmacologic methods used to aid sleep in patients with transient insomnia have substantial cognitive effects that are undesirable in this patient population.
- Sleep also has an internal architecture that can become disrupted as a consequence of neurodegenerative illness. Normal sleep contains several stages of slow-wave "deep" sleep alternating with "light" sleep associated with faster electroencephalographic (EEG) activity. Inserted into light sleep are periods of desynchronized, rapid eye movement (REM) essentially indistinguishable from wakefulness except for the presence of pervasive muscle atonia preventing behavioral expression during dreaming. REM sleep appears to be initiated, and muscle atonia maintained, by pontine and brainstem nuclei in association with higher brain structures. Each of these elements of sleep architecture can be disrupted by the presence of a neurodegenerative dementia with consequences to the patient and caregiver.

## CONSEQUENCES OF SLEEP DISTURBANCE

Most patients, particularly in the early and midstages of a neurodegenerative illness, have a caregiver, and the consequences of a sleep disturbance impact both members of this patient–caregiver dyad.

- For the caregiver, the ability to maintain a steady sleep schedule may become impossible due to the need to manage the patient's agitation and restlessness at night. These increased demands invariably lead to some degree of caregiver exhaustion and consequent institutionalization of the patient.

- For the patient, the impact of sleep loss may be severe in cognitive and behavioral domains. Since sleep deprivation leads to decrements in working memory, and executive functioning in normal adults in a dose-dependent fashion, cognitive and behavioral symptoms of AD or other dementias are likely to worsen as sleep deficit increases. The consequences of these additional decrements to the overall disease burden are likely to be substantial. There can also be increased physical danger from falls and physical injury resulting from the nocturnal wandering and agitation that frequently accompanies sleep disturbance in addition to the known increase in risk of physical injury resulting from chronic sleep deprivation.

- Decrements in cognitive performance can be substantial, not only from sleep deprivation or restriction resulting from the impact of the illness on the sleep homeostatic system or the circadian system, but also by circadian disruption alone without apparent sleep loss. Circadian misalignment induced through a forced desynchrony protocol (maintaining a sleep–wake rhythm significantly different from 24 h such that the sleep–wake rhythm and physiologic circadian rhythm become separate) has been demonstrated to impair performance on simple cognitive tasks, such as addition performance, during the period when the sleep–wake and circadian rhythms are out of alignment. Motivation also becomes quite impaired in normal subjects under these conditions. All of these outcomes are undesirable from the standpoint of a patient with a neurodegenerative illness.

## CHARACTERIZATION OF SLEEP DISTURBANCES

There are several progressive neurodegenerative dementias, and all are characterized by progressive cognitive and functional decline with increasing neuropathology over the course of the illness. However, while many of them share significant pathologic features, there are also substantial differences between them. Given this wide variety of neurodegenerative illnesses, their differing etiologies and courses of neural destruction, it would make sense that

although the sleep disturbances associated with them may appear superficially similar, there are likely to be vast differences in their expression.

- There are also great differences in our knowledge of sleep disturbance in these different neurodegenerative dementias. Some of the illnesses have a large quantity of information characterizing the polysomnography, circadian dysregulation, or other factors impacting sleep. However, for some of them, there is virtually no information available characterizing the sleep disturbance although it is known to be present.

### Dementia with Lewy Bodies

Dementia with Lewy bodies (DLB) has many pathologic similarities to AD, including the development of amyloid plaques in the brain. The phenotypic expression of sleep–wake disturbances is also quite similar between the diseases, although the severity of the disturbances may be more pronounced in DLB according to caregiver reports. To date, no polysomnographic study has compared the sleep architecture seen in DLB and AD. However, objective quantitative measures, such as locomotor activity monitoring, in pathologically confirmed cases, show differences between DLB and AD especially in the quantity of diurnal activity seen, with DLB patients showing markedly reduced diurnal activity.

- The most striking sleep-associated feature of DLB is the emergence of REM sleep behavior disorder (RBD) in a subpopulation of these patients. This finding of RBD is almost unique to DLB and often precedes the symptoms of dementia by more than 10 years. The only other neuropathologic diagnosis associated with RBD is multiple system atrophy, a synucleinopathy sharing the significant neuropathologic finding of intracellular inclusions composed of alpha synuclein. A recent estimate of the prevalence of RBD in pathologically confirmed DLB was placed at 50%, which yields significant diagnostic value to this parasomnia.

### Frontotemporal Dementia, Pick Disease, and Corticobasal Degeneration

Frontotemporal dementia (FTD) and Pick disease are now nosologically considered subtypes of a single diagnostic entity based on neuropathologic patterns of damage. They share the hyperphosphorylation of the *tau* protein and consequent development of neurofibrillary tangles with AD; however, these illnesses do not generate the amyloid plaques seen in AD. The sleep disturbances in patients diagnosed with Pick disease or other frontotemporal dementias have several features in common and can be quite devastating to the patients.

Polysomnographically, patients show significant loss in total sleep time, especially slow-wave sleep, and frequent awakenings throughout the night. While REM sleep was observed in all patients studied, it is remarkably fragmented and frequently occurred at sleep onset.

- Studies of time-series activity recordings of patients with FTD show a remarkable loss of diurnal-nocturnal rhythmicity with very high fragmentation of the rhythm. While the circadian rhythms of core body temperature in patients with FTD are indistinguishable from those of normal elderly subjects, suggesting that the circadian oscillator is unimpaired, the locomotor activity appears arrhythmic and chaotic. These results suggest that an uncoupling has occurred between the central circadian clock and the expression of that rhythm in a coherent pattern of rest and activity occurring over 24 h. Therefore, treatment approaches based on the altering circadian rhythmicity are unlikely to be effective in these patients.

### Huntington Disease

Until recently, very little attention has been paid to the clear circadian and sleep disturbances seen in Huntington disease (HD). Case reports have described deeply disturbed sleep in these patients but no quantitative work has been done until recently. A recent study shows deeply disrupted expression of circadian timing of the rhythm of locomotor activity in these patients. In addition, nocturnal activity was significantly increased in the HD patients, although it is difficult to tell whether this effect was due to a shift in the circadian rhythm or wakefulness not attributable to a circadian etiology.

### KEY POINTS

1. Tremendous progress has been made over the last decade in our understanding of the sleep disturbances in patients with different forms of neurodegenerative illnesses, so that this knowledge can be employed in developing innovative treatments for these patients. However, much work remains to be done, including elaborating the underlying mechanisms behind neurodegenerative damage in the brain and how this damage then leads to the phenotypic expression of sleep and/or circadian disturbances. Increasing our knowledge of these factors will ultimately lead to new insights for treatments.

2. Another important area for further research is the impact of ameliorating sleep and circadian disturbances on the severity and progression of the illness. It is possible that by treating sleep problems successfully, we can lower the cognitive burden of the disease and possibly impact the disease course.

### BIBLIOGRAPHY

Ancoli-Israel S, et al. Variations in circadian rhythms of activity, sleep, and light exposure related to dementia in nursing-home patients. *Sleep* 1997a; 20:18–23.

Ancoli-Israel S, et al. Use of wrist activity for monitoring sleep/wake in demented nursing-home patients. *Sleep* 1997b; 20:24–27.

Boeve BF, et al. REM sleep behavior disorder and degenerative dementia: An association likely reflecting Lewy body disease. *Neurology* 1998; 51:363–370.

Boeve BF, et al. REM sleep behavior disorder in Parkinson's disease and dementia with Lewy bodies. *J Geriatr Psychiatry Neurol* 2004; 17:146–157.

Gehrman PR, et al. Sleep-disordered breathing and agitation in institutionalized adults with Alzheimer disease. *Am J Geriatr Psychiatry* 2003; 11:426–433.

Goldberg R, et al. Sleep problems in emergency department patients with injuries. *Acad Emerg Med* 1999; 6:1134–1140.

Grace JB, et al. A comparison of sleep profiles in patients with dementia with Lewy bodies and Alzheimer's disease. *Int J Geriatr Psychiatry* 2000; 15:1028–1033.

Harper DG, et al. Differential circadian rhythm disturbances in men with Alzheimer disease and frontotemporal degeneration. *Arch Gen Psychiatry* 2001; 58:353–360.

Harper DG, et al. Dementia severity and Lewy bodies affect circadian rhythms in Alzheimer disease. *Neurobiol Aging* 2004; 25:771–781.

Harper DG, et al. Disturbance of endogenous circadian rhythm in aging and Alzheimer disease. *Am J Geriatr Psychiatry* 2005; 359–368.

Hatfield CF, et al. Disrupted daily activity/rest cycles in relation to daily cortisol rhythms of home-dwelling patients with early Alzheimer's dementia. *Brain* 2004; 127:1061–1074.

Jewett ME, et al. Interactive mathematical models of subjective alertness and cognitive throughput in humans. *J Biol Rhythms* 1999; 14:588–597.

Jones K, et al. Frontal lobe function, sleep loss and fragmented sleep. *Sleep Med Rev* 2001; 5:463–475.

Kersaitis C, et al. Regional and cellular pathology in frontotemporal dementia: Relationship to stage of disease in cases with and without Pick bodies. *Acta Neuropathol (Berl)* 2004; 108:515–523.

Lawlor BA. Behavioral and psychological symptoms in dementia: The role of atypical antipsychotics. *J Clin Psychiatry* 2004; 65:5–10.

Mishima K, et al. Melatonin secretion rhythm disorders in patients with senile dementia of Alzheimer's type with disturbed sleep-waking. *Biol Psychiatry* 1999; 45:417–421.

McCurry SM, et al. Sleep dysfunction in Alzheimer's Disease and other dementias. *Curr Treat Options Neurol* 2003; 5:261–272.

Morton AJ, et al. Disintegration of the sleep-wake cycle and circadian timing in Huntington's disease. *J Neurosci* 2005; 25:157–163.

Saper CB, et al. The sleep switch: Hypothalamic control of sleep and wakefulness. *Trends Neurosci* 2001; 24:726–731.

Shochat T, et al. Illumination levels in nursing home patients: Effects on sleep and activity rhythms. *J Sleep Res* 2000; 9:373–379.

Smith ME, et al. The impact of moderate sleep loss on neurophysiologic signals during working-memory task performance. *Sleep* 2002; 25:784–794.

Stopa EG, et al. Pathologic evaluation of the human suprachiasmatic nucleus in severe dementia. *J Neuropathol Exp Neurol* 1999; 58:29–39.

Tractenberg RE, et al. The Sleep Disorders Inventory: An instrument for studies of sleep disturbance in persons with Alzheimer's disease. *J Sleep Res* 2003; 12:331–337.

Van Someren EJ, et al. Indirect bright light improves circadian rest-activity rhythm disturbances in demented patients. *Biol Psychiatry* 1997; 41:955–963.

Vitiello MV, et al. Alzheimer's disease. Sleep and sleep/wake patterns. *Clin Geriatr Med* 1989; 5:289–299.

Wu YH, et al. Molecular changes underlying reduced pineal melatonin levels in Alzheimer disease: Alterations in preclinical and clinical stages. *J Clin Endocrinol Metab* 2003; 88:5898–5906.

# 45

## PARKINSON'S DISEASE

Michael H. Silber
Center for Sleep Medicine and Department of Neurology, Mayo Clinic College of Medicine, Rochester, Minnesota

### INTRODUCTION

Idiopathic Parkinson's disease (PD) is the commonest cause of Parkinsonism, a clinical syndrome characterized by rest tremor, rigidity, bradykinesia, and abnormal postural reflexes. It is associated with Lewy inclusion bodies in multiple nuclei, especially in the substantia nigra.

- The frequency of sleep disorders in PD is high and can best be conceptualized under the headings of insomnia, excessive daytime sleepiness, excessive motor activity at night, and nocturnal perceptual and behavioral abnormalities. (Table 45.1)

### INSOMNIA

Problems initiating or maintaining sleep in PD may be due to uncontrolled motor symptoms, the effects of medications, restless legs syndrome, depression, or circadian sleep–wake reversal in patients with superimposed dementia.

- Bradykinesia and rigidity may prevent patients from changing position in bed, a normal phenomenon that occurs two or three times an hour. This results in muscle pain and stiffness that may wake the patient from sleep. Parkinsonian tremor may occur during light sleep and periods of wakefulness during the night. Nocturia is common in PD patients, and painful early morning dystonia may also contribute to insomnia.
- Dopaminergic drugs, such as levodopa or dopamine receptor agonists, have alerting effects and thus may cause insomnia if taken before sleep. Patients will often describe feeling wide-awake or "wired" and can relate the start of insomnia to the initiation of medication.
- Restless legs syndrome (RLS) is probably more common in PD than in age-matched controls, although

case control data is not available. However, both conditions are common in older people and frequently coincide. High-dose levodopa therapy for PD may result in daytime augmentation of RLS, thus exacerbating the problem.

- Depression is a frequent occurrence in PD and may be more common compared to other disorders with similar degrees of disability. It may be difficult to diagnose, as the neuro-vegetative symptoms of depression may resemble the bradykinesia of PD.
- When dementia is present in advanced PD, disruption of circadian rhythms may result in sleep–wake reversal and apparent nocturnal insomnia.
- The mechanisms of insomnia in PD can usually be elucidated by a careful history from the patient and bed partner or caregiver. Difficulty turning over during the night and persistent tremor suggest undertreatment of the disorder at night and should be managed by addition of controlled release carbidopa/levodopa or a dopamine agonist before bed. If insomnia is believed due to the alerting effects of an evening dose of medication, then the dose should be reduced or a hypnotic such as a benzodiazepine or sedating antidepressant such as trazodone added. The management of RLS in PD can be challenging, especially if it appears that levodopa augmentation has occurred. Strategies include substituting a dopamine agonist such as pramipexole or ropinirole for levodopa or adding a dopamine agonist, gabapentin, an opioid or a benzodiazepine, especially in the evening. If depression is suspected, a trial of an antidepressant should be undertaken.

### EXCESSIVE DAYTIME SLEEPINESS

Clinic-based studies of consecutive PD patients have found an abnormal Epworth Sleepiness Scale (ESS) score of >10 in about 30–40% of patients. In one study, 76% reported

*Sleep Medicine Essentials*, edited by Teofilo L. Lee-Chiong
Copyright © 2009 John Wiley & Sons, Inc.

**Table 45.1   Mechanisms of Sleep Disturbances in Parkinson's Disease**

| Insomnia | Excessive movement at night |
|---|---|
| Motor symptoms of PD | REM sleep behavior disorder |
| Restless legs syndrome | Periodic limb movements of sleep |
| Effects of medication | PD tremor |
| Depression | Drug-induced dyskinesias |
| Circadian dysrhythmias | **Perceptual or behavioral disturbances** |
| **Excessive daytime sleepiness** | Effects of medication |
| Intrinsic to PD | Confusion with dementia |
| Effect of medication | REM sleep behavior disorder |
| Sleep-disordered breathing | |
| Depression | |
| Circadian dysrhythmias | |

feeling sleepy during the day with 21% falling asleep while driving. In a community-based study, 27% complained of excessive daytime sleepiness (EDS). Multiple factors interact to cause sleepiness in PD patients, with the three most important being somnolence intrinsic to the disorder itself, the effects of medication, and sleep-disordered breathing.

- It might intuitively be thought that disrupted nocturnal sleep due to undertreated PD might be an important cause of EDS. However, in several studies, nocturnal sleep complaints such as short sleep duration and frequent arousals did not correlate with daytime sleepiness. In objective studies of PD patients, polysomnography (PSG) measures such as total sleep time and sleep efficiency actually correlated negatively with the subsequent mean multiple sleep latency test (MSLT) latency and longer sleep latencies correlated positively. Shorter MSLT latencies were associated with longer duration of PD, lower cognitive functioning, hallucinations, and sleep-onset REM periods (SOREMPs) during MSLT naps. Hallucinating PD patients were more likely to have SOREMPs than nonhallucinators. Low cerebrospinal fluid (CSF) hypocretin-1 levels have been noted in PD patients compared to controls and extensive hypocretin cell loss found at autopsy in the brains of PD patients. These data have led to the hypothesis that an intrinsic, narcolepsy-like condition may occur in PD, especially as the disease progresses. However, proof of this concept has been difficult to achieve, as almost all advanced PD patients are taking medications that can themselves cause drowsiness, as discussed next.

- Concern has been raised that the newer Parkinsonian drugs such as pramipexole and ropinirole may cause patients to fall asleep while driving. Dopamine release is generally considered to have alerting effects, and thus hypersomnia induced by these drugs is paradoxical and little understood. However, it has become clear that all dopaminergic agents, including levodopa, can in certain patients induce sleep, sometimes but not always, linked in time to ingestion of a dose of the drug. Despite initial reports, it appears that the newer, non-ergot-based agonists do not have a greater propensity to induce sleepiness than the older ergot-based agonists such

as pergolide or bromocriptine. While sudden "sleep attacks" without preceding warnings of drowsiness may occasionally occur, this phenomenon is uncommon and nonspecific, also occurring in some patients with sleepiness due to narcolepsy, sleep apnea syndrome, and sleep deprivation. Most, but not all, studies using the ESS and MSLT have shown that total daily dose of dopaminergic agents correlates with severity of sleepiness.

- Pulmonary function tests indicate upper airway obstruction during wakefulness in PD patients, and thus one might predict a high prevalence of obstructive sleep apnea (OSA) in the disorder. Snoring and its severity correlate with ESS scores in PD patients. Two small controlled studies have shown contradictory results, one demonstrating a significant increase in obstructive apneas and hypopneas and the other showing no difference between patients and controls. Larger studies are needed to establish a definite association, but both conditions are common in the elderly. At the very least, the coincidental occurrence of OSA must be an important consideration in the sleepy PD patient.

- In addition to these three major factors, depression may mimic sleepiness in PD, and circadian disruption with day–night reversal may occur in PD patients with dementia.

- In assessing the sleepy PD patient, a careful history of snoring, snort arousals, and observed apneas should be taken from the patients and bed partner or caregiver. If OSA is suspected, PSG should be performed followed by appropriate treatment of sleep-disordered breathing. If OSA is not present, then consideration should be given to reduction of the dose of dopaminergic agents if this can be achieved without compromise of control of the movement disorder. If this is ineffective or not medically possible, then stimulant medication such as modafinil or methylphenidate should be considered.

- Trials of modafinil in sleepy PD patients have shown conflicting results with respect to improvement in the ESS scores but no change in maintenance of wakefulness or multiple sleep latency test results. Driving should be restricted in PD patients with uncontrolled sleepiness until the problem has been resolved.

## EXCESSIVE MOTOR ACTIVITY AT NIGHT

Rapid eye movement (REM) sleep behavior disorder (RBD) is characterized by often violent dream enactment behavior associated with an absence of the normal skeletal muscle atonia of REM sleep.

- Rapid eye movement sleep behavior disorder is closely linked to the alpha synucleinopathies, disorders characterized by neuronal inclusion bodies staining positive to alpha synuclein, and including PD and dementia with Lewy bodies (DLB). RBD is present in 15–33% of PD patients assessed in PD clinics and the PSG finding of REM sleep without atonia in 58%. Patients with PD comprise up to 27% of RBD patients diagnosed in sleep disorders centers.

- In the presence of dementia RBD, even without Parkinsonism, is highly suggestive of dementia with Lewy bodies. Of 18 reported autopsy studies of patients with RBD, 15 had Lewy body pathology.

- Symptoms of RBD often develop before the onset of Parkinsonism or dementia. In a retrospective study, RBD was recalled as the first manifestation by 52% of patients with RBD and PD with the median time from onset of RBD to onset of other symptoms of the neurologic disorder being 3–4 years. In a prospective study of 29 RBD patients greater than 50 years old with normal neurologic examinations, 65% had developed Parkinsonism or dementia after a mean of 13 years from onset. Another study showed the development of neurodegenerative disease in 45% of 40 idiopathic RBD patients after 2 years follow-up. These data suggest that Lewy body pathology may underlie many patients with apparently cryptogenic RBD and that RBD may be a very early manifestation of PD and DLB.

- A modified PSG with additional upper extremity surface electromyogram (EMG) derivation and time-synchronized video recording is usually needed to diagnose RBD. However, in clinical practice, the diagnosis can sometimes be inferred from a typical history in patients with PD.

- Management includes improving the safety of the bed environment by moving furniture away from the bedside and considering placing a mattress or large pillows on the floor next to the bed.

- The drug of choice is clonazepam, commencing at 0.25–0.5 mg before bed and increasing as needed and tolerated to 2 mg. Up to 80% of patients appear to respond to this drug in open-label trials. However, clonazepam is associated with side effects that may be harmful to PD and DLB patients, including gait disturbances and cognitive impairment, especially in the elderly.

- Other possible alternative treatments, tested in open-label studies, include melatonin (3–12 mg) and possibly pramipexole. Quetiapine may sometimes be useful, especially in DLB patients who also manifest nocturnal confusion.

- Other causes of excessive motor behavior during sleep in PD patients include persistent Parkinsonian tremor, levodopa-induced dyskinesias and periodic limb movements of sleep (PLMS). PLMS appear more frequent in PD patients compared to controls. While PLMS can sometimes fragment sleep, they are common in asymptomatic older subjects and should not be considered clinically significant unless most are accompanied by arousals.

## PERCEPTUAL AND BEHAVIORAL ABNORMALITIES AT NIGHT

Hallucinations and behavioral problems at night in PD usually result from one of three causes: the effects of dopaminergic drugs, RBD, and confusion from dementia that may develop in about one third of patients.

- Levodopa and the dopamine agonists can cause a spectrum of perceptual disturbances, ranging from vivid dreams through nightmares to complex visual hallucinations. These hallucinations may occur during the day but are especially common when sensory input is diminished at night. Initially, patient- may retain insight into their unreality, but later this insight is lost. They manifest as vivid, multicolor, sometimes oddly distorted images of animals or people and disappear when the light is switched on.

- Very similar complex nocturnal visual hallucinations may occur in DLB even without the use of dopaminergic drugs.

- Confusional wandering behavior may occur in demented patients with PD. This can usually be differentiated from RBD by careful questioning of an observer. Confusional wandering usually lasts hours while episodes of RBD last minutes. Confusional wandering occurs out of bed, while patients with RBD usually kick and flail their arms in bed. An observer usually describes the wandering patient as awake but confused, while the patient with RBD appears to be asleep but acting out dreams. If a PSG is performed, the behavior usually arises from non-REM (NREM) sleep and takes place during wakefulness, often with slow electroencephalographic (EEG) rhythms, in contrast to RBD in which the behavior arises from REM sleep without atonia. It should be recalled that 58% of PD patients have abnormal tone in REM sleep, and thus it is essential in PSG studies to record the actual behavior and not rely on the neurophysiologic findings alone.

- Reduction in dopaminergic therapy should be considered in PD patients who develop hallucinations or confusion, but often a careful balance is needed between control of motor symptoms and reduction of side effects. RBD should always be considered and a sleep study performed if there is clinical doubt. Often neuroleptic medication is required with the use of new generation agents such as quetiapine that do not worsen Parkinsonism. However, even these agents should be used with caution, as they have been associated with hyperglycemia and cardiovascular mortality.

## KEY POINTS

1. The frequency of sleep disorders is high in PD, and patients should always be questioned about symptoms related to sleep.

2. Most sleep disorders in PD can be elucidated by a careful history from the patient and a bed partner or caregiver; polysomnography is only needed in specific circumstances.

3. Depression should always be considered in a PD patient with insomnia and can be hard to diagnose as the neuro-vegetative symptoms of depression can mimic the motor symptoms of PD.

4. Restless legs syndrome may be challenging to treat in PD patients because of augmentation caused by levodopa; strategies include adding or substituting a dopamine agonist, or adding gabapentin, an opioid or a benzodiazepine.

5. Medication, sleep apnea, or PD itself may cause excessive daytime sleepiness in PD; sleep studies may be needed to rule out sleep apnea.

6. REM sleep behavior disorder may be present in up to a third of PD patients; treatment options include clonazepam and melatonin.

7. Confusional nocturnal wandering in Lewy body dementia can usually be differentiated from RBD by a careful history. Atypical neuroleptics may help nocturnal confusion, but physicians should be aware of their association with hyperglycemia and cardiovascular mortality.

## BIBLIOGRAPHY

Adler CH, et al. Randomized trial of modafinil for treating subjective daytime sleepiness in patients with Parkinson's disease. *Mov Disord* 2003; 18:287–293.

Boeve B, et al. Synucleinopathy pathology and REM sleep behavior disorder plus dementia or parkinsonism. *Neurology* 2003; 61:40–45.

Boeve BF, et al. Melatonin for treatment of REM sleep behavior disorder in neurologic disorders: Results in 14 patients. *Sleep Med* 2003; 4:281–284.

Brodsky MA, et al. Sleepiness in Parkinson's disease: A controlled study. *Mov Disord* 2003; 18:668–672.

Comella CL, et al. Sleep-related violence, injury, and REM sleep behavior disorder in Parkinson's disease. *Neurology* 1998; 51:526–529.

Fronczek R, et al. Hypocretin (orexin) loss in Parkinson's disease. *Brain* 2007; 130:1577–1585.

Gagnon J, et al. REM sleep behavior disorder and REM sleep without atonia in Parkinson's disease. *Neurology* 2002; 59:585–589.

Hobson DE, et al. Excessive daytime sleepiness and sudden-onset sleep in Parkinson disease. A survey by the Canadian Movement Disorders Group. *JAMA* 2002; 287:455–463.

Hogl B, et al. Modafinil for the treatment of daytime sleepiness in Parkinson's disease: A double-blind, randomized, crossover, placebo-controlled polygraphic trial. *Sleep* 2002; 25:905–909.

Hogl B, et al. Increased daytime sleepiness in Parkinson's disease: A questionnaire survey. *Mov Disord* 2003; 18:319–323.

Iranzo A, et al. Rapid-eye-movement sleep behaviour disorder as an early marker for a neurodegenerative disorder: A descriptive study. *Lancet Neurol* 2006; 5:572–577.

Maria B, et al. Sleep breathing disorders in patients with idiopathic Parkinson's disease. *Resp Med* 2003; 97:1151–1157.

Olson EJ, et al. Rapid eye movement sleep behavior disorder: Demographic, clinical and laboratory findings in 93 cases. *Brain* 2000; 123:331–339.

Ondo W, et al. Modafinil for daytime somnolence in parkinson's disease: Double blind, placebo controlled parallel trial. *J Neurol Neurosurg Psychiatry* 2005; 76:1636–1639.

Razmy A, et al. Predictors of impaired daytime sleep and wakefulness in patients with Parkinson disease treated with older (ergot) vs newer (nonergot) dopamine agonists. *Arch Neurol* 2004; 61:97–102.

Rye DB, et al. Daytime sleepiness in Parkinson's disease. *J Sleep Res* 2000; 9:63–69.

Schenck CH, et al. REM behavior disorder (RBD): Delayed emergence of Parkinsonism and/or dementia in 65% of older men initially diagnosed with idiopathic RBD, and an analysis of the minimum and maximum tonic and/or phasic electromyographic abnormalities found during REM sleep [abstr]. *Sleep* 2003; 26:A316.

Tandberg E, et al. Excessive daytime sleepiness and sleep benefit in Parkinson's disease: A community-based study. *Mov Disord* 1999; 14:922–927.

Thannickal T, et al. Hypocretin (orexin) cell loss in Parkinson's disease. *Brain* 2007; 130:1586–1595.

Wetter TC, et al. Sleep and periodic leg movement patterns in drug-free patients with Parkinson's disease and multiple system atrophy. *Sleep* 2000; 23:361–367.

# 46

## SEIZURES

Margaret N. Shouse
Department of Neurobiology, UCLA School of Medicine, Los Angeles, California

## INTRODUCTION

Sleep states have a potent effect on the expression or suppression of epileptic seizure manifestations. Epileptic seizure manifestations include various generalized or localized epileptic electroencephalographic (EEG) discharges. Epileptiform EEG activity may consist of interictal discharges (IIDs), which occur between seizures, or ictal discharges, which typically last longer than IIDs and are frequently associated with clinically evident behavioral seizure events.

## SEIZURES AND INTERICTAL DISCHARGES IN NREM VERSUS REM SLEEP

During nonrapid eye movement (NREM) sleep, focal and generalized epileptic discharges are common, even if clinical seizures do not occur. During rapid eye movement (REM) sleep, generalized epileptiform discharges are either infrequent or the degree of spread is restricted. Focal IIDs persist during REM and are highly localized. Clinically evident seizures rarely occur during REM. The differential effects of NREM versus REM sleep on interictal and ictal epileptiform discharge depend somewhat on the type and severity of the epileptic seizure syndrome.

## GENERALIZED EPILEPTIFORM DISCHARGES BY SLEEP STATES

| | Interictal Discharges | | Ictal Discharges | |
|---|---|---|---|---|
| Epilepsy Syndrome: Circadian Seizure Rhythm | NREM | REM | NREM | REM |
| Primary generalized epilepsies of idiopathic or hereditary origin: awakening epilepsies | Common | Rare | Rare[a] | Rare |
| Localization epilepsies with known or suspected local pathology: sleep epilepsies | Common | Rare[b] | Common | Rare |
| Symptomatic epilepsies with extensive encephalopathy: sleep and waking epilepsies | Common | Rare[c] | Common | Rare |

[a]Except stage 1 (> 5-s trains of spike-wave complexes would likely be associated with an absence of seizure in waking).

[b]Note maximal focalization.

[c]As long as REM is intact.

Source: From Shouse MN, et al. *Epilepsy: A Comprehensive Textbook* (1997), Lippincott-Raven. Philadelphia, Pennsylvania.

*Sleep Medicine Essentials*, edited by Teofilo L. Lee-Chiong
Copyright © 2009 John Wiley & Sons, Inc.

## CHARACTERISTICS OF EPILEPSY SYNDROMES

| Epilepsy Syndrome | Main IID Type | Seizure Type | Age at Onset | Response to Medications | Spontaneous Remission |
|---|---|---|---|---|---|
| *Primary Generalized Epilepsies (PGEs): Awakening Epilepsies* | | | | | |
| Childhood absence with or without generalized tonic-clonic convulsions (GTCs) | 3/s spike and wave during transitional arousal states | Absence seizure (↓ responsiveness with behavioral arrest) | ~ 4 years | Good; ethosuximide for absence; valproate or benzodiazepines for GTCs | May convert to primary GTC at ~12 years with remission ~25–50 years |
| Juvenile absence and/or myoclonus | Multi- or poly-spike-wave on awakening | Absences and/or bilateral myoclonus | Puberty | Good; e.g., valproate | Frequent seizures may require continued medication |
| GTCs on awakening | 4–5/s spike and wave with frontal maximum | GTCs within 2 h of awakening | 10–20 years | Good, e.g., phenobarbital or benzodiazepines | Frequently remits at ~25 years |
| *Localization Related Epilepsies: Sleep Epilepsies* | | | | | |
| Benign epilepsy with centrotemporal spikes (BECTs) | Centro-temporal slow spikes or sharp waves | Vocalize, salivate, jaw and/or limb clonus, > 50% in NREM | 1–13 years, more male than female | Good, if needed; carbamazepine or valproate | ~Puberty |
| Electrical status epilepticus during sleep (ESES) | Fronto-central focal spikes and 1.5–3 c/s spike and wave; < 25% in waking; > 85% generalized spike and wave during NREM sleep | Partial motor (mostly nocturnal), and atypical absence | ~8 years (range 4–14 years) | Good; prednisone | ~12 years with possible residual intellectual, other cognitive, and behavior disorders |
| Landau–Kleffner (acquired epileptic aphasia) | Temporal (50%) or parietal-occipital foci (30%); otherwise resembles ESES in NREM sleep | Partial motor, GTC or atypical absences; few clinical seizures even in sleep | ~ 6.5 years (range 3–9 years) | Good; prednisone | ~Puberty, with possible residual aphasia |
| Secondary generalized temporal and/or frontal lobe epilepsies | Temporal or frontal spikes, multi-spike-wave and/or sharp waves | Partial complex or typical automatisms with or without secondary GTCs | Any age, frequently 15–30 years | Good to intractable; e.g., carbamazepine, phenytoin, or gabapentin | Unlikely, especially with documented pathology |
| *Symptomatic Generalized Epilepsies: Diffuse (Sleep and Waking) Epilepsies* | | | | | |
| West syndrome (infantile spasms) | Hypsarrhythmia; IIDs most frequent and have a burst-suppression pattern in NREM sleep | "Jack-knife" seizures; rare in sleep | 6 months–1 years | Poor; adrenocorticotropic (ACTH), benzodiazepines, vigabatrin | No; often converts to Lennox-Gastaut |
| Lennox–Gastaut | 1.5–2.5 slow spike and wave; tonic seizure pattern of 10–25 c/s bursts lasting of 1–30 s | Tonic, atonic, myoclonic, GTC, atypical absence; "tonic" EEG seizure patterns (often subclinical) are very likely to increase in sleep | 1–10 years | Poor; valproate, benzodiazepines, felbamate; lamotrigine; best response if seizures are state dependent | No; seizures and mental retardation are less likely with a discernible state-dependent seizure pattern |

| Epilepsy Syndrome | Main IID Type | Seizure Type | Age at Onset | Response to Medications | Spontaneous Remission |
|---|---|---|---|---|---|
| Progressive (essential hereditary) myoclonus, Lafora–Unverricht–Lundborg syndrome | Generalized spike and wave, and multispike and wave | Myoclonus and GTCs *plus* numerous other subclinic epileptic or nonepileptic symptoms | Childhood to adolescence | Poor; autosomal recessive genetic syndrome complicated by numerous cerebellar and mental symptoms | No; death within 2 years of onset or later depending on age at onset; worst prognosis with earliest onset |

## PRIMARY GENERALIZED EPILEPSIES OF GENETIC OR IDIOPATHIC ORIGIN: AWAKENING EPILEPSIES

In the primary generalized epilepsies (PGEs), interictal and ictal EEG discharges begin simultaneously virtually everywhere in the brain. Most PGEs are thought to be genetic with age-related penetrance. The prognosis is good, and PGEs respond well to antiepileptic medications and tend to remit spontaneously. Included in this category are childhood and juvenile absence epilepsy and juvenile myoclonic epilepsy (JME). These disorders can occur with or without GTCs. GTCs can also occur as the only seizure type.

- Primary generalized epilepsies are considered "awakening" epilepsies because massive myoclonus and GTCs occur on awakening from sleep in about 90% of the cases. Nocturnal awakening, naps, and evening relaxation may also be associated with increases in ictal seizure events.
- Frequently IIDs are detected during transitional arousal states to and from NREM sleep, and, occasionally, between NREM and REM sleep. IIDs are most often detected in relation to "arousal"-related events during NREM sleep.

## NONRAPID EYE MOVEMENT SLEEP

Interictal discharges, such as typical spike-and-wave (3/s) and multi-spike-and-wave or poly-spike-and-wave complexes, are most frequently detected during NREM stages 1 and 2 sleep. It is also easier to provoke behavioral arousal from light NREM stages 1 and 2 sleep than from deep NREM stage 3 or REM sleep.

- The longest trains of spike-and-wave complexes (> 5 s) occur in NREM stage 1 sleep. Discharges of similar duration in an awake patient are typically accompanied by clinically evident absence seizures.
- The next most prominent time for spike-and-wave and multi-spike-and-wave complexes is NREM stage 2 sleep. During this stage, IID complexes are frequent but of short duration. They usually coincide with sleep transients, which have an EEG configuration similar to epileptiform potentials and

include sleep spindles, K complexes, vertex waves, and bursts of slow waves. These events are thought to reflect aborted arousals during sleep, in part, because they can be evoked by exogenous stimulation (e.g., a noise) during NREM sleep.

- Stage 3 NREM sleep is usually considered least likely to activate spike-and-wave and multi-spike-and-wave complexes. However, some evidence suggests that deep NREM sleep is equally, if not more, conducive than light NREM sleep to activate these IIDs. IID trains are briefer and less organized during deep NREM sleep than in light NREM sleep. This probably results from prolonged hyperpolarization of thalamocortical cells that generates the delta-wave oscillation of deep NREM sleep, and disrupts the rhythmic burst–pause discharge pattern and morphology of IIDs seen in light NREM sleep.
- "Cyclic alternating patterns" of arousal, or CAPs, which pervade sleep, provide compelling evidence linking PGEs to sleep-related arousal events.

## RAPID EYE MOVEMENT SLEEP

Generalized IIDs can occur during REM sleep but are uncommon. "Breakthrough" generalized IIDs are less diffuse in REM than NREM sleep. Even when epileptic EEG potentials do occur in REM sleep, there is rarely any clinical accompaniment.

## LOCALIZATION-RELATED EPILEPSIES: SLEEP EPILEPSIES

This group of seizure disorders is thought to result from one or more focal regions of cerebral dysfunction, and usually reflects a more severe pathophysiology than PGE. However, there is significant variation in severity defined by medical refractoriness, spontaneous remission, and organicity. Partial epilepsies that secondarily generalize are often most likely to display IIDs and to generate clinically evident seizures, especially GTCs, during sleep.

- The category of "benign" localization-related seizure disorders includes benign epilepsy with centrotemporal spikes (BECT, also called benign rolandic partial epilepsy), benign occipital localization epilepsies, electrical status epilepticus during sleep (ESES), and Landau–Kleffner (acquired epileptic aphasia).

- Like seizure disorders of deep temporal or frontal lobe origin, these epilepsies are associated with diffuse IIDs during NREM sleep, and maximal localization during REM sleep. Unlike seizure disorders of temporal or frontal lobe origin, ESES, and Landau–Kleffner are childhood seizure disorders and are considered benign because they are likely to remit spontaneously. Patients may be referred for a variety of reasons other than seizures (e.g., slow progress in school in ESES, or sudden deterioration of language skills related to auditory aphasia in Landau–Kleffner), and the seizure disorder may only be noted during polysomnography. In both ESES and Landau–Kleffner, cognitive, social, and linguistic anomalies tend to mitigate with seizure remission, but residual "nonepileptic" effects often persist and significantly interfere with quality of life. Many patients can never live on their own.

- Temporal and frontal lobe epilepsies comprise the largest group of partial seizure disorders and the largest group of "sleep epilepsies." Onset can occur at any age, and the response to treatment is variable. Most clinicians agree that NREM sleep activates seizure events. About 45–78% of patients exhibit IIDs, and up to 58% present with partial complex seizures and GTCs only or mostly during sleep. IIDs, such as anterior spikes or sharp waves, have higher amplitudes, longer durations, and rounder peaks in NREM sleep than in other sleep or waking states.

- Clinically evident seizures and IIDs can occur at any time during NREM sleep. Some evidence suggests that transitions to or from REM sleep and deep NREM are the most vulnerable periods for both IID and clinical seizures. Seizure activity may be associated with arousal-related sleep EEG transients and/or CAPs, although seizure onset may induce rather than follow behavioral arousal during sleep. With some exceptions (notably neocortical foci), IID and clinically evident seizures rarely occur during REM sleep. Some authors suggest that optimal "focalization" of IID occurs during REM, and the possibility of localizing epileptogenic foci during REM sleep may assist in targeting the epileptogenic region for surgical resection.

- Unlike PGEs in which "awakening" seizure patterns rarely switch to a sleep and waking seizure pattern, localization-related seizures that initially occur only during sleep often develop a random seizure pattern in the sleep–wake cycle later in their clinical course. Localization-related epilepsies without documented lesions are most likely to retain nocturnal clinical seizure patterns. Frequent seizures may exacerbate cell dysfunction at the seizure focus and can ultimately influence cell discharge patterns in extrafocal brain areas.

## SYMPTOMATIC GENERALIZED EPILEPSIES: SLEEP AND WAKING EPILEPSIES

This group of seizure disorders is associated with severe, diffuse cerebral encephalopathy, is medically refractory, and does not remit spontaneously. The underlying pathology can disrupt sleep, dissociate its components, and disperse IIDs and ictal discharges throughout the sleep–wake cycle. Epilepsies included in this category are West syndrome, Lennox–Gastaut syndrome, and progressive myoclonic epilepsies such as Lafora–Unverricht–Lundborg syndrome.

- When NREM and REM sleep can be differentiated from waking, there is sleep-state modulation of IID and ictal seizure manifestations. Hypsarrhythmia, the characteristic EEG manifestation associated with infantile spasms or West syndrome, as well as the atypical or slow spike-and-wave discharges and multiple clinical seizures of Lennox–Gastaut, show a peak during NREM sleep and subside during REM sleep. Response to medical treatment is improved if IID or clinical seizures exhibit a sleep–waking state dependency, even if modulation is confined to suppression of seizure activity during REM sleep.

## SLEEP ABNORMALITIES

Sleep abnormalities are common in epileptic patients of all ages, may arise from multiple sources, and may require different interventions. Epileptic patients may have disorganized nocturnal sleep as a result of the effects of recent seizures, or the use of antiepileptic medications. Epileptic patients may, in addition, have a comorbid sleep disorder such as nocturnal myoclonus or sleep apnea. These disorders may produce hypersomnolence, insomnia, or parasomnias.

- Disorganized and disrupted sleep may lead to complaints of poor sleep quality, excessive daytime sleepiness, and a general decline in the quality of life, including mood, cognitive, and memory deficits. Sleep abnormalities can also increase refractoriness of the seizure disorder.

- Several diagnostic tools, including sleep logs, diaries, questionnaires, and polysomnography (PSG) with simultaneous video recordings. It may be helpful to include a full EEG array during the sleep study in order to detect and differentiate ictal and IID abnormalities from other nocturnal disorders, particularly in patients with epilepsy and complicated histories, or when the differential diagnosis of nocturnal events is an issue.

- Questionnaires may provide important data that may lead to referral for PSG. Patients with evidence of disordered sleep or a confusing clinical picture are candidates for a PSG, particularly when complaints of excess daytime sleepiness occur in epilepsy patients on monotherapy, with low antiepileptic drug serum levels or with poor seizure control.

- Simultaneous video can be particularly valuable in cases where EEG seizure events are difficult to record or are absent in the waking EEG, clinical seizures are subtle, and distinguishing seizures from sleep disorders or pseudoseizures is difficult. For example, epileptic seizures originating from mesio-orbito-frontal areas may have bizarre manifestations (e.g., screaming, sleepwalking, and complex automatisms during sleep) and ambiguous EEG correlates leading to a misdiagnosis of parasomnia. Most patients with paroxysmal dystonia have sleep-related frontal lobe seizures, but EEG alone is inconclusive. In other cases, parasomnias coexist with limbic epilepsy without a common etiology.

- The most frequently reported sleep abnormalities are increased sleep-onset latency; increased number and duration of awakenings after sleep onset; reduced sleep efficiency; reduced or abnormal K complexes and sleep spindles; reduced or fragmented REM sleep; and increased stage shifts. One or more of these sleep abnormalities have been observed in patients with juvenile myoclonic epilepsy, primary generalized tonic-clonic seizure disorders, and localization-related epilepsies of frontal or temporal lobe origin. There are conflicting reports about the presence of sleep anomalies in patients with pure absence seizures. No sleep abnormalities have been reported in BECT.

- Some sleep abnormalities, especially delayed REM sleep onset, can occur as a result of recent convulsions or acute administration of anticonvulsant drugs. Sleep abnormalities are more common in patients with generalized convulsive seizures than in those with simple or partial complex seizures. Sleep disruption is also prominent in patients with frequent or medically refractory seizures. Severe sleep abnormalities occur in symptomatic epilepsies that are associated with significant neurologic deficits. The sleep abnormalities described above are exaggerated, and sleep cycles may be poorly organized. In very serious epileptic disorders, sleep cycles may not even be discernible.

- There are chronic, deleterious effects of seizure-related or non-seizure-related sleep disorders on daytime activities, including exacerbation of seizure activity. It is appropriate and essential to consider treating the sleep abnormality and the seizure disorder as separate but related entities; however, both must be addressed before the patient will be able to perform at his or her best.

## ANTIEPILEPTIC DRUGS

It is often difficult to disentangle the effects of antiepileptic drugs (AEDs), sleep, and seizure disorders. However, the degree to which seizure patterns are state dependent may predict response to medication. Frequent seizures that are entrained to a specific sleep or arousal state usually respond better to medical treatment than epilepsies in which seizures are randomly distributed across the sleep–wake cycle. However, AEDs that reduce seizure frequency may also cause seizures to be randomly dispersed in the sleep–wake cycle. While a correlation between AED effects on sleep and seizure improvement has long been hypothesized, effective AEDs need not improve short- or long-term sleep quality, as indexed by sleep-onset latency, sleep time, sleep efficiency, nocturnal arousals, or percentages of NREM or REM sleep.

- Vagus nerve stimulation (VNS) has been accepted for use in intractable seizure conditions. VNS has been shown to improve daytime alertness, but it can also induce obstructive respiratory events in sleep.

## SLEEP DEPRIVATION

Sleep deprivation can precipitate seizures and increase activation of IIDs in all seizure types, regardless of the state-dependent or random distribution of seizures in the sleep–wake cycle. Increased activation has been detected at all ages; some report that children under 10 years old are more responsive than 11- to 30-year-old children, who are in turn more responsive than adults greater than 30 years of age.

## KEY POINTS

1. Nonrapid eye movement sleep, awakening from sleep, and other transitional arousal states are conducive to electrographic and clinically evident seizures, whereas REM sleep is not. Epileptic discharges are most focal during REM sleep.

2. The timing of epileptic discharges is to some extent dependent on the type of seizure disorder. Increased severity of the seizure disorder, indexed by degree of encephalopathy, is associated with increased dispersion of seizure manifestations across the sleep–wake cycle, increased refractoriness to medication, and reduced likelihood of spontaneous remission.

3. A combination of diagnostic techniques ranging from questionnaires to PSG video monitoring can assess disturbances in nocturnal sleep or excessive daytime sleepiness. Sleep disturbances often parallel the severity of seizure disorders.

4. Antiepileptic drugs can ameliorate seizure-related sleep disturbances, but improvement in sleep architecture is not a critical factor in seizure control.

5. Sleep deprivation may be superior to routine waking EEGs and to natural or drug-induced sleep for activation of epileptic discharges.

6. The incidence of interictal discharges (IIDs) is usually more closely affiliated with sleep stage, particularly NREM vs. REM sleep stages, than with either the timing of clinical seizures in the sleep–wake cycle or chronobiologic factors such as circadian rhythms. Antiepileptic drugs can affect sleep variables, such as overall sleep time, sleep stage percentages, sleep-onset latencies, and wakefulness after sleep onset,

but there is no short- or long-term correlation between AED effects on sleep and seizure activity.

## BIBLIOGRAPHY

Halasz P, et al. Spike-wave discharge and the microstructure of sleep-wake continuum in idiopathic generalized epilepsy. *Neurophysiol Clin* 2002; 32:38–53.

Malow BA, et al. Relationship of temporal lobe seizures to sleep and arousal: A combined scalp-intracranial electrode study. *Sleep* 2000; 23:231–234.

Marzec ML, et al. Approaches to staging sleep in polysomnographic studies with epileptic activity. *Sleep Med* 2003; 4:409–419.

Mendez M, et al. Interactions between sleep and epilepsy. *J Clin Neurophysiol* 2001; 18:106–127.

# 47

## SCHIZOPHRENIA

Rachel J. Norwood and Teofilo Lee-Chiong
National Jewish Health Denver, Colorado

## INTRODUCTION

The psychiatric symptoms of schizophrenia are amplified and aggravated by sleep disruption, while, at the same time, the pathology of schizophrenia may contribute to worsened sleep. Schizophrenia is a disabling, chronic disorder with a worldwide lifetime prevalence of approximately 1% and a median age of onset between 15 and 25 years of age.

- Clinical manifestations can include "positive symptoms" (hallucinations and delusions) as well as "negative symptoms" (disorganized speech and behavior, affective flattening, avolition, and alogia). Schizophrenia typically leads to deterioration in self-care, interpersonal relations, and work performance.

## SLEEP DISTURBANCE

Sleep disturbance is an integral symptom of schizophrenia. Approximately 25% of schizophrenic patients experience "postpsychotic depression" or a "secondary depression" often associated with the extrapyramidal symptoms imposed by antipsychotic medications. Just as with primary depression, these affective symptoms are associated with increased sleep disturbance.

- Poor sleep is associated with lower quality of life scores, greater depression, more adverse effects to medications, and more profound subjective suffering.

## POLYSOMNOGRAPHIC FEATURES

### REM Sleep

There is a significant variation in rapid eye movement (REM) sleep in schizophrenics compared to normal subjects, with shortened REM sleep latencies and a greater percent of total sleep time spent in REM.

- The changes in sleep architecture vary over the natural history of the illness. There is a marked reduction in total sleep time, and a disproportionately larger reduction in REM sleep during the waxing of psychotic symptoms; these normalize during the waning and persevere at normal levels during the postpsychotic and remission phases of schizophrenia.

- In unmedicated, recently hospitalized schizophrenics, REM latency is markedly shortened, likely the result of a deficit of slow-wave sleep seen in the first non-REM (NREM) period. As treatment progresses, patients may demonstrate a modest increase in REM latency about 4 weeks postpresentation. At one year, there are further increases in REM latency, REM time, and REM density. REM sleep latency correlates with the duration of wakefulness in the first cycle in patients suffering from chronic schizophrenia.

- Similarly, short REM latencies that are significantly different from controls are seen in patients with major depressive disorder, schizophrenia, and schizoaffective disorder, suggesting that changes in sleep architecture are quite common across psychiatric diagnoses.

### REM Deprivation Studies

Actively symptomatic schizophrenic patients have a reduced total REM sleep and percent REM sleep rebound following sleep deprivation.

### REM Sleep and Cognitive Function

In schizophrenic patients, the minutes of the first period REM sleep and REM density show a negative correlation with neuropsychologic performance. REM latency of drug naïve and previously medicated, now drug-free,

*Sleep Medicine Essentials*, edited by Teofilo L. Lee-Chiong
Copyright © 2009 John Wiley & Sons, Inc.

schizophrenics is inversely correlated with negative schizophrenic symptoms.

- Significantly increased REM activity and duration has been described in actively psychotic patients with suicidal behavior.

### Slow-Wave Sleep

Generally, patients with schizophrenia have a deficit of slow-wave sleep compared to normal individuals. Interestingly, slow-wave sleep deficits correlate inversely with negative symptoms but not with positive symptoms.

- When deprived of sleep for extended periods of time, schizophrenic patients have, in some instances, been shown to fail to generate the slow-wave sleep rebound characteristic of normal subjects.

### SPECIFIC SLEEP DISORDERS

### Insomnia

Insomnia, either sleep onset or sleep maintenance, is common in schizophrenia and often intensifies during exacerbations of psychiatric symptoms.

- The atypical antipsychotic agents, olanzapine, risperidone, and clozapine, significantly increase total sleep time and may be helpful. Moreover, olanzapine and risperidone enhance slow-wave sleep. The typical antipsychotics—haloperidol, thiothixene, and flupentixol—increase sleep efficiency.

### Narcolepsy

Patients with narcolepsy accompanied by unusually prominent hypnagogic hallucinations may mistakenly be diagnosed with schizophrenia. The use of amphetamines may increase the risk of psychotic symptoms in patients with narcolepsy.

### Obstructive Sleep Apnea

Patients with schizophrenia on long-term neuroleptic treatment may have higher rates of obstructive sleep apnea (OSA), due, in part, to the weight gain common with such medications. Obesity, male gender, and chronic neuroleptic administration are risk factors for OSA in psychiatric patients. In one study, patients with schizophrenia were significantly heavier and had higher rates of OSA than did other psychiatric patients.

### DREAM CONTENT OF PATIENTS WITH SCHIZOPHRENIA

The presence of psychopathology may be associated with impoverishment of dream content, and negative, rather than positive, schizophrenic symptoms may influence the dream content of schizophrenic patients.

- The dream content of schizophrenics differs both in the frequency and intensity of anxious and hostile affects. Patients experience themselves in their dreams more frequently as victims of hostility, while value anxieties (guilt and separation) are found less frequently in their dreams.

### BIOLOGY OF SLEEP DISRUPTION IN SCHIZOPHRENIA

The "dopamine hypothesis of schizophrenia" was the starting point for current understanding of the chemical contributors to schizophrenia, positing that schizophrenia was the result of excessive dopaminergic activity. Other neurotransmitters including other monoamines, particularly serotonin, and hormonal influences have also been postulated to contribute to the pathogenesis of schizophrenia.

- Abnormalities in neuroendocrine release and their consequent impact on sleep have been observed in patients with schizophrenia. One study demonstrated low melatonin levels in subjects with schizophrenia; melatonin replacement improved rest-derived sleep efficiency, especially in low-efficiency sleepers.
- It is most likely that schizophrenia results from a pathologic interplay between genetic predisposition, environmental stress, and neurobiologic insult. Imaging studies have shown enlarged ventricles and generalized reduction in brain volume with magnetic resonance imaging and diminished neuronal content by magnetic resonance spectroscopy.

### MEDICATION EFFECTS ON SLEEP IN SCHIZOPHRENIA

Sleep quality and duration as well as levels of daytime alertness are influenced by the use of psychotropic medications. The goals of antipsychotic medications are to control daytime agitation and positive symptoms and improve negative symptoms and sleep.

- Antipsychotics are divided into two groups, the "typical" and "atypical" agents. The newer atypical antipsychotics have greater clinical effects and less problematic side effects compared to the typical agents, which include chlorpromazine and haloperidol. In general, antipsychotic medications improve sleep continuity and quantity of NREM stage N3 sleep. They increase REM sleep latency. Sedation is a common side effect that can be minimized by gradual dose escalation.
- Atypical agents generate significantly more stages N2 and N3 sleep and less N1 sleep compared to the typical agents. Olanzepine improves sleep efficiency

and increases stages N3 and REM sleep. Clozapine increases mean total sleep time, sleep efficiency, and stage N2 sleep.

- Sleep quality can progressively deteriorate following antipsychotic discontinuation. Schizophrenic patients with sleep disturbances are at a greater risk for worsening of positive symptoms after antipsychotic discontinuation.

- Neuroleptic withdrawal reduces REM sleep and shortens REM latency. The insomnia that develops during discontinuation of antipsychotic medication or when switching from low- to high-potency agents can be attributed to either medication withdrawal effects or exacerbation of schizophrenia. Abrupt neuroleptic withdrawal induces a transient reduction in total sleep time, which typically stabilizes 2–4 weeks after withdrawal to levels between the values observed during chronic treatment and withdrawal periods.

- The effects of antipsychotic medications on sleep appear not to be limited to sedation alone, and rebound insomnia arising from neuroleptic discontinuation has been hypothesized to have a contribution from cholinergic hypersensitivity.

## NEUROLEPTIC SIDE EFFECTS ON SLEEP

Akathisia shares similarities with restless legs syndrome (RLS), both clinically and pathophysiologically, since the two conditions involve alterations in dopamine and iron metabolism. Akathisia is distinguished from RLS primarily by the sensation of inner restlessness rather than leg discomfort, and by the absence of the pronounced circadian variability in symptoms that are seen with patients with RLS, who tend to be more restless in the evening and during repose. Neuroleptic-induced akathisia (NIA) generally causes less sleep disruption than RLS.

- Long-term use of neuroleptics might contribute to insomnia in elderly patients by giving rise to nocturnal myoclonus or periodic leg movement disorder (PLMD). PLMD and/or RLS have been reported following administration of olanzapine and haloperidol.

## USE OF HYPNOTIC MEDICATION AS ADJUNCTS IN SCHIZOPHRENIA THERAPY

Reduction in slow-wave sleep secondary to benzodiazepine use may be of concern in schizophrenics, who usually already have decreased slow-wave sleep. Newer nonbenzodiazepine benzodiazepine receptor agonists may have less effect on slow-wave sleep.

- In some cases, the sedating effect of the antipsychotic agent may be sufficient, if taken at bedtime, for sleep induction, thereby eliminating the need for a separate hypnotic medication.

## KEY POINTS

1. Sleep disruption is a common and very debilitating comorbid symptom of schizophrenia. Sleep disruption can aggravate psychosis; conversely, increased susceptibility to external stimuli in schizophrenia will lead to greater sleep disruption.

2. For the most part the medications used to treat schizophrenia improve sleep disturbance. However, their discontinuation can worsen sleep symptoms.

## BIBLIOGRAPHY

Adams CE, et al. Depot fluphenazine for schizophrenia. *Cochrane Database Syst Rev* 2000; (2):CD000307.

Auslander LA, et al. Perceptions of problems and needs for service among middle-aged and elderly outpatients with schizophrenia and related psychotic disorders. *Commun Ment Health J* 2002; 38:391–402.

Benes FM, et al. A reduction of nonpyramidal cells in sector CA2 of schizophrenics and manic depressives. *Biol Psychiatry* 1998; 44:88–97.

Cecil KM, et al. Proton magnetic resonance spectroscopy in the frontal and temporal lobes of neuroleptic naïve patients with schizophrenia. *Neuropsychopharmacology* 1999; 20:131–140.

Chemerinski E, et al. Insomnia as a predictor for symptom worsening following antipsychotic withdrawal in schizophrenia. *Compr Psychiatry* 2002; 43:393–396.

Garcia-Rill E. Disorders of the reticular activating system. *Med Hypotheses* 1997; 49:379–387.

Hadjez J, et al. Dream content of schizophrenic, nonschizophrenic mentally ill, and community control adolescents. *Adolescence* 2003; 38:331–342.

Jeste DV, et al. Hippocampal pathologic findings in schizophrenia: A morphometric study. *Arch Gen Psychiatry* 1989; 46:1019–1024.

Kato M, et al. Association between delta waves during sleep and negative symptoms in schizophrenia. Pharmaco-eeg studies by using structurally different hypnotics. *Neuropsychobiology* 1999; 39:165–172.

Kubicki M, et al. Voxel-based morphometric analysis of gray matter in first episode schizophrenia. *Neuroimage* 2002; 17:1711–1719.

Lee JH, et al. Effects of clozapine on sleep measures and sleep-associated changes in growth hormone and cortisol in patients with schizophrenia. *Psychiatry Res* 2001; 103:157–166.

McConville BJ, et al. Treatment challenges and safety considerations for antipsychotic use in children and adolescents with psychoses. *J Clin Psychiatry* 2004; 65:20–29.

Monti JM, et al. Sleep in schizophrenia patients and the effects of antipsychotic drugs. *Sleep Med Rev* 2004; 8:133–148.

Muller MJ, et al. Subchronic effects of olanzapine on sleep EEG in schizophrenic patients with predominantly negative symptoms. *Pharmacopsychiatry* 2004; 37:157–162.

Nishimatsu O, et al. Periodic limb movement disorder in neuroleptic-induced akathisia. *Kobe J Med Sci* 1997; 43:169–177.

Poyurovsky M, et al. Actigraphic monitoring (actigraphy) of circadian locomotor activity in schizophrenic patients with acute neuroleptic-induced akathisia. *Eur Neuropsychopharmacol* 2000; 10:171–176.

Ritsner M, et al. Perceived quality of life in schizophrenia: Relationships to sleep quality. *Qual Life Res* 2004; 13:783–791.

Rotenberg VS, et al. REM sleep latency and wakefulness in the first sleep cycle as markers of major depression: A controlled study vs. schizophrenia and normal controls. *Prog Neuropsychopharmacol Biol Psychiatry* 2002; 26:1211–1215.

Rye DB. Contributions of the pedunculopontine region to normal and altered REM sleep. *Sleep* 1997; 20:757–788.

Saletu-Zyhlarz GM, et al. The key-lock principle in the diagnosis and treatment of nonorganic insomnia related to psychiatric disorders: Sleep laboratory investigations. *Methods Find Exp Clin Pharmacol* 2002; 24 (Suppl D):37–49.

Salin-Pascual RJ, et al. Olanzapine acute administration in schizophrenic patients increases delta sleep and sleep efficiency. *Biol Psychiatry* 1999; 46:141–143.

Serretti A, et al. Depressive syndrome in major psychoses: A study on 1351 subjects. *Psychiatry Res* 2004; 127:85–99.

Shamir E, et al. Melatonin improves sleep quality of patients with chronic schizophrenia. *J Clin Psychiatry* 2000; 61:373–377.

Staedt J, et al. Can chronic neuroleptic treatment promote sleep disturbances in elderly schizophrenic patients? *Int J Geriatr Psychiatry* 2000; 15:170–176.

Stompe T, et al. Anxiety and hostility in the manifest dreams of schizophrenic patients. *J Nerv Ment Dis* 2003; 191:806–812.

Vourdas A, et al. Narcolepsy and psychopathology: Is there an association? *Sleep Med* 2002; 3:353–360.

Winkelman JW. Schizophrenia, obesity, and obstructive sleep apnea. *J Clin Psychiatry* 2001; 62:8–11.

Woo TU, et al. A subclass of prefrontal gamma-aminobutyric acid axon terminals are selectively altered in schizophrenia. *Proc Natl Acad Sci USA* 1998; 95:5341–5346.

# 48

## MOOD DISORDERS

MELYNDA D. CASEMENT, J. TODD ARNEDT, AND ROSEANNE ARMITAGE
University of Michigan, Ann Arbor, Michigan

### INTRODUCTION

Mood disorders are among the most prevalent psychiatric illnesses, with an estimated lifetime prevalence in the United States of 17% for major depressive disorder (MDD) and 5% for bipolar illness.

- Young- to middle-aged adults, non-Hispanic whites, and females are at the greatest risk for developing mood disorders. During the reproductive years, from adolescence through menopause, females are at about twice the risk of males for developing MDD. Mood disorders have a slightly lower prevalence in children, estimated to occur in 8–15 % of the population. However, there is evidence of a secular trend in depression with an increasingly younger age of onset.

- Sleep abnormalities are key features of unipolar and bipolar mood disorders and are included in most diagnostic and symptom-severity classification instruments. Sleep complaints such as insomnia and hypersomnia are reported by a majority of adults and children with MDD, and sleep disturbances that persist beyond clinical remission of depressive symptoms increase the risk of suicide as well as the risk of relapse and recurrence of depression.

- Reciprocally, individuals with insomnia are 9 times more likely to have mood disorders compared to healthy individuals, and insomnia of at least 2 weeks duration increases the lifetime risk of developing depression.

### POLYSOMNOGRAPHIC FEATURES

Laboratory sleep studies consistently demonstrate sleep abnormalities in unipolar and bipolar mood disorders. Studies of depressive disorders that use visual stage scoring to examine sleep macroarchitecture commonly find abnormalities in:

1. Sleep efficiency, including increased in sleep latency (sleep-onset insomnia), nighttime awakening (middle insomnia), and early awakening (terminal insomnia)

2. Nonrapid eye movement (NREM) sleep, including increased stage 1 sleep and decreased slow-wave sleep (SWS)

3. Rapid eye movement (REM) sleep, including decreased REM latency and increased REM duration, amount, and activity.

- Laboratory findings in childhood and adolescent depression are much more equivocal, with about half of the literature demonstrating shortened REM latency, most frequently in in-patient populations. Prolonged sleep latency tends to be the most stable finding in young depressed patients. Research on bipolar disorder is less common and the results are varied, but the most common abnormalities are in sleep efficiency and REM sleep.

- Studies of depressive disorders that examine sleep microarchitecture using quantitative electroencephalographic (EEG) analyses such as power spectral and digital period analysis commonly find:
  1. Increased fast-frequency beta and alpha activity;
  2. Decreased slow-wave activity (SWA; delta in NREM sleep), especially in males
  3. Reduced synchrony of fast and slow activity between brain hemispheres (spatial coherence) and across the night (temporal coherence), especially in females

- Sleep microarchitecture often differentiates patients from controls even when sleep macroarchitecture does not (with some exceptions), and it also appears to identify prospectively individuals at greatest risk for developing depression in the future. However, no single sleep architectural variable is likely to reliably distinguish patients from controls, or individuals with MDD from those with other psychiatric disorders.

- Studies have also found an increased prevalence of sleep-disordered breathing (SDB) in depressed individuals, and abnormal respiration distinguished individuals with MDD from controls with 80% accuracy in a recent study.

## MECHANISMS UNDERLYING SLEEP DISTURBANCES

The mechanism of sleep disturbance in mood disorders is generally identified as one or more of the following: REM sleep disinhibition, homeostatic drive reduction, or circadian rhythm dysregulation. Most theories assume that there is a reciprocal relationship between REM and NREM sleep, but the primary cause of disturbance in unknown.

- The REM sleep disinhibition hypothesis suggests that individuals with mood disorders have early onset of REM sleep and an overall increase in REM activity due to an imbalance in cholinergic/aminergic neurotransmission. This theory is largely based on animal research, but it has fairly robust support from cholinergic challenge studies in individuals with mood disorders.
- Another leading theory is the two-process model of sleep regulation, which posits that individuals with mood disorders have less daily accumulation of homeostatic sleep drive (process S) and dysregulated circadian rhythms (process C) compared to controls. Reductions in homeostatic sleep drive are reflected by the lower accumulation and faster dissipation of SWA in depression, but this only appears to be true for males. Circadian rhythm disturbance is reflected by desynchrony between homeostatic sleep drive and circadian rhythm, irregular circadian phase, and damped circadian amplitude in adults and children with mood disorders.

## EVALUATION OF MOOD DISORDERS

The high comorbidity between sleep and mood disorders indicates that mood should be regularly assessed in individuals with sleep complaints. Diagnostic symptoms of unipolar and bipolar mood disorders are presented in Table 48.1.

- A diagnosis of MDD requires that either low mood or anhedonia, plus five or more additional depressive symptoms, be present for at least 2 weeks.
- A diagnosis of bipolar disorder requires that elevated or irritable mood, plus at least three additional symptoms of mania, be present for either 4 days (for bipolar II) or at least a week (for bipolar I), and depressive symptoms may or may not be present.
- Screening for symptoms of depression can be accomplished through self-report questionnaires such as the Quick Inventory for Depressive Symptomatology (QIDS-SR, Beck Depression Inventory (BDI-II), or Patient Health Questionnaire (PHQ-9), but follow-up by a mental health clinician is necessary for formal diagnosis.
- Assessment of sleep in individuals with mood disorders is also important. Subjective evaluations of sleep disruption correspond to many polysomnographic measures in patients with mood disorders, but laboratory assessment is clearly indicated where there is suspicion of SDB.

## THERAPY OF SLEEP DISRUPTION IN MOOD DISORDERS

First-line treatments for sleep disruption in mood disorders can include medications for mood and/or sleep symptoms and cognitive behavioral therapy for insomnia. Alternative treatments may include sleep deprivation and light therapy. These treatment approaches can also be combined to good effect in many cases.

- The effects of antidepressant medications on sleep in individuals with MDD are summarized in Table 48.2. Consistent with the cholinergic hypotheses of REM sleep disinhibition, most antidepressant medications suppress REM sleep. REM sleep suppression is especially pronounced for monoamine oxidase inhibitors (MAOIs) and tricyclic antidepressants (TCAs), where MAOIs result in dramatic but delayed effects and TCAs have immediate effects. However, REM sleep inhibition is not a necessary condition for antidepressant efficacy, and changes in NREM sleep architecture may also be relevant to antidepressant effects.

Table 48.1   Symptoms of Mood Disorders

| Depressive Symptoms | Manic Symptoms |
| --- | --- |
| Persistent low mood | Elevated or irritable mood |
| Anhedonia | Increased self-esteem or grandiosity |
| Weight change | Decreased need for sleep |
| Insomnia or hypersomnia | Increased or pressured speech |
| Psychomotor agitation or retardation | Racing thoughts |
| Loss of energy | Distractibility |
| Feelings of worthlessness or guilt | Increased activity or psychomotor agitation |
| Change in appetite | Excessive risk taking |
| Impaired concentration or decision making | |
| Recurrent thoughts of death or suicide | |

**Table 48.2    Effects of Antidepressant Medications on Sleep in MDD**

| Drug | Sleep Efficiency | REM Sleep | Other |
|---|---|---|---|
| MAOIs | ↓ Sleep efficiency | ↑ REM latency<br>↓ REM sleep | ↑ Stage 2 sleep/NS |
| TCAs | Mixed results | ↑ REM latency<br>↓ REM sleep | ↑ Periodic limb movements |
| SSRIs | ↓ Sleep efficiency | ↑ REM latency<br>↓ REM sleep | ↑ Stage 1 sleep<br>↓ SWS<br>↑ Limb movements<br>↑ Bruxism<br>↑ Eye movement in NREM sleep |
| Venlafaxine | ↓ Sleep continuity | ↑ REM latency<br>↓ REM sleep | NS |
| Mianserin | ↑ Sleep efficiency | ↓ REM latency | ↑ Stage 2 sleep |
| Trazodone | ↑ Sleep efficiency | ↑ REM latency/NS<br>↓ REM sleep/NS | ↑ SWS<br>↑ SWA (delta) |
| Nefazodone | ↑ Sleep efficiency | ↓ REM latency/NS<br>↑ REM sleep/NS | ↓ Stage 1 sleep/NS<br>↑ Stage 2 sleep/NS<br>↓ SWS/NS |
| Mirtazapine | ↑ Sleep efficiency | ↑ REM latency/NS | ↑ Stage 2 sleep/NS<br>↑ SWS/NS |
| Bupropion | ↑ Sleep latency/NS | Mixed results | ↑ SWS/NS<br>↓ periodic limb movement |

*Note*: NS, no significant effect; SSRI, selective serotonin reuptake inhibitor; TCA, tricyclic antidepressant; MAOI, monoamine oxidase inhibitor. Reversible MAOIs, such as moclobemide, may enhance REM. Iprindole and trimipramine do not suppress REM. Trimipramine improves sleep efficiency.

- Note that sleep difficulties do not always remit with antidepressant medications, and some antidepressants actually exacerbate sleep difficulties. This is of particular concern given the heightened risk of suicide as well as depression relapse and recurrence in patients with persistent sleep problems. Comparatively little is known about the sleep effects of pharmacologic treatments for bipolar disorder, but existing evidence indicates that lithium carbonate suppresses REM sleep.

- Benzodiazepine receptor agonists (BzRAs), including zolpidem, zolpidem-CR, eszopiclone, and zaleplon, are considered first-line treatments for sleep disturbances in mood disorders based on the quality of the scientific evidence and their favorable side effect profiles. A recent study found that individuals with depression and insomnia who were treated with a combination of fluoxetine and eszopiclone showed greater sleep and mood improvements than those who received fluoxetine and placebo. The fluoxetine–eszopiclone group also had more treatment responders and remitters after 8 weeks of treatment.

- Despite evidence favoring BzRAs as first-line treatments, trazodone is the most commonly prescribed hypnotic for depressed patients with sleep problems. However, trazodone's therapeutic efficacy is commonly offset by impairments in next-day functioning, such as sedation, and the efficacy of trazodone over the longer term is unclear.

- Atypical antipsychotics, such as olanzapine and quetiapine, have limited efficacy data for sleep and are associated with a variety of adverse effects, including extrapyramidal and cardiovascular abnormalities, that limit their indications in most mood-disordered patients with sleep disturbance.

- Cognitive behavioral therapy (CBT) for insomnia can also improve sleep and mood in individuals with MDD. CBT for insomnia targets cognitive (e.g., worry, beliefs, apprehension about sleep) and behavioral (e.g., maladaptive sleep habits, irregular sleep scheduling) factors that are believed to perpetuate insomnia. For patients with chronic insomnia without psychiatric comorbidity, this therapy demonstrates moderate to large treatment effects across most subjective sleep parameters, with treatment gains maintained over follow-up periods ranging from 3 weeks to 3 years. Although few well-controlled studies have been conducted in patients with comorbid insomnia and depression, preliminary evidence indicates that CBT for insomnia improves mood and sleep in individuals with MDD. Moreover, a recent controlled trial published in abstract form found that combination treatment with CBT for insomnia and escitalopram improved sleep and mood in individuals with comorbid MDD and insomnia. To date, no studies evaluating nonpharmacologic approaches to sleep disturbances in bipolar disorder have been conducted. Alterations in format and/or content of cognitive–behavioral insomnia therapy may be important to optimize outcomes in mood disorder populations.

- Other sleep-focused treatments for mood disorders include sleep deprivation and light therapy. Sleep deprivation has long been known to benefit approximately 60% of mood disorder patients, but its clinical utility has been limited by a reversal of treatment effects with subsequent sleep. Light therapy, which is thought to increase mood by modifying circadian rhythms, is also an effective MDD treatment, especially when used in conjunction with SSRIs.

## KEY POINTS

1. Mood disorders are extremely common, and they are usually accompanied by sleep disruption. The mechanisms of sleep disturbance in mood disorders warrant further inquiry, but leading theories point to decreased REM inhibition, decreased homeostatic sleep drive, and/or disrupted circadian rhythms as important factors. Although the laboratory studies are not always in agreement, the clinical relevance of sleep disturbances in depression is clear.

2. Microarchitectural measures of sleep disruption can often distinguish patients from controls when macroarchitectural measures cannot, and they can also prospectively identify patients at risk for developing mood disorders.

3. Sleep difficulties that persist after the remission of depression are associated with increased risk of suicide as well as depression remission and recurrence.

4. Patients reporting sleep difficulties should be screened for mood disorders, and vice versa.

5. Combined treatment of mood and sleep with SSRIs plus BzRAs or cognitive behavioral therapy for insomnia may be more effective than treating mood or sleep in isolation.

## BIBLIOGRAPHY

Argyropoulos SV, et al. Correlation of subjective and objective sleep measurements at different stages of the treatment of depression. *Psychiatry Res* 2003; 120:179–190.

Argyropoulos SV, et al. Sleep disturbances in depression and the effects of antidepressants. *Int Rev Psychiatry* 2005; 17:237–245.

Armitage R. The effects of antidepressants on sleep in patients with depression. *Can J Psychiatry* 2000; 45:803–809.

Armitage R. Sleep and circadian rhythms in mood disorders. *Acta Psychiatr Scand* 2007; 115(Suppl 433):104–115.

Asnis GM, et al. Zolpidem for persistent insomnia in SSRI-treated depressed patients. *J Clin Psychiatry* 1999; 60:668–676.

Birmaher B, et al. Biological studies in depressed children and adolescents. *Int J Neuropsychopharmacol* 2001; 4:149–157.

Deldin PJ, et al. A preliminary study of sleep-disordered breathing in major depressive disorder. *Sleep Med* 2006; 7:131–139.

Fava M, et al. Eszopiclone co-administered with fluoxetine in patients with insomnia coexisting with major depressive disorder. *Biol Psychiatry* 2006; 59:1052–1060.

Gursky JT, et al. The effects of antidepressants on sleep: A review. *Harv Rev Psychiatry* 2000; 8:298–306.

Jindal RD, et al. Treatment of insomnia associated with clinical depression. *Sleep Med Rev* 2004; 8:19–30.

Kessler RC, et al. Lifetime prevalence and age-of-onset distributions of DSM-IV disorders in the National Comorbidity Survey Replication. *Arch Gen Psychiatry* 2005; 62:593–602.

Kroenke K, et al. The PHQ-9: Validity of a brief depression severity measure. *J Gen Intern Med* 2001; 16:606–613.

Mendelson WB. A review of the evidence for the efficacy and safety of trazodone in insomnia. *J Clin Psychiatry* 2005; 66:469–476.

Morawetz D. Insomnia and depression: Which comes first? *Sleep Res Online* 2003; 5:77-81.

Morehouse RL, et al. Temporal coherence in ultradian sleep EEG rhythms in a never-depressed, high-risk cohort of female adolescents. *Biol Psychiatry* 2002; 51:446–456.

Ohayon MM, et al. Comorbidity of mental and insomnia disorders in the general population. *Compr Psychiatry* 1998; 39:185–197.

Peterson MJ, et al. Sleep in mood disorders. *Psychiatr Clin North Am* 2006; 29:1009–1032.

Rush AJ, et al. The 16-Item Quick Inventory of Depressive Symptomatology (QIDS), clinician rating (QIDS-C), and self-report (QIDS-SR): A psychometric evaluation in patients with chronic major depression. *Biol Psychiatry* 2003; 54:573–583.

Sharafkhaneh A, et al. Association of psychiatric disorders and sleep apnea in a large cohort. *Sleep* 2005; 28:1405–1411.

Smith MT, et al. Comparative meta-analysis of pharmacotherapy and behavior therapy for persistent insomnia. *Am J Psychiatry* 2002; 159:5–11.

Taylor DJ, et al. A pilot study of cognitive-behavioral therapy of insomnia in people with mild depression. *Behav Ther* 2007; 38:49–57.

Tsuno N, et al. Sleep and depression. *J Clin Psychiatry* 2005; 66:1254–1269.

Wirz-Justice A. Biological rhythm disturbances in mood disorders. *Int Clin Psychopharmacology* 2006; 21(Suppl 1):S11–15.

# 49

## ANXIETY DISORDERS

MICHAEL WEISSBERG
Department of Psychiatry, University of Colorado School of Medicine Denver, Colorado

## INTRODUCTION

Anxiety disorders are among the most prevalent psychiatric conditions worldwide, and people who experience excessive anxiety utilize health services at a much higher level than those who are not anxious. The anxious patient is both aware of altered physiologic sensations while also cognitively experiencing anxiety, fear, or dread. In general, anxiety has two components, cognitive and the physiologic state of hyperarousal. The experience of anxiety is associated with a reduction in the ability to think clearly, to plan, and to learn.

- Anxiety, the response to real or imagined danger, is a normal and necessary part of life. Anxiety, if manageable, gets us to act and to deal with a perceived threat. However, in some, anxiety persists, does not recede, and begins to overwhelm.

- Excessive anxiety is not conducive to sleep. The cognitive and physiologic changes associated with excessive anxiety alter sleep and are made worse by the sleeplessness that anxiety can cause, thus setting up a vicious cycle. Sleepiness, for instance, increases the likelihood of panic.

- Anxiety may either cause or complicate the course of a number of sleep complaints, including sleep onset or maintenance insomnia and awakenings with choking, gasping, chest pain, fear, and dread. In addition, "worriers" or individuals who are generally hyperaroused will also frequently develop psychophysiologic insomnia, and the fear of not sleeping increases the hyperarousal in those so prone.

## GENERALIZED ANXIETY DISORDER

The symptoms of generalized anxiety disorder (GAD) include complaints of excessive fear, worry, and apprehension and are often associated with somatic worries and

trouble with concentration. Physical complaints predominate for long periods of time (usually at least 6 months) and can consist of muscle tension, fatigue, irritability, restlessness, trouble falling or staying asleep, or nonrestorative sleep.

- Frequently GAD is comorbid with other psychiatric disorders, particularly depression, panic disorder, and social phobia.

- The usual onset of GAD is during young adulthood, between the ages of 20 and 35 years, with a slight predominance in women. Patients usually report that they have been anxious for "most" of their lives. It is not uncommon to see significant life stressors at the onset of GAD. It tends to be a chronic condition.

- Chronic daytime anxiety and insomnia are common, and patients may complain of daytime fatigue and/or excessive sleepiness. Polysomnography may demonstrate an increased sleep latency, decreased efficiency, decreased stage N3, and increased stages N1 and N2.

## PANIC DISORDER WITH AND WITHOUT AGORAPHOBIA

Persons with panic disorder experience both physical (precipitated by the "flight-or-fight" sympathetic reaction) and cognitive symptoms (intense dread, fears of dying, and/or fears of going crazy). Panic episodes are fairly common in the general population and only become a problem if they increase in frequency and patients begin to anticipate further attacks. Onset is generally during young adulthood and panic is more prevalent in women.

- The physical symptoms associated with panic are worrisome and consist of a racing heart and possible palpitations, shortness of breath, numbness and

*Sleep Medicine Essentials*, edited by Teofilo L. Lee-Chiong

tingling around the mouth and fingers, and feelings of choking accompany the cognitive changes. Attacks can last for minutes to over an hour. As panic recurs, patients may begin to associate attacks with specific activities such as crossing bridges, heights, crowds, or being outside.

- Panic can also occur at night in about a third of patients; in some, they occur exclusively at night, and patients can become phobic about going to sleep for fear of experiencing further episodes. It can manifest as sudden awakening with choking, anxiety, dread, fears of death, and the like and associated with moderate autonomic arousal. There are commonly no formed dreams. Nocturnal panic episodes occur mainly in stage N2 sleep toward the transition to stage N3 sleep. There appear to be differences in patient characteristics between those who panic during the day and those who panic also at night. It might be that night panic patients have more severe levels of anxiety and experience longer attacks.

- There is a higher incidence of suicide in those suffering from panic disorder than the general population. Many patients develop frank depression, alcohol, or substance abuse often with short-acting benzodiazepines. Obsessive–compulsive disorder is also seen in a significant number of patients with panic disorder.

- Panic disorder may be associated with increased hippocampus and locus ceruleus activity, increased adrenergic tone, abnormal benzodiazepine receptors, and a tendency to catastrophize when dealing with life events.

- Other mechanisms may contribute to panic. High-altitude exposure may precipitate symptoms analogous to panic such as breathlessness, palpitations, dizziness, headache, and insomnia. Similar mechanisms are found in three models of panic disorder: hyperventilation (hypoxia leads to hypocapnia), suffocation false alarms (hypoxia counteracted to some extent by hypocapnia), and cognitive distortions (symptoms from hypoxia and hypocapnia interpreted as dangerous). High-altitude exposure also produces respiratory disturbances during sleep analogous to changes found in panic disorder at low altitudes. However, the evidence for the role of altitude in panic or the development of anxiety is minimal at this time.

## OBSESSIVE–COMPULSIVE DISORDER

This disorder is characterized by obsessions—unwelcome, recurring, and upsetting thoughts usually having to do with cleanliness, sexuality or aggression, and compulsions—behaviors that patients resort to in order to avoid intense anxiety. Sufferers hope that these rituals—for instance, hand washing—will control the obsessive thoughts.

- Obsessive–compulsive disorder (OCD) "spectrum" consists of other syndromes where obsessions and compulsions are apparent such as compulsive exercising, hair pulling (trichotillomania), nail biting, eating disorders, and Tourette's syndrome.

- Adult patients, but not children, realize at some point in their illness that their obsessions and compulsions are unreasonable. Two to three percent of the general population suffers from OCD.

- Depression and bipolar depression are highly comorbid with OCD, and sleep disturbance in patients with OCD might actually be due to bipolar illness. Common polysomnographic features include reduced rapid eye movement (REM) sleep latency, decreased sleep efficiency, and prolonged sleep latency.

- Pathophysiology appears to involve serotonin dysregulation, which results from abnormal brain functioning, particularly in the striatum.

- Therapy includes high doses of selective serotonin reuptake inhibitors (which can precipitate mania or a rapid cycling downhill course in susceptible individuals), or behavior therapy, particularly response prevention and exposure techniques.

## PHOBIC DISORDER

Phobic people develop fears of a specific object or behavior, such as embarrassing themselves in public (social phobia), speaking in groups, snakes, or heights.

- Agoraphobia, or the fear of public places, is often a later development of panic disorder.

- Performance anxiety may be involved in the genesis of social phobia as well as psychophysiologic insomnia.

- Patients with nocturnal panic may become phobic about going to sleep since they are frightened of an ensuing attack.

## ANXIETY IN CHILDREN

Besides the usual disorders seen in adults, such as panic disorder with or without agoraphobia, obsessive–compulsive disorder, generalized anxiety disorder, social phobia, children experience anxiety and worry in other areas, particularly associated with bedtime.

- Delayed sleep phase syndrome may be confused with anxiety as the child struggles unsuccessfully to fall asleep. Limit-setting sleep disorder and sleep-onset association disorder are also associated with worry and anxiety in the child and parents.

- Co-sleeping raises some interesting issues. In one study, healthy school-aged children who still co-slept where more likely than non-co-sleeper controls to suffer from bedtime resistance, sleep anxiety, night awakenings, and parasomnias than solitary sleepers. However, no significant behavioral problems were found in co-sleepers.

## DIFFERENTIAL DIAGNOSIS

The differential diagnosis of nocturnal anxiety and panic include sleep-related breathing disorders (obstructive and central sleep apnea), gastroesophageal reflux disease, sleep-related abnormal swallowing syndrome, sleep choking syndrome, sleep-related laryngospasm, Munchausen's stridor, sleep terrors, nightmares, posttraumatic stress disorder (PTSD), REM sleep behavior disorder, seizures, and nocturnal cardiac ischemia.

- Symptoms of nocturnal choking, gasping, or coughing that can be seen with anxiety disorders need to be distinguished from sleep-related breathing disorders, gastroesophageal reflux disease, sleep terrors, seizures, nocturnal asthma, and chronic obstructive pulmonary disease.

## BIOLOGY OF ANXIETY

Anxiety disorders result from the interplay of genes and experience. Areas of concern are the role of genetic transmission, locus ceruleus activity, neurotransmission, and cognitive styles. While there is evidence that early stress and loss can sensitize children to the later development of anxiety syndromes such as panic, PTSD, and depression, one's genetic makeup also influences the likelihood of developing anxiety disorders later in life.

- One area of interest is the function of neuropeptide $\gamma$ (NP$\gamma$). NP$\gamma$ appears to act as a neuromodulator of circadian, endocrine, and behavioral circadian processes. It is a potent antianxiety agent. On the other hand, corticotropin-releasing factor (CRF) plays a role in hyperarousal associated with anxiety and depression. It is postulated that a balance between the two agents plays a role in state regulation, and that dysregulation of the sleep and arousal states seen with depression or anxiety is consistent with an imbalance of the hypothalamic neuropeptide systems.

## EFFECT OF ANXIETY ON SLEEP

Anxiety can lead to nocturnal awakenings due to panic or insomnia due to excessive nighttime worry.

- Stress is likely the most frequent cause of temporary sleeplessness and has been shown to be linked with a reduction of stage N3 sleep. The trepidation concerning a "difficult" next working day is associated with decreased stage N3 sleep, increased stage N2 sleep, bedtime state anxiety, and poor subjective sleep.
- Chronic morning headaches have been found to have a greater correlation to comorbid anxiety and depressive and insomnia disorders and not specifically related to sleep-related breathing disorders. Confusional arousals, or sleep drunkenness, have

been found to be strongly associated with bipolar depression and anxiety disorders as well as obstructive sleep apnea (OSA).

- One study found that recurrent isolated sleep paralysis is more common among anxious African Americans than among anxious Caucasians who are similarly diagnosed with panic disorder or other anxiety disorders.

## TREATMENT

Pharmacotherapy, especially selective serotonin reuptake inhibitors (SSRIs), and behavioral treatments are useful first-line approaches.

- Benzodiazepines, both long- and short-acting agents, offer immediate relief for panic disorder and GAD but have also been associated with problems such as dependency, tolerance, and addiction. For this reason, antidepressants, especially SSRIs and novel antidepressants such as venlafaxine, and psychotherapeutic treatments, particularly behavioral treatments such as cognitive behavioral treatment for panic disorder and GAD should be considered first.

## KEY POINTS

1. The categorical diagnostic problems most likely to affect sleep are panic disorder, generalized anxiety disorder, posttraumatic stress disorder and acute stress disorder, performance anxiety that is part of social phobia, psychophysiologic insomnia, and obsessive–compulsive disorder.
2. Anxiety disorders can cause insomnia and recurrent nighttime awakenings.

## BIBLIOGRAPHY

Flavia C, et al. Co sleeping and sleep behavior in Italian school-aged children. *J Dev Behav Pediatr* 2004; 25:28–33.

Gillin JC. Are sleep disturbances risk factors for anxiety, depressive and addictive disorders? *Acta Psychiatr Scand* 1998; 393:39–43.

Goran K, et al. Apprehension of the subsequent working day is associated with a low amount of slow wave sleep. *Biol Psychol* 2004; 66:169–176.

Hamilton SP, et al. Evidence for genetic linkage between a polymorphism in the adenosine 2A receptor and panic disorder. *Neuropsychopharmacology* 2004; 29:558–565.

Merritt-Davis O, et al. Nocturnal panic: Biology, psychopathology, and its contribution to the expression of panic disorder. *Depress Anxiety* 2003;18:221–227.

O'Mahony JF, et al. Differences between those who panic by day and those who also panic by night. *J Behav Ther Exp Psychiatry* 2003; 34:239–249.

Roth WT, et al. High altitudes, anxiety, and panic attacks: Is there a relationship? *Depress Anxiety* 2002;16:51–58.

# 50

## ALCOHOL, ALCOHOLISM, AND SLEEP

MAREN HYDE,[1] TIMOTHY A. ROEHRS,[1,2] AND THOMAS ROTH[1,2]
[1]Henry Ford Health System, Sleep Disorders and Research Center, Detroit, Michigan
[2]Department of Psychiatry and Behavioral Neurosciences, School of Medicine, Wayne State University, Detroit, Michigan

## INTRODUCTION

Ethanol has far-reaching effects on sleep and sleep disorders. The sleep of healthy normal individuals initially improves with both low and high doses of ethanol, but becomes disturbed in the second half of the sleep period at high doses, whereas lower doses appear to be beneficial across the night in individuals with insomnia. Nevertheless, tolerance to any beneficial effects of ethanol on sleep develops quickly.

- Individuals with alcoholism commonly have sleep problems that may occur during active ingestion, acute ethanol discontinuation, and prolonged abstinence. Although most sleep disturbance improves with time, there are some abnormalities that may take months to years to return to baseline levels after prolonged abstinence.

- Individuals with insomnia may have an increased likelihood of ethanol use, and ethanol is more reinforcing in people with insomnia compared with people without insomnia. Additionally, persons with insomnia have used ethanol as a sleep aid, and a majority views it as being beneficial.

- Ethanol is a small, water-soluble molecule that quickly distributes throughout the body, and its effects are widespread. It has a negative effect on many organ systems and disrupts almost all neurobiologic mechanisms in some way. It has, therefore, been difficult to determine the specific mechanisms by which ethanol affects the various aspects of sleep and sleep disorders. It is recognized that ethanol's effects on sleep may play a role in the initiation and maintenance of alcoholism.

## EFFECTS OF ETHANOL ON SLEEP OF HEALTHY NORMAL PERSONS

### Ethanol Measurement and Dosing

The measurement and dosing of ethanol is complex and varies from study to study, making comparisons among studies quite difficult. A dose of ethanol that is administered on a gram/kilogram basis can produce various breath ethanol concentrations (BrEC). There are a number of factors that contribute to this, namely type of beverage administered, concentration of ethanol in the beverage, rapidity with which the beverage is consumed, contents of the gastrointestinal tract, and the body's total amount of water, the latter varying with age, height, and sex. Estimated ethanol doses and BrEC conversions at peak concentrations are as follows:

| Dose (g/kg) | Number of BrEC (%) at Its peak | 12-oz U.S. beers |
|---|---|---|
| 0.2 | 0.02 | 1–2 |
| 0.4 | 0.03 (0.011) | 2–3 |
| 0.6 | 0.05 (0.008) | 3–4 |
| 0.8 | 0.07 (0.015) | 4–5 |
| 1.0 | 0.09 (0.005) | 5–6 |

- The United States considers legal intoxication in most states to be between 0.08 and 0.10% BrEC, and, in a minority of states, a 0.05% BrEC is considered to be impairing. All European countries consider 0.05% or lower BrECs to be the level of legal intoxication. Breath analyzers used in the United States have been calibrated to give a BrEC of 0.10% for a blood ethanol concentration (BEC) of 100 mg per 100 mL blood.

## Ethanol's Effects on Sleep Physiology

In order to observe the effects of ethanol on sleep, researchers typically administer ethanol to their subjects about 30–60 min before bedtime, resulting in peak breath or blood concentrations of ethanol at the time of "lights out." Ethanol's effects on healthy normal individuals have been studied extensively at doses ranging from 0.16 to 1.0 g/kg of body weight. These doses correspond to approximately one to six standard drinks, which can produce BrECs as high as 0.105%. A standard drink is defined as one 12-ounce bottle of beer or wine cooler, one 5-ounce glass of wine, and 1.5 ounces of 80 proof distilled spirits. Studies using ethanol doses in this range have typically reported reduced sleep latency compared to controls without ethanol consumption. One study noted an increased sleep time at a low ethanol dose of 0.16 g/kg, but no effects at higher ethanol doses of 0.32 and 0.64 g/kg.

- Increased wake time and light nonrapid eye movement (NREM) stage 1 sleep occurs during the second half of the sleep period, especially at higher ethanol doses. Sleep disruption during the second half of the sleep period is generally ascribed to a "rebound effect" once ethanol has been completely metabolized. With "rebound," worsening of certain sleep variables, such as amount of rapid eye movement (REM) sleep or slow-wave sleep, occurs and might even exceed baseline levels once ethanol is completely eliminated. In most experiments, the typical peak BrECs measured at lights out are 0.06–0.08%, and ethanol metabolism decreases BrEC by 0.01–0.02% per hour. At this rate, ethanol is completely metabolized within 4–5 h of sleep onset.

- In addition to its effects on sleep induction and sleep maintenance, ethanol consistently affects the proportions of the various sleep stages. Most studies report a dose-dependent suppression of REM sleep, at least in the first half of the sleep period, and some studies have found increased slow-wave sleep in the first half of the sleep period. REM suppression during the first half of the sleep period, if present, is typically followed by a REM rebound during the second half of the night. Thus, overall REM percentage for the entire night does not differ significantly from placebo controls. REM rebound is also related to ethanol's metabolism and elimination from the body.

- Over repeated nights of administration, tolerance to ethanol's sedative and sleep stage effects develops within as little as three nights, during which percentages of slow-wave sleep and REM sleep return to basal levels.

- Discontinuation of nightly ethanol administration may result in a REM sleep rebound. Not all studies have found a REM rebound following cessation of ethanol use; this variability may be related to several factors, including, degree of REM suppression, dose and duration of ethanol administration, basal level of REM sleep, and extent of prior tolerance to REM suppression.

## EFFECTS OF ETHANOL ON SLEEP OF INSOMNIACS

Approximately 30% of individuals in the general population with persistent insomnia have reported using ethanol during the previous year to help them sleep, and 67% of these have reported that ethanol was effective in inducing sleep.

- A recent study evaluated the effects of an ethanol dose (0.5 g/kg) typically used by insomniacs for their sleep and age-matched healthy normal individuals. The sleep of individuals with insomnia improved with ethanol administration compared with placebo, and there was no sleep disruption during the second half of the night that is seen in normal individuals at higher ethanol doses. Ethanol consumption in individuals with insomnia increased slow-wave sleep to levels comparable to age-matched controls.

- The beneficial effects of ethanol on sleep of individuals with insomnia are also supported by self-administered studies. When the opportunity to choose between a previously experienced color-coded ethanol or placebo beverage was presented before sleep, individuals with insomnia tend to choose ethanol, while normal individuals chose placebo. The average self-administered nightly dose in individuals with insomnia is 0.045–0.06 g/kg.

- In summary, the relationship between ethanol use and sleep is dynamic. Disturbed nocturnal sleep increases the likelihood of ethanol use, while ethanol use also has the potential to disturb sleep.

## EFFECTS OF ETHANOL ON SLEEP OF ALCOHOLICS

Polysomnographic studies have measured sleep characteristics in patients with alcoholism after acute ethanol administration and withdrawal (Figure 50.1). Measures of sleep continuity (i.e., total sleep time and sleep latency) are disturbed during both alcohol ingestion and withdrawal nights in patients with alcoholism. In contrast, decreases in sleep latency are found in healthy normal men after drinking ethanol, suggesting that tolerance has developed to the sleep-inducing effects of ethanol among individuals with alcoholism, although they remain sensitive to its stimulating effects. Slow-wave sleep percentage increases with drinking and returns to baseline levels during withdrawal. Lastly, REM sleep is generally suppressed with drinking and either returns to baseline levels (e.g., REM sleep latency), or exceeds baseline levels secondary to a rebound (e.g., percentage of REM sleep) during withdrawal.

## ACUTE ETHANOL ABSTINENCE

The acute ethanol withdrawal phase lasts about 1–2 weeks. Some of the symptoms of withdrawal, such as mood instability, insomnia, and craving, however, can persist beyond this period, a phenomenon that has been called "subacute

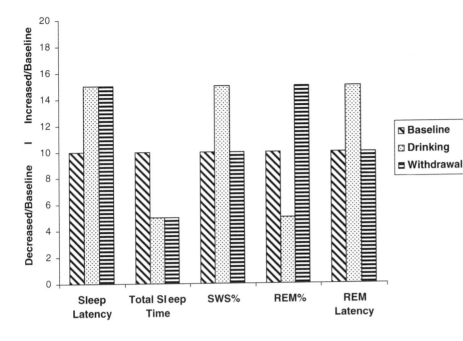

**Figure 50.1** Sleep characteristics of alcoholics at baseline, after drinking, and during acute ethanol withdrawal. (Adapted from Brower KJ. Alcohol's effects on sleep in alcoholics. *Alcohol Res Health* 2001; 25:110–125.)

withdrawal," "protracted withdrawal," or "protracted abstinence."

- Acute ethanol abstinence is characterized by a decrease in the percentage of slow-wave sleep. REM sleep is also altered, with more frequent REM episodes and shorter NREM–REM cycles, but without increasing duration of REM periods.

- It has been hypothesized that hallucinations related to alcohol withdrawal are intrusions of REM sleep into wakefulness as a result of REM rebound and REM sleep fragmentation. This rebound is not found in all subjects studied, however, even if they demonstrate severe ethanol withdrawal syndrome, including hallucinations. It has also been hypothesized that REM suppression and the subsequent REM rebound is indicative of physical dependency on ethanol.

## SUSTAINED ETHANOL ABSTINENCE

Polysomnographic studies have found that some sleep abnormalities (e.g., brief arousals and REM sleep disruption) can persist as long as 1–3 years after the cessation of ethanol consumption. Most of the other sleep disturbances that are observed during acute abstinence (e.g., decreased total sleep time, percentage of slow-wave sleep, and increased sleep latency) appear to normalize with sustained abstinence.

- There is considerable variability with regards to the return of REM sleep to basal levels across several studies. REM sleep latency may remain abnormal for 9–27 months, and the return of percentage REM sleep to basal levels can take from 3 to 27 months. However, many of these studies are based on small sample sizes, include only men, do not include control groups, do not specify their methodology for determining abstinence,

and do not take into consideration comorbid mental disorders with alcoholism making date interpretation difficult. Evidence suggests that patients with alcoholism who have good prognoses tend to sleep better than patients at a high risk for relapse. As a result, good sleepers may be selected for prolonged-abstinence studies, which may, thus, underestimate sleep problems among individuals with alcoholism.

- Three possible mechanisms may explain the persistence of sleep problems in individuals with alcoholism despite sustained abstinence, namely (1) some sleep abnormalities could precede the development of alcoholism and therefore continue into abstinence; (2) the chronic use of ethanol may result in either slowly reversible or irreversible damage to the systems that regulate sleep; and (3) the chronic use of ethanol may be related to persisting medical and psychiatric disorders that interrupt sleep during periods of abstinence.

## KEY POINTS

1. Ethanol has far-reaching effects on sleep and sleep disorders. The sleep of healthy normal individuals appears to be disturbed with acute high ethanol doses, whereas in individuals with insomnia, lower doses appear to be beneficial. However, healthy normal individuals develop tolerance to the beneficial effects of ethanol quickly, which, in turn, may result in excessive hypnotic ethanol use and excessive daytime use as well.

2. Individuals with alcoholism commonly have sleep problems, which may occur during active drinking, acute ethanol discontinuation, or prolonged abstinence. Although most sleep abnormalities improve with time, there are some sleep disturbances that take months to years to return to baseline levels.

3. Sleep disturbances can develop both before and after the start of alcoholism. It is unknown whether sleep disturbances predispose individuals to develop patterns of drinking that are excessive. An increased likelihood of ethanol use in people with insomnia has been suggested by evidence that ethanol is more reinforcing in nonalcoholic people with insomnia compared to controls. In addition, ethanol is more likely to be used as a sleep aid by people with insomnia rather than people without insomnia.

## BIBLIOGRAPHY

Ancoli-Israel S, et al. Characteristics of insomnia in the United States: Results of the 1991 Nation Sleep Foundation Survey. I. *Sleep* 2000; 22:S347–S353.

Brower KJ. Alcohol's effects on sleep in alcoholics. *Alcohol Res Health* 2001; 25:110–125.

Dougherty DM, et al. Effects of moderate and high doses of alcohol on attention, impulsivity, discriminability, and response bias in immediate and delayed memory task performance. *Alcohol Clin Exp Res* 2000; 24:1702–1711.

National Institute on Alcohol Abuse and Alcoholism (NIAAA). *Alcohol Alert No. 41: Alcohol and Sleep.* NIAAA, Bethesda, MD, 1998.

Roehrs T, et al. Ethanol as a hypnotic in insomniacs: Self administration and effects of sleep and mood. *Neuropsychopharmacology* 1999; 20:279–286.

Roehrs T, et al. Sleep, sleepiness, sleep disorders and alcohol use and abuse. *Sleep Med Rev* 2001a; 5:287–297.

Roehrs T, et al. Sleep, sleepiness, and alcohol use. *Alcohol Res Health* 2001b; 25:101–109.

Vitiello MV. Sleep, alcohol, and alcohol abuse. *Addict Biol* 1997; 2:151–158.

# 51

## DRUGS OF ABUSE AND SLEEP

Maren Hyde,[1] Timothy A. Roehrs,[1,2] and Thomas Roth[1,2]
[1]Henry Ford Health System, Sleep Disorders and Research Center, Detroit, Michigan
[2]Department of Psychiatry and Behavioral Neurosciences, School of Medicine, Wayne State University, Detroit, Michigan

### INTRODUCTION

Psychoactive substances from a number of drug classes, including stimulants, analgesics, and sedative-hypnotics, are used routinely for social or medical purposes in many cultures. These drugs can also be used excessively and compulsively for nonmedical purposes, leading to personal and social harm. Surveys have found that 18% of the general population in the United States experiences a substance abuse disorder within their lifetime.

- Scientists have hypothesized that there may be common biological mechanisms that underlie the reinforcing effects of these drugs, leading to their excessive use. Drug abuse can be analyzed from the perspective of the behavioral mechanisms of positive and negative reinforcement. *Positive reinforcement* occurs when the presentation of the drug increases the likelihood of a response to obtain the drug again. *Negative reinforcement* occurs when the drug reduces an existing aversive state, or lessens a drug-induced aversive state (e.g., withdrawal).

- Nearly all drugs of abuse have considerable effects on sleep and wakefulness and on particular stages of sleep. The sleep stage most typically affected by these drugs is rapid eye movement (REM) sleep. It has been hypothesized that sleep and wake changes, although not the primary reinforcing mechanisms, function as contributing factors in maintaining the compulsive and excessive drug use, and in increasing the risk for relapse.

### STIMULANTS

Stimulants, such as amphetamine and its derivatives, cocaine, caffeine, and nicotine, are associated with an extremely high abuse liability. These drugs produce arousal and excitation and have important therapeutic effects for attention deficit disorder, obesity, depression, narcolepsy, and other sleep disorders characterized by excessive sleepiness.

- Stimulants enhance the activity of the neurotransmitters, dopamine and norepinephrine, by blocking their reuptake and increasing their release. When taken for a short period of time and in moderation, these stimulants are able to counteract excessive daytime sleepiness and sleep loss, and improve performance, mood, and endurance. Direct physiological measures, as well as measures of mood and performance, have documented the daytime alerting effects of amphetamines.

*Amphetamine* and its derivatives, when administered before sleep, delay sleep onset, increase wakefulness during the sleep period, and suppress REM sleep. An increase in slow-wave sleep during the first recovery night, and increased amounts of REM sleep and reduced latency to REM sleep on subsequent nights occur with cessation of chronic amphetamine use.

*Ecstasy* or (±)3,4-methylenedioxymethamphetamine (MDMA) is an amphetamine derivative that has become increasingly popular as a recreational and drug of abuse. This drug has hallucinogenic properties and acts indirectly by stimulating the release of brain monoamines. Exposure to MDMA decreases total sleep time with a decrease in non-rapid eye movement (NREM) sleep (primarily stage 2 sleep, but no significant changes in stage 1 or slow-wave sleep), but no significant effects on REM sleep.

*Anorectics*, or drugs used to suppress appetite, also enhance central catecholamine activity. They, too, are amphetamine derivatives with central nervous system (CNS) stimulant activity. The appetite suppression and stimulant effects of these drugs are inseparable, so insomnia is a frequent side effect of anorectic use.

*Cocaine*, which is used medically as a local anesthetic, also has CNS stimulant effects, which foster its abuse.

Cocaine increases fast-frequency electroencephalogram (EEG) activity, which suggests an alerting effect. The use of cocaine during the late afternoon and early evening is linked with reduced nocturnal sleep time and REM sleep, as well as an increased latency to REM sleep. Cessation of chronic cocaine abuse results in increased sleep time and REM rebound, characterized by reduced REM latency and increased REM sleep.

*Caffeine* is the most widely used stimulant in the world. In North America, 80–90% of adults report using caffeine on a regular basis. Among caffeine consumers in the United States, the mean daily intake is approximately 280 mg, and soft drinks and coffee are the major sources of caffeine; nearly half of caffeine consumers ingest caffeine from multiple sources, including tea and chocolate.

- Individuals have very different responses to caffeine, with as little as 250 mg causing overstimulation in some people. Others may be less affected, especially chronic caffeine users who appear to develop tolerance to its stimulating effects. Restlessness, nervousness, insomnia, excitement, gastrointestinal disturbances, and facial flushing characterize caffeine intoxication. Although caffeine has a half-life of about 3–7 h, its effects may last as long as 8–14 h, which can have significant effects on nighttime sleep, even if caffeine is consumed in the late afternoon. Insomnia can result following consumption of six or more cups of coffee throughout the day, even if it is not taken shortly before bedtime. This may lead to a vicious cycle of consuming caffeine during the day to remain alert, which will end up disrupting sleep at night, therefore perpetuating daytime sleepiness the following day. Many people develop tolerance to the stimulating effects of caffeine.

*Nicotine* is an addictive, legal, stimulating drug found in tobacco products. Approximately 20% of the adult population in the United States currently smokes cigarettes, 4% smoke cigars or pipes, and 3% use smokeless tobacco. It has been estimated that 20–50% of smokers meet the diagnostic criteria for nicotine dependency. The plasma half-life of nicotine is about 2 h, so the average smoker who consumes nicotine throughout the day has increasing plasma concentrations that fall throughout the night. A simple measure of dependency is how long a smoker can go in the morning before his or her first cigarette.

- Nicotine has sedating effects at low doses and alerting effects at high doses. Both questionnaire and polysomnographic (PSG) studies have reported an increased sleep latency, increased arousals, and difficulty staying asleep at night. Some studies have suggested that smoking is a risk factor for sleep-disordered breathing.
- Acute withdrawal from nicotine tends to worsen sleep in smokers, and increase arousals at night, followed by sleepiness the next day on the Multiple Sleep Latency Test (MSLT).

## ANALGESICS

Analgesics are drugs that reduce pain, and opiate analgesics have a fairly high abuse liability. The term *opiate* was derived originally from opium, which was acquired from the poppy plant. Although the word *opioid* initially referred to synthetic drugs, the term now refers to natural, semisynthetic, and synthetic substances with opiatelike activity.

- Opiates influence a number of neurotransmitter systems in the brain, including those involved with sleep and wakefulness. They produce sedative-like effects on waking EEGs, and individuals taking these drugs have impaired performance.
- Opioids decrease REM sleep and reduce total sleep time. However, tolerance to most of these effects develops quickly with chronic administration of opioids. Cessation of opioid use leads to REM rebound, an increase in REM sleep, and a shortened latency to the first REM episode.
- Opioids have been used for the treatment of restless legs syndrome (RLS) with and without periodic leg movements of sleep (PLMS).

*Morphine* is the primary active ingredient of opium and was originally named after Morpheus, the Greek god responsible for dreams. Ironically, research has shown that short-term administration of the drug actually reduces REM sleep rather than increase it, and also reduces total sleep time, slow-wave sleep, and sleep efficiency.

*Heroin* is a semisynthetic opiate that is metabolized within the body to morphine, thereby producing the same sleep disturbances as morphine, but with greater effects.

*Methadone* is a synthetic opiate that has similar effects on sleep and wakefulness as morphine. It is rarely abused, and due to its relatively long half-life, it has been used for the treatment of chronic opioid addicts. Immediately after opiate administration before sleep onset, isolated EEG bursts of delta waves are seen on the waking EEG. These findings have been correlated with the behavior of head nodding, which may refer to the street term *being on the nod*.

## HALLUCINOGENS

The characteristic pharmacologic effect of hallucinogens is to modify perceptions. Mescalin, psilocybin, and LSD (*d*-lysergic acid diethylamide) are the three classic hallucinogens. A state similar to dreaming is experienced after using hallucinogens. The only hallucinogen that has been studied for its effects on sleep is LSD; this agent increases REM sleep early in the night, although the total amount of REM sleep for the night remains unchanged.

*Marijuana* is another drug of abuse with hallucinogenic properties. Its active ingredient is tetrahydrocannabinol (THC), and the effects of this substance on the waking EEG are quite different from those of classic hallucinogens. The sedating effects of THC occur at much lower doses than the hallucinatory effects. Administration of marijuana or THC to humans is associated with an increase in slow-wave sleep and a reduction in REM sleep. When administered chronically, the effects on REM and slow-wave sleep decrease, which indicates the presence of tolerance. Upon discontinuation, increased wakefulness and increased REM sleep time are seen.

## SEDATIVE-HYPNOTICS

Sedative-hypnotic drugs including barbiturates, benzodiazepine receptor ligands, and $H_1$ antihistamines have a mixed picture regarding their abuse liability. The barbiturates are well-known drugs of abuse, while the scientific evidence regarding the abuse liability of benzodiazepine receptor ligands is less compelling. The anxiolytic and sedative effects of barbiturates and benzodiazepine receptor ligands are associated with the facilitation and enhancement of gamma amino butyric acid (GABA)a receptor function, which is the major inhibitory neurotransmitter system in the CNS. When the GABAa receptor is occupied, the chloride channel is opened on the neuronal membranes, which allows the negatively charged chloride ions to cross the cell membrane, and hyperpolarize the postsynaptic cell.

- In clinical use, the benzodiazepines are not strongly reinforcing or pleasurable for most individuals. Sedative-hypnotic abuse occurs most often in the context of polysubstance abuse, most notably to reduce the adverse effects of stimulants, to self-medicate withdrawal from alcohol or heroin, or to produce intoxication when no other drugs of abuse are available. Other individuals who are at high risk for sedative-hypnotic abuse include those with a history of sedative-hypnotic abuse, dependency, or alcoholism; those who are current substance abusers; and those who are seeking relief from anxiety and depression through pharmacologic therapy.
- All hypnotics effectively induce and maintain sleep. The barbiturates suppress REM sleep, but tolerance develops rapidly. The benzodiazepine receptor ligands, at clinical doses, have little impact on REM sleep. On barbiturate discontinuation, a REM rebound, evident as increased REM percent and reduced REM latency, occurs.
- $H_1$ antihistamines are occasionally found to be drugs of abuse. These drugs, which are used for the treatment of allergy, have been associated with sedative effects because they easily pass into the brain and affect the neural structures that are associated with sleep. Although not as potent in hypnotic effects as the traditional benzodiazepine receptor ligands, the sedative potential of $H_1$ antihistamines has made them the most common ingredient of over-the-counter sleeping pills. Overnight sleep studies on antihistamines do not typically show increased sleep times or decreased wakefulness. Daytime studies

that use the MSLT clearly demonstrate the sedative potential of these drugs, which have also been shown to impair daytime performance. Impairment of daytime performance is most likely modulated by the sedative effects of these drugs.

- Gamma-hydroxybutyrate (GHB) acts on the GABAb receptor, producing CNS depressant effects, in many ways similar to the classical sedative-hypnotics such as barbiturates and benzodiazepines. GHB is increasingly being used as a growth promoter and mild sedative without medical supervision. It has also been labeled as the new recreational "club drug" due to its intoxicating effects, as well as its use in combination with alcohol to leave women more vulnerable to sexual assault. GHB has also been used as a sleep-inducing agent, and there have been reports that it is used as a sleep aid for improvement of the after effects of methamphetamine. GHB-induced sleep is easily reversed by external stimuli and is virtually identical to normal sleep. Behavior, subjective evaluations, and EEG patterns all suggest that GHB-induced sleep mimics physiologic sleep and increases both slow-wave sleep and REM sleep. This differs from the classic sedative-hypnotics, which suppress slow-wave sleep. GHB does not result in REM rebound with nightmares, as is observed with discontinuation of barbiturates. GHB is currently used for the symptomatic treatment of sleepiness and cataplexy in narcoleptic patients. Although this may seem counterintuitive, the ability for GHB to produce physiologic sleep during the night allows for the alleviation of narcolepsy symptoms (daytime sleepiness, cataplexy, sleep paralysis, and hallucinations) during the day.

## KEY POINTS

1. The drugs of abuse all appear to have common biological mechanisms that explain their reinforcing effects as well as sleep and wakefulness altering effects. These psychoactive substances affect the neurotransmitters that control sleep and wakefulness. Most drugs with high abuse liability change the amount and timing of REM sleep—barbiturates and stimulants decrease REM sleep, whereas the hallucinogen LSD hastens the onset of REM sleep and increases the amount of REM during the first half of the sleep period. Tolerance occurs during the chronic use of most of these drugs, leading to dose escalation and dependence.

2. Upon discontinuation of the drugs of abuse, a withdrawal syndrome occurs, with a characteristic REM rebound. Some studies have indicated that the occurrence and intensity of the REM sleep rebound is predictive of the relapse of drug use.

3. Stimulants, which have alerting effects, increase alertness and wakefulness at night, and suppress REM sleep.

4. Analgesics decrease REM sleep and total sleep time and increase daytime sleepiness.

5. Hallucinogens have varying effects on sleep. LSD reduces the onset to REM sleep and increases REM sleep in the first half of the sleep period. Marijuana decreases REM sleep and increases slow-wave sleep.

6. Sedative-hypnotics, which have a low abuse liability, have little effect on REM sleep.

## BIBLIOGRAPHY

Galloway GP, et al. Gamma-hydroxybutyrate: An emerging drug of abuse that causes physical dependency. *Addiction* 1997; 92:89–96.

Grozinger M, et al. Effects of Lorazepam on the automatic online evaluation of sleep EEG data in healthy volunteers. *Pharmacopsychiatry* 1998; 31:55–59.

Hughes JR, et al. A systematic survey of caffeine intake in Vermont. *Exp Clin Psychopharmacol* 1997; 5:393–398.

James JE. Acute and chronic effects of caffeine on performance, mood, headache, and sleep. *Neuropsychobiology* 1998; 38:32–41.

Juliano LM, et al. A critical review of caffeine withdrawal: Empirical validation of symptoms and signs, incidence, severity, and associated features. *Psychopharmacology* 2004; 176:1–29.

Koob GF, et al. Drug abuse: Hedonic homeostatic dysregulation. *Science* 1997; 278:52–58.

Koob GF, et al. Drug addiction, dysregulation of reward, and allostasis. *Neuropsychopharmacology* 2001; 24:97–129.

Nicholson KL, GHB: A new and novel drug of abuse. *Drug Alcohol Depend* 2001; 63:1–22.

# 52

## POLYSOMNOGRAPHY

Nancy A. Collop
Johns Hopkins University, Baltimore, Maryland

### INTRODUCTION

Polysomnography (PSG) continues to be the usual method for diagnosis of most sleep disorders, including obstructive sleep apnea. The most important recent development regarding polysomnography has been the publication of *The AASM Manual for the Scoring of Sleep and Associated Events* with the companion articles published in the *Journal of Clinical Sleep Medicine* entitled: "Review Articles for the AASM Manual for the Scoring of Sleep and Associated Events: Rules, Terminology and Technical Specifications."

- These publications include updated processes for properly conducting polysomnography as well as revised rules for scoring all the events that occur during polysomnography, including sleep staging and arousals, respiratory events, movement during sleep, and cardiac events.

### DIGITAL AGE

Polysomnography in the twenty-first century is predominately digital. Considerations for digital polysomnography include impedance, sampling rates, calibrations, filtering, video monitoring, filing, and storage.

- Impedance measurement of the electrodes should ideally be done individually. Many of the current systems do not provide the option of measuring impedence of individual electrodes. The current recommended maximum electrode impedance is 5 kΩ.
- Sampling rates are no longer as limited as in the past because present computers have extremely rapid processing and storage capabilities. Now individual signals can have different sampling rates based on their qualities. The current recommended sampling rates and the minimal acceptable rates are shown in Table 52.1.

### FILTERING

Filtering is an important aspect of PSG as amplification of the physiologic signals often results in unwanted artifacts. However, overfiltering can result in lack of appropriate detail.

- It is recommended that current PSG systems include the capability for setting a notch filter (50/60 Hz) on each signal. Notch filters should be used on an as-needed basis for situations in which there may be unwanted electrical interference (such as an inpatient setting). Recommended filter settings for the common PSG signals are shown in Table 52.1.

### BIOCALIBRATIONS

Machine and biocalibrations are required to test signal quality. Ideally, a digital PSG system should have the capability of applying a 50-µV direct current (dc) signal for all channels to allow visual inspection of polarity, amplitude, and time constant settings on the computer screen.

- Calibrations should be performed at both the beginning and the end of each study.
- Issues regarding display include a recommended screen resolution of $1600 \times 1200$ pixels and synchronization of the video recording with the actual PSG signals.
- Polysomnography data should be stored in the exact manner in which it was collected. This data must be rigorously protected against manipulation and should be backed up to prevent data loss. The unmanipulated file should be retained until all scoring and interpretations have been completed.

*Sleep Medicine Essentials*, edited by Teofilo L. Lee-Chiong
Copyright © 2009 John Wiley & Sons, Inc.

**Table 52.1  Sampling and Filtering Recommendations**

| Signal | Recommended (Hz) | Minimum (Hz) | LFF (Hz) | HFF (Hz) |
|---|---|---|---|---|
| EEG | 500 | 200 | 0.3 | 35 |
| EOG | 500 | 200 | 0.3 | 35 |
| EMG | 500 | 200 | 10 | 100 |
| ECG | 500 | 200 | 0.3 | 70 |
| Airflow—Th | 100 | 25 | 0.1 | 15 |
| Airflow—NPT | 100 | 25 | 0.1 | 15 |
| Oximetry | 25 | 10 | — | — |
| Effort | 100 | 25 | 0.1 | 15 |

*Note*: LFF: low-frequency filter; HFF: high-frequency filter; airflow—Th: airflow measured by thermal sensor; airflow—NPT: airflow measured by nasal pressure transducer.

**Table 52.2  Recommended Montage for PSG**

| Lead | Name | Signal |
|---|---|---|
| 1 | C4-M1 | Electroencephalogram (EEG) |
| 2 | F4-M1 | Electroencephalogram |
| 3 | O2-M1 | Electroencephalogram |
| 4 | E1-M2 | Electrooculogram (EOG) |
| 5 | E2-M2 | Electrooculogram |
| 6 | Chin muscle | Electromyogram (EMG) |
| 7 | Right anterior tibialis muscle | Electromyogram |
| 8 | Left anterior tibialis muscle | Electromyogram |
| 9 | Lead II | Electrocardiogram (ECG) |
| 10 | Oronasal airflow | Oronasal thermistor |
| 11 | Nasal airflow | Nasal pressure transducer |
| 12 | Thoracic effort | Inductance plethysmography |
| 13 | Abdominal effort | Inductance plethysmography |
| 14 | Oxygen saturation | Oximetry |

## RECOMMENDED MONTAGE

The recommended montage is slightly different from what was typically used in the past (see Table 52.2).

- The most prominent change includes the addition of a frontal EEG lead to improve recognition of arousals, and the concurrent use of an oronasal thermal sensor and a nasal pressure transducer.
- It is recommended that both legs be individually monitored with EMG to detect the maximal number of leg movements.

## KEY POINTS

1. Considerations for digital polysomnography include impedance, sampling rates, calibrations, filtering, video monitoring, filing, and storage.

2. Filtering is an important aspect of polysomnography as amplification of the physiologic signals often results in unwanted artifacts.

3. Machine and biocalibrations should be performed at both the beginning and the end of each study.

4. The montage should include the addition of a frontal EEG lead to improve recognition of arousals, and the concurrent use of an oronasal thermal sensor and a nasal pressure transducer to detect respiratory events.

## BIBLIOGRAPHY

Iber C, et al. *The AASM Manual for the Scoring of Sleep and Associated Events: Rules, Terminology and Technical Specifications*, 1st ed., American Academy of Sleep Medicine, Westchester IL, 2007a .

Iber C, et al. Review articles for the AASM Manual for the Scoring of Sleep and Associated Events: Rules, Terminology and Technical Specifications. *J Clin Sleep Med* 2007b; 3(2):99–246.

# INDEX